INBORN ERRORS
of METABOLISM

INBORN ERRORS
of METABOLISM

DAVID YI-YUNG HSIA, M.D.

Associate Professor of Pediatrics, Northwestern University Medical School; Attending Biochemist and Director of Research, Children's Memorial Hospital, Chicago; Associate Attending Physician, Cook County Hospital and Evanston Hospital

Director, Genetic Clinic, Children's Memorial Hospital, Chicago.

THE YEAR BOOK PUBLISHERS • INC.

200 EAST ILLINOIS STREET • CHICAGO

To MY PARENTS

Foreword

TO THE AVERAGE physician the diseases included in most textbooks under the heading of "inborn errors of metabolism" have represented an esoteric group unlikely to be encountered in clinical practice. A true understanding of these disorders is made doubly difficult because two disciplines are required: a knowledge of genetics and an acquaintance with fairly specialized biochemistry. However, during the past few years so many additions have been made to the known inborn errors of metabolism that the group can no longer be considered a rarity and the physician must expend the effort required to understand the problems involved. The present volume has been designed to review basic concepts and clinical aspects for the physician who is neither geneticist nor enzyme chemist.

The evolution of the author's interest in this field is worthy of reconstruction. His investigative work dealt originally with physiological jaundice and later with the problem of jaundice in erythroblastosis and its relationship to kernicterus. Problems of obstructive jaundice next engaged his interest, and at this time he encountered infants with galactosemia, an inborn error of metabolism which frequently presents with obstructive jaundice. Shortly afterward he became involved in the study of constitutional hepatic dysfunction and congenital, familial nonhemolytic icterus. It became obvious to both Dr. Hsia and his friends that a basic understanding of these disorders could be obtained only through a knowledge of both human genetics and enzyme chemistry, and so he embarked on a program which would furnish him with such knowledge. This book is the culmination of these studies.

Despite the exciting recent advances in knowledge regarding inborn errors of metabolism, it is clear that we have only begun to explore a

7

field with apparently unlimited possibilities. In the near future not only will we acquire additional understanding of the diseases reviewed here but we will also see the addition of numerous conditions not previously considered to be inborn errors of metabolism.

SYDNEY S. GELLIS

Preface

IN RECENT YEARS, unprecedented progress in the field of biochemical genetics has permitted, for the first time, a logical approach to the various inborn errors of metabolism in man. The present volume is an attempt to present this approach in a simple and understandable form for physicians, but it should be emphasized that the book does not in any way represent a comprehensive or complete survey of the field. The investigative worker in biochemistry, genetics, or medicine should consult the excellent reviews which are marked by an asterisk in each section. However, despite its limitations, it is hoped that this volume will be helpful to the general practitioner and the house officer when they next come face to face with a patient who has a hereditary disease. In the same way, it is hoped that the Appendix will act as a readily available laboratory manual for their use in the detection of these conditions.

In looking back over the past eight years, I realize that it would be impossible to acknowledge all of the many friends and colleagues who have helped in the preparation of the manuscript. Of those in the Department of Pediatrics at Harvard University, I would first like to express my deep gratitude to Dr. Charles A. Janeway. It was largely through his influence that I first went into the field of enzyme chemistry, and throughout the years he not only has provided the necessary financial support for this work but has also been a constant source of personal guidance and support. To no less degree, I would like to express my sincere thanks to Dr. Sydney S. Gellis. Through him I first became interested in pediatric research, and he has remained a loyal colleague and friend.

Among those at the Department of Biological Chemistry at Harvard University to whom I owe acknowledgment, I wish to express my personal debt to Dr. W. Eugene Knox. It was while working with him that the idea of preparing such a volume arose, and he was most helpful in outlining the approaches to be taken during the early phases. I am also grateful to Dr. A. Baird Hastings and his M. D. Luncheon group, who devoted their meetings during the spring of 1955 to discussing various phases of the material covered in this book. It is largely through their encouragement that the manuscript was initiated.

Recalling my stay at the Galton Laboratory in London, I wish to acknowledge first the kindness of Professor L. S. Penrose. His mature philosophy and understanding of biochemical genetics were most helpful in clarifying many points. I also want to acknowledge the many helpful ideas and detailed information given to me by Dr. H. Harris during our many talks together. Finally, it was a real privilege to get to know and learn from Professors J. B. S. Haldane and H. Gruneberg and Drs. H. Kalmus, Sylvia Lawler, J. Renwick, and C. A. B. Smith—all of the University College, London.

I would also like to acknowledge my indebtedness to Dr. Arthur Steinberg for his many suggestions and to Drs. John A. Bigler and Joseph D. Boggs of the Children's Memorial Hospital of Chicago for giving me the moral support and necessary time to complete the manuscript.

During the period of preparation of the manuscript the author was the recipient of a fellowship from the Playtex Park Research Institute and a traveling fellowship from the Elizabeth McCormick Memorial Fund, and also was a Wellcome Associate of the Royal Society of Medicine. All of this assistance is gratefully acknowledged.

I would like to express my appreciation to the following for giving suggestions on specific chapters: Dr. H. Kalmus (Chapter 1), Dr. Aaron Josephson (Chapter 2), Dr. John Hartmann (Chapter 5), Dr. Albert Renold (Chapter 7), Dr. Matthew Steiner (Chapter 8), Dr. Allen Crocker (Chapter 12), and Dr. Robert Dowben (Chapter 13). Their contributions have added greatly to the book, but the responsibility for any mistakes lies with the author.

Finally, I wish to express my thanks to Dr. Shirley Driscoll for the pathological descriptions and Dr. Jean Naylor for proofreading the manuscript; to Dr. Harvey White for preparing the roentgenograms; to Miss Grace Lawrence for checking the section on laboratory procedures; to Mr. Hsio-Chang Shih and my wife, Mrs. Hsio-Hsuan Hsia, for preparing the illustrations; to Miss Marilyn Holmquist for typing the manuscript; and to the Year Book Publishers for their helpful co-operation in completing the volume in such a satisfactory manner.

DAVID YI-YUNG HSIA

Table of Contents

PART III. DISTURBANCES IN MOLECULAR FUNCTION
(ENZYME DEFECTS)

1

General Considerations

THE CONCEPT OF "inborn errors of metabolism" was first suggested by Sir Archibald Garrod in 1908. In the Croonian Lectures delivered at the Royal College of Physicians he suggested that four metabolic disorders—albinism, alkaptonuria, cystinuria, and pentosuria—had certain features in common. First, in all four conditions the onset of the particular abnormality could be dated to the first days or weeks of life, especially when a special effort was made to do so. A second characteristic was their familial occurrence in a considerable number of cases. A third feature was that the conditions were relatively benign and compatible with a normal life-expectancy. A fourth feature, noted by other clinicians in his day, was the frequency with which these disorders occurred among the offspring of consanguineous marriages.

Garrod made the following comments about the pathogenesis of these conditions:

Nowadays very different ideas are in the ascent. The concept of metabolism in blocks is giving place to that of metabolism in compartments. The view is daily gaining ground that each successive step in the building up and breaking down, not merely of proteins, carbohydrates, and fats in general, but even of individual fractions of proteins and of individual sugars is the work of special enzymes set apart for each particular purpose. . . .

It may well be that the intermediate products formed at the several stages have only momentary existence as such, being subjected to further changes almost as soon as they are formed and that the course of metabolism along any particular path should be pictured as in continuous movement rather than as series of distinct steps. If any one step in the process fails, the intermediate product in being at this point of arrest will escape further change, just as when the film of a biograph is brought to a standstill, the moving figures are left foot in air. All that is known of catabolism tends to show that in such circumstances, the intermediate product is being wont to be excreted as such rather than that it is further dealt with along abnormal lines. Indeed it is an arguable

15

question whether, under abnormal conditions, the metabolic processes are ever thrown out of their ordinary lines into entirely fresh paths with the result that products are formed which have no place in the normal body chemistry. It is commonly assumed that this happens, but if the concept of metabolism in compartments, under the influence of enzymes, be a correct one, it is unlikely a process, that alternative paths are provided which may be forbred when for any reason the normal paths are blocked. It is far easier to suppose in such circumstances, normal intermediate products are excreted without further changes.

Half a century later, rapid progress in the basic sciences has given body and substance to what was, by necessity, supposition in Garrod's time. The original four inborn errors of metabolism have now been increased to well over fifty. We know more not only about how these conditions are transmitted from one generation to another but also about the very biochemical processes responsible for these changes. Much of this information is highly technical and known only to the biochemist, geneticist, or clinical investigator working on specialized studies in this field. The present volume attempts to make this knowledge available to the practicing physician.

This will be done first by formulating in general terms what we know today about how a gene produces its effect in a person. We shall then review each of the hereditary disorders, taking up first those conditions in which the pathogenesis is fairly well understood and then those clearly genetic entities about whose etiology we know little. A final chapter will consider how these concepts might be extended to other situations in which heredity may play a role. The chemical procedures which are useful in the diagnosis and treatment of these inborn errors of metabolism will be given in the Appendix. The failure to include morphologically inherited differences does not imply that they do not represent examples of inborn errors of metabolism and do not ultimately have a biochemical basis. Their bases will become known only when we eventually understand enough embryology to know how chemistry affects structure.

It is hoped that, by summarizing here the information that we do have, this work not only will be helpful to the clinician in treating his patients but will also point out to him the gaps in our knowledge of these patients' conditions which will have to be filled out by proper clinical and laboratory observations as the opportunities arise. We should take the view that the study of such disorders in human beings can contribute valuable information to the development of biochemical and genetic knowledge. In the same way, the latter can be of immense help in the diagnosis and management of patients with clinical disease.

We might well start off by considering three basic problems which concern all inborn errors of metabolism: (1) How do they arise? (2) How are they transmitted? (3) How is the abnormality expressed in the affected individual? Since this is not a textbook on genetics, the discussion will, of necessity, appear to be oversimplified; however, it is hoped that it will provide some of the necessary background for a proper understanding of the subsequent chapters.

How Do the Inborn Errors of Metabolism Arise?

It has been well established that all of us are endowed with *chromosomes,* small bodies of various sizes and shapes located in the cell nuclei. The chromosomes can be easily identified because they take up certain dyes with avidity and appear quite dark in the usual stained preparation of a cell. With a few exceptions, every cell in the human body contains 23 pairs of chromosomes, one member of each pair being derived from the father and the other member from the mother. A *gene* is a submicroscopic substance on the chromosome which determines the inherited characteristics of an organism. For instance, there is a gene which determines the character of the MN blood groups; another that determines whether a person develops thalassemia; and yet a third that determines whether he or she will show homogentisic acid in the urine; and so on. Suitable experiments have shown that the genes are arranged in a linear sequence along the length of the chromosomes and that the sequence in which the genes are arranged tends to be the same for all individuals of a particular species.

During fertilization the father contributes one of each pair of his chromosomes and the mother contributes one of each pair of her chromosomes, and these two make up the pair of chromosomes in their offspring. Since the genes are located along the length of the chromosome, usually there is for each gene on a maternal chromosome a corresponding homologous gene on the paternal chromosome in the same position. Most of the time, the two homologous genes are identical and of the type most common to the species—and that is "normal," as we say. For example, most of us have the normal form of the gene for sickle cell anemia, and therefore we have normal hemoglobin in our blood. But, here and there along the line of genes on a chromosome there is likely to be found an "abnormal," or, as we say, a *mutant,* gene. If this should occur in the gene for sickle cell anemia, the individual carrying the abnormal gene would have some Type S hemoglobin as well as Type A hemoglobin; and if both genes in that position should be abnormal, the person would have only Type S hemoglobin (Hgb S). All inborn errors of metabolism are the result of mutations of one or another of the genes.

The exact reason why a normal gene becomes a mutant gene is not known. Investigators have suggested that environmental factors, such as temperature, atmospheric oxygen, and nutrition, may play a role. There is considerable evidence that radiation from x-rays or ultraviolet light can cause fresh mutations. Regardless of the cause, once a mutation occurs, the abnormal characteristic will be transmitted to future generations. Mutant genes may, however, be removed from the general population by one of several means. The mutant gene may have a lethal effect on the affected individual and he will fail to reproduce, thereby permanently removing that gene from circulation. Environmental circumstances may favor the reproduction and survival of normal genes over the reproduction and survival of abnormal genes. Finally, a mutant gene may spontaneously revert back to normal. This is a rare event, but it has been known to occur.

Medically, we have tended to emphasize the similarity of the characteristics of a given hereditary disease. For instance, the clinical manifestations of one patient with the adrenogenital syndrome are very similar to those of another. Chemically, all such patients excrete excessive amounts of 17-ketosteroids. Finally, the condition is usually transmitted as an autosomal recessive. It is not surprising, therefore, that we have always regarded the adrenogenital syndrome as one uniform entity. During the past 2 or 3 years, careful studies have revealed that there are at least two or three different varieties of the adrenogenital syndrome. Although the patients appear to be quite similar clinically, they show definite chemical differences; and genetic studies have shown that, in any given family, only one of the three types of the condition appears. This is not surprising if one remembers that fresh mutations are occurring constantly; also, it seems unlikely that all of the present cases of the adrenogenital syndrome stem from a single mutation that occurred many generations ago. Instead of thinking of the syndrome as a single homogeneous entity, one should think of it in terms of the occurrence of many separate fresh mutations. Some of these may involve the same genes and will give an identical laboratory and clinical picture; others may involve entirely separate genes, located in different positions on perhaps other chromosomes. It is only our inability to determine these differences clinically, or even in the laboratory, that has led us to believe they were all a single homogeneous entity. Other examples of probable differences in mutations are the dominant and recessive forms of alkaptonuria, the several different forms of cystinuria, and the three different types of methemoglobinemia. If one appreciates the fact that every inborn error of metabolism encountered may represent a fresh mutation, this will lead to a more flexible approach to their study.

HOW ARE THE INBORN ERRORS OF METABOLISM TRANSMITTED?

We turn next to the problem of how abnormal genes are transmitted from one generation to the next. Classically, a genetic defect has been

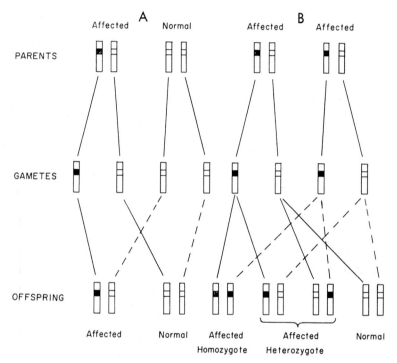

FIG. 1.—Dominant inheritance. *A*, only one parent affected with the defect. *B*, both parents affected.

shown to be transmitted by one of three modes: dominant, recessive, or sex linked. We shall, therefore, discuss these modes first.

CONDITIONS TRANSMITTED AS AN AUTOSOMAL DOMINANT.—A *dominant* condition, such as renal glycosuria, is transmitted in the manner shown in Figure 1, *A*. Let us assume that the father of such a mating has one abnormal gene for renal glycosuria. Since he has two genes which are different, he is described as a *heterozygote* for the trait. The mother, on the other hand, has two genes which are both normal, and she is described as being *normal* for the trait. Since the condition is a dominant one, the character will show up in the heterozygote and the father will have sugar in his urine; however, the mother, being normal, will not have renal glycosuria.

When two such individuals mate, the father can contribute either a normal or an abnormal gene as gametes, while the mother can only contribute two normal genes as gametes. Two types of offspring can arise from such a mating. Half of the offspring would have one normal and one abnormal gene for renal glycosuria and be heterozygotes like the father; the other half will have two normal genes and be normal like the mother.

In dominant inheritance, most of the affected individuals are heterozygotes for the abnormality and the trait is carried through each successive generation. Thus, the mode of transmission of a dominant defect is an indication of how the chromosomes actually behave, just as if we could observe the chromosomes themselves at each reduction division and at each fertilization. If an investigator can study only one family properly, he can describe the way the abnormal gene is transmitted.

Very rarely, two affected individuals will mate and produce an offspring with two abnormal genes, the offspring being a *homozygote* for the trait (Fig. 1, *B*). Such an individual usually has a more severe form of the disease than either of his affected parents. In many disorders the homozygote may die either before birth or shortly thereafter.

CONDITIONS TRANSMITTED AS AN AUTOSOMAL RECESSIVE.—A *recessive* gene, such as the one for phenylketonuria, can be transmitted in the manner shown in Figure 2. If one of the parents is a heterozygote and the other is completely normal, half of the offspring will be heterozygotes and the other half completely normal, as shown in Figure 2, *A*. Since the condition is a recessive one, the heterozygote cannot usually be identified by simple means, and the abnormal gene is passed from one generation to another without the condition being known.

However, when two such heterozygotes mate, a rather different picture emerges, as shown in Figure 2, *B*. Each of the heterozygotes will contribute one normal and one abnormal gene at the gamete stage. Three types of offspring will result. One quarter of them will receive one normal gene from the father and a similar normal gene from the mother and will be completely normal, in the genetic sense. One half of the offspring will receive one normal and one abnormal gene from each of the parents and be heterozygotes, just like their parents. The final quarter of the offspring will receive one abnormal gene from the father and one abnormal gene from the mother; they will be homozygotes with two abnormal genes for the trait and will have the full-blown clinical picture of phenylketonuria.

As a general rule, a recessive mode of inheritance is suggested by the following genetic findings: (1) the great majority of affected persons are

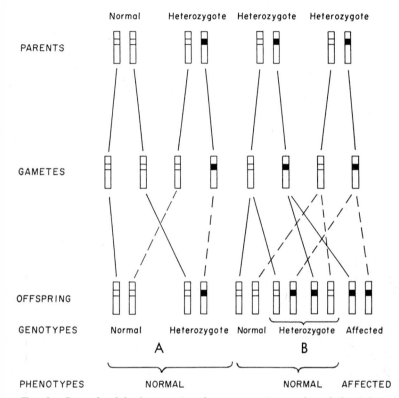

FIG. 2.—Recessive inheritance. *A,* only one parent a carrier of the defect. *B,* both parents carriers.

the offspring of parents who are normal to all outward appearances; (2) the condition tends to affect the siblings in a family (with a ratio of 1 affected to 3 unaffected) but does not usually affect parents or offspring unless there is intermarriage between close blood relatives; and (3) there is usually an undue proportion of consanguineous marriages among the parents of affected persons. The reasons for this increased incidence can be shown as follows:

Let us say that there is a marriage between two first cousins, where the father of the woman and the mother of the man are brother and sister, as shown in Figure 3. If one assumes that the woman (A) is heterozygous for phenylketonuria, she must have received the abnormal gene either from her father or from her mother, so that the chance of her father (B) also being a heterozygote is 1 in 2, or ½. If the father (B) is heterozygous, then he must have received the abnormal gene from his father or mother; and if so, the chance of his sister (C) being heterozygous is ½×½, or 1 in 4. Finally, if C is a heterozygote, the chance of her son (D) being a heterozygote is ½×½×½, or 1 in 8. Therefore, one

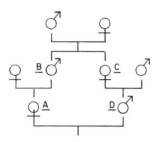

Fig. 3.—Genetic tree of a marriage of two first cousins.

can say that the probability of a heterozygote mating another heterozygote for the same trait in a first-cousin marriage is 1 in 8.

Estimates have shown that about 1 out of every 100 persons in the general population is a heterozygote for the phenylketonuria trait. Assuming random mating, the chance of a case of phenylketonuria occurring among unrelated marriages is $1/100 \times 1/100$, or less than 1 in 10,000. On the other hand, if first cousins were to marry each other, the chance would be increased by $1/100 \times \frac{1}{8}$, or 1 in 800. In other words, there is a 12.5 times greater likelihood of such a mating's getting an affected child than would a union from the general population. In the same way, consanguinity occurs in about 8 per cent of the parents of phenylketonurics, which is considerably higher than the 1 per cent seen in the population as a whole. Generally, the more rare the defect, the higher the proportion of consanguineous marriages.

CONDITIONS THAT ARE SEX LINKED.—In most cells in the human body the members of each of the 23 pairs of chromosomes are identical in appearance with one exception. Males possess one unequal pair of chromosomes, termed the "XY pair." The chromosomes in this pair differ in that the length of the X-chromosome is appreciably longer than that of the Y-chromosome, a difference which is easily detectable under the ordinary microscope. Females, on the other hand, possess two chromosomes of the X type and none of the Y type. Because of this difference, these chromosomes are described as *sex-chromosomes,* in contrast to the other chromosomes, which are called *autosomes.*

The sex-linked genes are carried on the X-chromosomes. We can illustrate this by describing the mode of inheritance of the gene for hemophilia, which is probably carried in the upper portion of the X-chromosome, as shown in region *A* in Figure 4. When a female who is hetero-

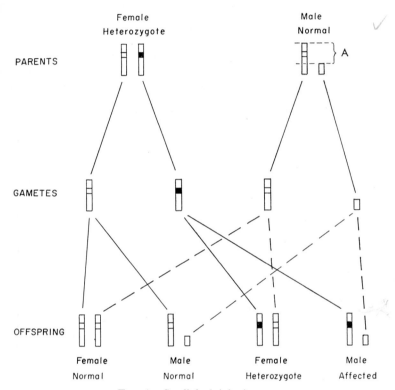

Fig. 4.—Sex-linked inheritance.

zygous for this gene mates with a normal male, one of four situations can occur: (1) the female and male can each contribute one normal X-chromosome and produce a normal female offspring; (2) the female can contribute one normal X-chromosome and the male a Y-chromosome and produce a normal male offspring; (3) the female can contribute an abnormal X-chromosome and the male a normal X-chromosome and produce a female offspring who is a heterozygous carrier just like her mother. Since hemophilia is a recessive trait, this offspring will show no clinical disease but can transmit the abnormality to her male offspring;

and (4) the female can contribute an abnormal X-chromosome and the male a Y-chromosome and produce an affected male. If this male hemophiliac mates with a normal female, he can transmit the trait to his daughters, who will be carriers. There is also the possibility that he will mate with a female who is a heterozygote and that both male and female hemophiliacs can result from such a marriage. However, the probability of this occurring is so small that only one or two such instances have been reported.

FACTORS THAT INFLUENCE GENE EXPRESSION.—Before leaving the question of how genes are transmitted, we should consider the factors that influence the proper expression of genes. First, we must remember

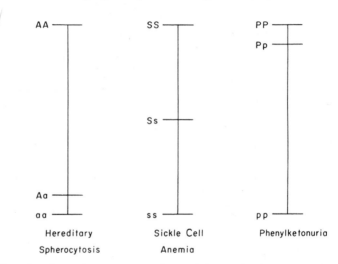

FIG. 5.—Illustrating gene expression. It is incompletely dominant in hereditary spherocytosis; neither dominant nor recessive in sickle cell anemia; and incompletely recessive (where the heterozygotes are detectable) in phenylketonuria.

that genetic conditions are seldom completely dominant or completely recessive. Rather, they appear to be relatively so, depending upon how well one can distinguish between the heterozygote and the normal, and also between the heterozygote and the homozygote with two abnormal genes. This can be illustrated by three examples, as shown in Figure 5.

In hereditary spherocytosis, the heterozygote (Fig. 5, Aa) has anemia, spherocytosis, increased fragility of erythrocytes, and all of the characteristics of the clinical disease. The homozygote with the two abnormal genes (aa) occurs rarely; but when such an individual is investigated, his or her condition is little different from that of the heterozygote except that he hemolytic process may be a little more severe. Yet, genetically the heterozygote and the homozygote are quite different. As a result, we regard the condition as being transmitted as a "dominant," or at least almost completely so. In sickle cell anemia, the heterozygote (Ss) has about 40% Hgb S and 60% Hgb A in the blood. This places it as intermediate between the affected homozygote (ss) and the normal (SS). Such conditions are regarded as being neither completely dominant nor completely recessive. Finally, in phenylketonuria, the heterozygote (Pp) is almost normal in every way except that he has some difficulty in handling large amounts of phenylalanine, as compared with the normal individual (PP). We classify this condition as a "recessive," although it is not completely so. By viewing most of the inborn errors of metabolism as being neither completely dominant nor recessive, we get a truer picture of the disease process and how it is transmitted.

Second, we should mention that genes are regularly transmitted but may not be regularly expressed. For instance, in a dominant mode of inheritance, one would expect the abnormality to be transmitted from parent to child to grandchild. In some families the abnormality is well documented in the first generation, skips the second generation, and reappears in several members of the third generation, indicating that the abnormal gene was transmitted but not expressed. In such instances, careful studies have shown that the individual in the "missed" generation did, in fact, show a minor degree of the abnormality but that it was too slight to be detected. In other instances, no abnormalities of any kind could be detected. For some unknown reason, the abnormal gene was not expressed in the second generation but reappeared in the typical manner in the third generation.

Third, one has to remember that a trait which is truly inherited need not necessarily be present at birth. In some cases, it may appear later in life. Huntington's chorea will serve as an example. This disease is characterized by the development, at about age 30 or 40, of mental deterioration, accompanied by involuntary movements of the face, body, and extremities. These symptoms are due to an actual degeneration of certain brain centers; and family studies have shown that, when the age of onset is taken into consideration, this disorder meets all the requirements of a dominant mode of inheritance.

Another problem to be faced is the fact that in some disorders only a few of the affected individuals actually show clinical signs and symptoms of disease. For instance, there are published pedigrees which show that many individuals in the family have hyperuricemia but that only a few of these develop gout clinically. Diabetes mellitus is probably another exam-

ple of a condition in which only a few of the affected individuals show
the full clinical picture.

INFLUENCE OF ENVIRONMENT.—Although geneticists prefer to deal
with characteristics that are relatively unaffected by the environment
this is frequently not possible, especially when one is dealing with human
genetics. Therefore, no data regarding the genetic behavior of a trait are

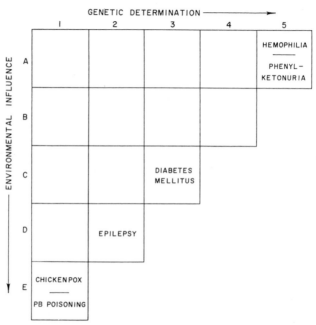

FIG. 6.—Method for delineating hereditary and environmental factors in the
pathogenesis of disease.

adequate without a specification of the environmental circumstances in
which the trait has developed.

The environmental events which may intervene between the basic
biochemical activities of a gene and the resulting finished characteristics
in man run a wide gamut. They may be overtly traumatic or subtly psychological; they may be related to geographical location, to climate, to
socioeconomic status or to rural or urban habitat; they may be infectious
in nature or they may involve immunological response to invasions; they
may be nutritional or they may relate to the psychological status of the
mother.

One convenient method for delineating hereditary and environmental
influences is illustrated in Figure 6. The horizontal axis shows the extent

f genetic influences, and the vertical axis shows the role played by en-
ronmental influences. Thus, a disease like hemophilia or phenylketonu-
a, which is entirely genetically determined, would fit in position $A5$.
Most workers would agree that diabetes mellitus is at least in part geneti-
ally determined. Yet, diet and mode of living may play a major role in its
athogenesis, and hence it should properly be placed in position $C3$. A
ondition like epilepsy cannot be considered as a hereditary disease in
the classical sense; yet, similar abnormal electroencephalogram tracings
re noted with great frequency among families, and especially among
the twins of affected individuals. This would probably place epilepsy in
osition $D2$. Finally, chickenpox and lead poisoning, although they may
in in families, are almost certainly due only to environmental factors,
id these diseases should be placed in position $E1$.

How Are the Inborn Errors of Metabolism Expressed?

We might start off by speculating on what happens to a fresh mutation.
i some instances the abnormality may be so severe as to be lethal while
ie fetus is still in utero. This could occur when the embryo is at the 4- or
- or 16-cell stage, or it may occur close to term. Careful studies with
ice have shown that death can occur and the fetuses become absorbed
: any stage of gestation and that only the unaffected members of a litter
ill be born. Early miscarriages among humans must in part be due to
thal genes.

In addition, certain mutant genes exert a definite but usually not
thal effect upon the fetus during the early stages of embryonic develop-
ent. This accounts for the long list of structural disorders which we
now to be determined on a genetic basis. How the genes affect morphol-
gy is not entirely clear at the present time. It is believed that most
obably they induce chemical abnormalities during the early stages of
nbryonic development and that this in turn causes structural malforma-
ons. If this is the case, then these conditions should also be included
nong the inborn errors of metabolism. However, such disorders will not
: discussed here because so little is known about the chemical changes
at a discussion of the pathogenesis of the disorders would be fruitless.

Finally, we come to the group of conditions caused by abnormal genes
here the biochemical abnormalities are relatively minor. As a result,
e fetus can survive to term, permitting us to make proper clinical and
ochemical observations. Garrod quite correctly defined such conditions
"inborn errors of metabolism"; however, we should extend that defini-
on to include any genetically determined condition where there is clear-

cut evidence of a chemical disturbance, and even include those condition
which are likely in the future to have a chemical basis. This means that th
term "inborn errors of metabolism" should include such things as hemat
logical abnormalities, renal-clearance disturbances, and such morpholo
ically characterized entities as the lipidoses.

Let us return once more to the fundamental question of how a ge
acts. Although we know a good deal about how a gene determines th
inherited characteristics of an organism, we know relatively little abo
its physical or chemical properties, and even less about how genes repr

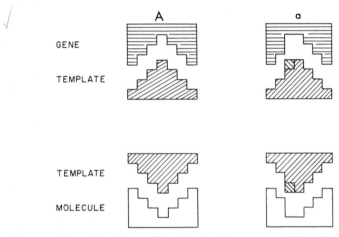

Fig. 7.—Illustrating the template theory of gene transmission. On the left,
normal gene (A) stamps a normal template, which in turn produces a norm
molecule. On the right, a slight abnormality in the gene (a) causes a slight a
normality in the template, which in turn produces a molecule that is abnorm

duce and act inside the body. Careful studies have shown that a gene is
submicroscopic particle made up of desoxyribose nucleic acid and pr
teins. Although genes cannot be seen on human chromosomes, they ha
been localized on the fruitfly chromosome, and there is little doubt th
they exist as physical entities. The mode of action of these small partic
is not known. One theory is that they act as a model consisting of standa
residues, nucleotides, amino acids, and perhaps other prosthetic grou
and are copied by another chain. These chains then float away and b
come the *primary gene products*. Another theory is that the gene and th
whole chromosome are "copied" into a completely different structur
much like antigens with an antibody. The "template" or "negative"
again copied, giving two new positions, and so on (Fig. 7). Since va
numbers of molecules have to be created each day to replace those whi

egenerate and disappear, it is apparent that one copying process would
robably not be sufficient to do the job. Instead, several such processes
must go on in separate stages, and we are only observing the end-results of
his mechanism.

While we know relatively little about gene reproduction, we do know
good deal about the primary effect which the gene exerts on specific
molecules in the body. *This primary gene effect represents the first direct
result of the action of the gene which can be shown by physical or chemical means.* We can illustrate this by considering sickle cell anemia. We
now from genetic studies that, when the gene for sickle cell anemia is
resent in the abnormal form, some or all of the hemoglobin present is in
he form of Hgb S instead of the normal Hgb A. As a result, sickling
occurs; and when the process is severe, a hemolytic process takes place.
In the laboratory we cannot identify the exact gene which brings about
his abnormality. But recent studies have shown that, if the globulin por-
on of the hemoglobin molecule is broken down into 30 or more peptides,
ne of these stays positively charged in Hgb S and not charged in Hgb A.
his difference is due to a slight difference in the arrangement of the
equence of amino acids in a small part of one of the polypeptide chains.
his is sufficient to cause a difference in the isoelectric point by electro-
horesis and the decreased solubility in the reduced state of Hgb S as
ompared with Hgb A.

With this information on the primary gene effect, it is possible to con-
ruct a "pedigree of causes" of sickle cell anemia, for example, starting
ith the known primary gene effect and continuing with the secondary
ene effects, as illustrated in Chart 1. Not so many years ago, it was commonly believed that the renal changes, sickling, and abdominal pain in
ckle cell anemia were caused by different mechanisms. Even when it was
hought that these disturbances might be caused by a single gene abnor-
ality, it was concluded that the gene must exert its effect directly on
everal different systems within the body. The concept of a "unitary gene
ypothesis" was largely an article of faith. Today we can say with rea-
onable certainty that each of the inborn errors of metabolism must re-
ult from mutations of single genes and that these exert a primary gene
fect, which can, in principle, be shown by physical means. These
mutant genes, in turn, are responsible for all of the signs and symptoms
f clinical disease.

The importance of each of the secondary gene effects relative to that
f the primary gene effect can sometimes be placed on a mathematical
asis, as illustrated by the example shown in Figure 8. It is apparent in
his illustration that the disturbance in phenylalanine or phenylpyruvic

CHART 1

SICKLE CELL ANEMIA

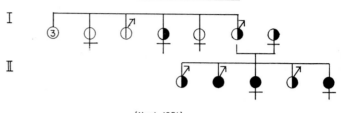

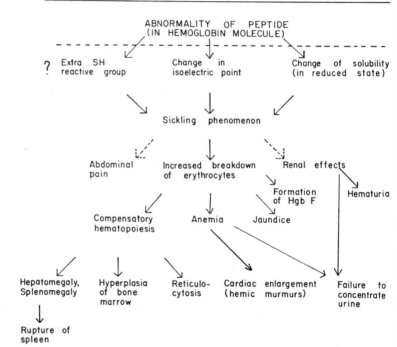

A "pedigree of causes" of sickle cell anemia. The mode of transmission of t abnormal gene is given at the top of the chart. A thick line then separates t genetic information, which can only be deduced mathematically from the chemic properties, which can be measured by physical means. The primary gene eff is given, in capital letters, immediately under the family data; and the seconda gene effects follow from the primary gene effect. For symbols, see Figure 9; a for further description of charts, see text, page 32. (This pedigree is tak from Neel, J. V.: The inheritance of the sickling phenomenon, with particu reference to sickle-cell disease, Blood 6:389, 1951.)

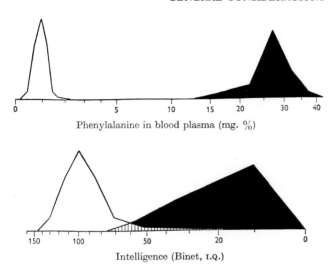

Phenylalanine in blood plasma (mg. %)

Intelligence (Binet, I.Q.)

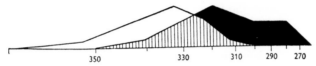

Head size. Length + breadth in mm. (corrected for sex)

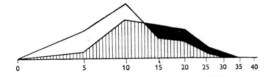

Hair colour. Reflectance % at 700 mμ (corrected for age)

FIG. 8.—Distribution of plasma phenylalanine levels, intelligence, head size, and hair color in normal persons (*left*) and in those with phenylketonuria (*right*). (From Penrose, L. S.: Measurement of pleiotropic effects in phenylketonuria, Ann. Eugenics [London] 16:134, 1951.)

acid is more important than, say, intelligence, where there is some overlap between normal and abnormal; and certainly more so than something like hair color, where the correlation is only on the order of 0.2-0.3.

Rapid biochemical progress during the past decade has made it possible for us to name the primary gene changes of many of the hereditary disorders. Up to the present, the changes seem to involve only protein molecules; however, it is probable that other types of molecules will also be involved in the future. The disturbances in protein molecules may be divided into four types:

1. Disturbances in the structure of the protein molecules, where there appears to be a change in the actual shape or arrangement of the molecules themselves.
2. Disturbances in the synthesis of the protein molecule, where the protein is not being made properly or may be entirely absent.
3. Disturbances in the function of the protein molecule, where an enzyme does not appear to be functioning properly. In such conditions we are often not certain as to whether the protein is completely absent or is abnormal and hence cannot function.
4. Disturbances in renal transport mechanisms, which probably are similar to enzyme disturbances.

It should be emphasized that this classification is highly tentative. Also, it should be remembered that, since we know so little about how a gene acts, the observed "primary" gene effect may, in fact, be several stages removed from the fundamental action of the gene. As we acquire more information, what we now regard as primary gene action may turn out to be very secondary after all. The very fact that we see the gene acting in different ways—by causing a disturbance in protein structure, in protein synthesis, and in protein function—is a clear indication that we have not reached the ultimate stage of understanding how a gene acts.

We shall now discuss each of the disorders individually, illustrating the disorder by means of a specially prepared chart. At the TOP of each chart (see Chart 1, p. 30) will be shown the pertinent information on the *gene* and how it is transmitted. Whenever possible, a typical family with the condition has been chosen from the literature to illustrate the heredity of the condition. The symbols used in the charts are shown in Figure 9.

The MIDDLE portion of the chart will be devoted to the *primary gene effect*. As discussed above, this reflects the first effect of the gene which is detectable by physical or chemical means. While it is not the purpose of the present book to take up all of the biochemical background of each disorder, clinical formulas and the site of the metabolic block will be shown whenever possible. Also, useful laboratory procedures for the diagnosis of each condition will be given in the Appendix.

The LOWER portion of each chart will be devoted to *secondary clinical signs and symptoms* which result from the primary gene effect. Where there is doubt as to how the mechanism operates, a question mark is placed along that pathway.

In the discussion of the disorder, particular emphasis will be placed upon clinical features, heredity, pathogenesis, diagnosis, and treatment. A list of the most useful references, including reviews (marked with an asterisk), will be given at the end of each section.

A book of this nature must, of necessity, be incomplete, and many important things have had to be left out. It is hoped, however, that it will

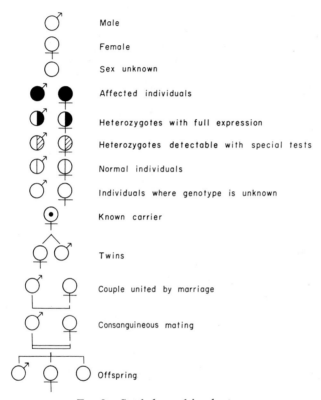

Male

Female

Sex unknown

Affected individuals

Heterozygotes with full expression

Heterozygotes detectable with special tests

Normal individuals

Individuals where genotype is unknown

Known carrier

Twins

Couple united by marriage

Consanguineous mating

Offspring

FIG. 9.—Symbols used in charts.

be of some help to the general practitioner and the house officer when they are next confronted with a disorder that seems to "run in the family."

Beadle, G. W.: Biochemical genetics, Chem. Rev. 37:15, 1945.
Childs, B., and Sidbury, J. B., Jr.: A survey of genetics as it applies to problems in medicine, Pediatrics 20:178, 1957.
*Garrod, A. E.: *Inborn Errors of Metabolism* (London: Henry Frowde, 1909).
Gruneberg, H.: *Animal Genetics and Medicine* (New York: Paul B. Hoeber, Inc., 1947).
Haldane, J. B. S.: *The Biochemistry of Genetics* (London: George Allen & Unwin, Ltd., 1954).

34 INBORN ERRORS OF METABOLISM

*Harris, H.: *An Introduction to Human Biochemical Genetics* (London: Cambridge University Press, 1953).

Hsia, D. Y. Y.: The laboratory detection of heterozygotes, Am. J. Human Genet. 9:98, 1957.

Knox, W. E.: The hereditary molecular diseases in man, Bull. New England Center Hosp. 2:1, 1956.

Neel, J. V.: The inheritance of the sickling phenomenon, with particular reference to sickle-cell disease, Blood 6:389, 1951.

—— and Schull, W. J.: *Human Heredity* (Chicago: University of Chicago Press, 1954).

Pauling, L.: Abnormalities of hemoglobin molecules in hereditary hemolytic anemias, Harvey Lect. 49:216, 1954.

Roberts, J. A. F.: *An Introduction to Medical Genetics* (London: Oxford University Press, 1940).

Sorsby, A. (ed.): *Clinical Genetics* (St. Louis: C. V. Mosby Company, 1953).

Snyder, L. H.: Human heredity and its modern application, Am. Scientist 43:391, 1955.

*Symposium on inborn errors of metabolism (Dent, C. E., guest editor), Am. J Med. 22:671-783, 1957.

PART I

Disturbances in
Molecular Structure

A NUMBER OF THE inborn errors of metabolism result from abnormalities of molecular structure and arrangement. These defects
are particularly important because they probably reflect closely the
direct action of the abnormal gene. In fact, some workers believe
that the specific protein molecules concerned are actual direct
products of the gene itself. In any event, the study of structural
disturbances is likely to give us information on how a gene acts.
Ultimately it may be found that all inborn errors of metabolism
involve some disturbance of molecular structure.

The structural disturbances may be of two kinds. First we have
the group of conditions where there is clearly a disturbance of structure within the molecule itself. This group would include *sickle cell
anemia* and the *other abnormal hemoglobins*. The finding of a
structural abnormality first in hemoglobin is not surprising, since
hemoglobin is the protein most readily available in the body and has
been intensively studied for years.

Then we have the group of conditions in which there is a difference in the make-up of the "stroma," or wall of cells. It is not clear
at present whether these changes represent a disturbance of structure within the molecule itself or an abnormality in the arrangement
of the molecules in relation to each other. However, these conditions
have many features in common with the abnormal hemoglobins
and should be considered together; they include: *thalassemia,*

hereditary elliptocytosis, acanthrocytosis, erythropoietic porphyria, and the *Pelger-Huet anomaly of the leukocytes.*

Finally, it should be mentioned that all of the blood groups, such as Rh, ABO, and MN, represent structural differences of molecules in individuals. Some of the serum protein groups described by Smithies and his co-workers probably should be regarded as molecular differences also. These variations, however, affect all human beings and probably should not be regarded as examples of errors of metabolism.

2

Sickle Cell Anemia and the Other Abnormal Hemoglobins

In 1949, Pauling, Itano, Singer, and Wells made the fundamental discovery that the erythrocytes of patients with sickle cell anemia contain hemoglobin with an isoelectric point which is significantly different from that of normal individuals. This provided the first positive evidence that adult human hemoglobin exists in more than one molecular form, and it implied for the first time that many of the hereditary diseases of a biochemical nature may be caused by genetically determined abnormalities

TABLE 1.—Physical Characteristics of the Abnormal Hemoglobins

Name	Alkali Denatur- ation	Iso- elec- tric Point	Anodic Mobil- ity on Paper Electropho- resis (Rela- tive) (pH 8.6)	Solubility of Reduced Hgb (Relative to Hgb A)	Amino Acid Composition	Sick- ling
Hgb A	Normal	6.87	4	High	Normal	No
Hgb F	Alkali resistant	6.98	5	Higher than Hgb A	Abnormal	No
Hgb S	Normal	7.09	7	Very low	Normal*	Yes
Hgb C	Normal	7.30	10	Higher than Hgb A	Abnormal	No
Hgb D	Normal	7.09	8	Same as Hgb A	Unknown	No
Hgb E	Normal	7.09?	9	Same as Hgb A	Normal	No
Hgb G	Normal	6.98	6	Same as Hgb A	Unknown	No
Hgb H	Normal	5.60	1	Low	Unknown	No
Hgb I	Normal	....	2	High	Unknown	No
Hgb J	Normal	....	3	High	Unknown	No

*Evidence of difference in charges of one peptide.

of protein synthesis. Since then, additional examples of abnormal hemoglobins have been described; together, they may be described as a "family of hemoglobin disorders" (Table 1).

At the present time, there appear to be at least three separate loci responsible for hemoglobin production: (1) It has been shown that the genes responsible for Hgbs S and C are alleles, or closely linked. These have been designated h_1^S for Hgb S, h_1^C for Hgb C, and h_1^A for its normal allele. (2) The production of Hgb G is inherited independently of the genes mentioned above. This state has been designated h_2^G for Hgb G, and h_2^A for its normal allele. (3) Finally, evidence has been presented showing that the genes responsible for Hgbs S and G and for thalassemia are not allelic. Therefore, the thalassemia gene has been designated h_t^T, and its normal allele as h_t^A. The relationship of the genes responsible for Hgbs D, E, H, I, J, and K to these three loci remains to be worked out. These genes could be alleles of those responsible for Hgbs S and C or for Hgb G, or they may occur at independent loci. For the present purposes, they will be defined as h^D, h^E, h^H, h^I, h^J, and h^K.

The abnormal hemoglobins will be discussed under the following headings: (1) *sickle cell anemia,* (2) *other abnormal hemoglobin variants,* (3) *mixed heterozygous hemoglobin diseases,* (4) *the thalassemia syndrome,* and (5) *other mixed disturbances.*

I. SICKLE CELL ANEMIA

The red blood cells of certain individuals possess the peculiar property of undergoing a reversible alteration in shape in response to changes in the partial pressure of oxygen within the cell. When oxygen tension is lowered, these cells change from their normal biconcave form to elongated filamentous or crescentic forms. The peculiar shape of such cells in man was first recognized by Herrick. However, in retrospect, the same phenomenon had been noted in 1840 by Gullivar in some blood films prepared from deer in the London Zoo. This peculiar ability of red cells to sickle under conditions of reduced oxygen tension is the primary feature of sickle cell disease.

CLINICAL FEATURES.—Patients with *sickle cell anemia* (h_1^S/h_1^S) normally show only a moderate anemia, a subicteric tint of the scleras, and little or no enlargement of the spleen. Some changes in the tissues such as extramedullary hematopoiesis, hemosiderosis, and hyperplasia of the bone marrow, are sometimes found, depending on the severity of the anemia.

From time to time, the patients develop recurrent attacks of weakness, fatigue, anorexia, abdominal pain, icterus of the scleras, and pallor. Examination during or shortly after such a hemolytic crisis will show an icteric tinge to the scleras, increased pallor of the lips and mucous membranes, and enlargement of the liver and spleen; and, as the anemia becomes more severe, enlargement of the heart with hemic murmurs occurs. Such hemolytic crises are frequently precipitated by an acute infection.

The course and prognosis of patients with sickle cell anemia vary with the severity of the sickling tendency, the frequency and duration of the hemolytic crises, and the age of the patient. Younger patients seem to fare less well, since recurrent severe anemia often interferes with proper growth and nutrition and thus restricts general activity. Older individuals frequently suffer from arthritic symptoms, leg ulcers, and aseptic necrosis

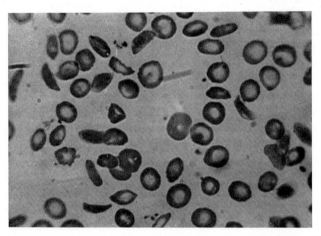

FIG. 10.—Smear from the peripheral blood of a patient with sickle cell anemia.

of the hip. Hematuria and hyposthenuria are not infrequent complications. Death may result from a rapidly developing severe anemia or intercurrent infection.

A relatively benign condition is *sickle cell trait* (h_1^S/h_1^A), which is characterized only by the ability of the erythrocytes to sickle under reduced oxygen tension. Two complications have occasionally been noted among those with the sickle cell trait. Hematuria may occur, especially during periods of low oxygen tension. Also, splenic infarction has been known to occur during flights at high altitude. When this occurs, massive hemorrhages and infarctions are found and the sinusoids in the spleen are packed with masses of sickled erythrocytes.

Sickling may be demonstrated by preparing a fresh blood film and excluding air by sealing with oil or petrolatum or by replacing the air with carbon dioxide (Fig. 10). Patients with sickle cell anemia usually have erythrocyte levels which are below normal, and during a sickle cell crisis the level will frequently drop to less than 1,000,000/mm³. In most cases, there is no reduction of the hemoglobin content within the cells. The life span of the sickle cell is shorter than normal; and such patients have to compensate for this by increasing their erythropoietic activity, as shown by the large number of reticulocytes, nucleated red cells, and hyperplasia of the bone marrow.

HEREDITY.—In 1949, Beet and Neel independently demonstrated that the sickle cell trait was the heterozygous manifestation of a gene which, when homozygous, resulted in sickle cell anemia. This manifestation can be shown in the laboratory as follows: (1) a normal individual, having only normal genes at the sickle cell locus (h_1^A/h_1^A) will have only normal adult hemoglobin (Hgb A); (2) the heterozygote with one normal and one abnormal gene (h_1^S/h_1^A) has about 40% sickle cell hemoglobin (Hgb S) and 60% normal adult hemoglobin (Hgb A); and (3) the patient with two abnormal genes (h_1^S/h_1^S), who has sickle cell anemia, produces only sickle cell hemoglobin (Hgb S).

Hemoglobin S trait occurs in 7-9% of the American Negroes, and the rate may increase up to 45% among certain African tribes. The trait is limited almost entirely to the Negro race. The occasional reports of sickle cell disease among Caucasians have almost always risen in areas where admixture with Negro blood could not be completely ruled out. At the present time, Hgb S trait can be found in three areas outside of America and Africa: (1) in Greece, in the vicinity of Lake Copais and in northern Greece; (2) among the primitive Veddoids of southern India; and (3) among the Achdam of southern Arabia. The spread of this trait can be attributed to people from Africa being transported to the Mediterranean area and the Americas through invasion, the use of African mercenaries, and the slave trade.

The genetics of Hgb S trait is of special interest because of the possibility that persons with the sickle cell trait may have increased resistance to falciform malaria. These observations are based on several pieces of evidence: (1) there seems to be a different rate of parasitemia by the malaria parasite among sicklers and nonsicklers in the same region; (2) there seems to be a difference in susceptibility to experimental malaria among sicklers and nonsicklers in two small studies; and (3) a correlation exists between the distribution of malaria and the distribution of the sickle cell trait in Africa. Against this hypothesis is the finding that malaria occurs in certain regions where sickle cell disease is unknown. Also, we know very little about the normal pathogenesis of malaria without sickle cell disease complicating the picture. Nevertheless, the possible relation between the two is an attractive hypothesis and could be of great significance clinically.

PATHOGENESIS.—Sickle cell anemia occurs as a result of an abnormality in the structure of the hemoglobin molecule. Ingram has recently shown that if the globin portion of the hemoglobin molecule is broken down by tryptic digests, some 28 peptides, each with an average chain length of 9-10 amino acids, will result. These can then be separated on paper first by electrophoresis and then by chromatography. The peptides prepared from Hgb S differ from those of Hgb A only in the location of one peptide group. Studies on the arrangement of amino acids within this abnormal peptide revealed that in sickle cell hemoglobin a valine unit had replaced the glutamic acid unit (Fig. 11).

This difference is useful in interpreting the differences in the physical properties of Hgbs S and A, which are as follows:

1. Hemoglobin S has a distinctive electrophoretic pattern. In the epoch-making discovery of Pauling and his co-workers it was found that Hgb S migrates as a positive ion, whereas Hgb A migrates as a negative ion in a 0.1 M phosphate buffer, pH 6.9. These variations in mobility correspond to a difference of 0.22 pH units in the isoelectric point of the two compounds. A difference in the rate of migration in an electric field can also be shown by the more simple technique of paper electrophoresis.

2. In their reduced form, crystals of Hgb S are birefringent, whereas those of Hgb A are not.

3. The difference in solubility between oxygenated Hgbs S and A is not striking. If one assigns an arbitrary value of 1 (one) to the solubility of oxyhemoglobin A, oxyhemoglobin S is found to have the same solubility. Reduced Hgb A has only half the solubility of its corresponding oxy-compound. Reduced Hgb S, on the other hand, has approximately 50 times less the solubility of reduced Hgb A and has only one one-hundredth the solubility of its oxy-compound.

As a consequence of this insolubility, a marked increase of viscosity takes place as concentrated solutions of Hgb S are reduced. Indeed, after sufficient reduction the entire hemoglobin mass forms a semisolid gel, which can be liquefied and solidified at will by the alternative use of oxygen and carbon dioxide. These Hgb S crystals have the appearance of crescents and strongly resemble sickled erythrocytes. Harris has described the sickled erythrocyte as "a hemoglobin tactoid thinly veiled and somewhat distorted by a red-cell membrane." Upon this unique biochemical phenomenon—the striking insolubility of reduced Hgb S with the subsequent formation of sickle-shaped tactoids—depends all the clinical tests for the demonstration of sickling and all the signs and symptoms of sickle cell disease which are shown in Chart 1 on page 30.

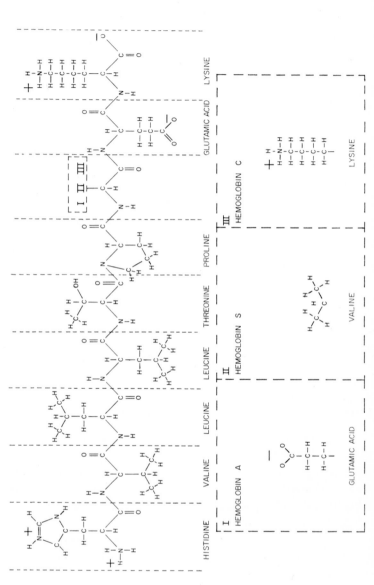

FIG. 11.—Short section of the hemoglobin molecule. The amino acid units of the molecule are set off by the vertical lines. The name of each amino acid is given below the diagram. There is a difference in the amino acid in the seventh position from the left. In the case of normal adult hemoglobin the amino acid is glutamic acid; in Hgb S the amino acid is valine; and in Hgb C the amino acid is lysine. (After Ingram, 1958.)

Sickling is probably responsible for the abdominal pain and specific renal effects, including hematuria and the inability to concentrate urine, which occur during hemolytic crises. The excessive breakdown of sickled cells causes anemia, formation of fetal hemoglobin (Hgb F), cardiac enlargement, icterus, and hyposthenuria, which are characteristic. The body tries to compensate for this anemia by extramedullary hematopoiesis, and the latter accounts for the hepatosplenomegaly, hyperplasia of the bone marrow, and reticulocytosis. Thus, the whole picture of sickle cell anemia can ultimately be attributed to the peptide abnormality in the hemoglobin molecule itself.

DIAGNOSIS.—Sickle cell anemia may be diagnosed by the detection of sickling in the peripheral blood (see Procedure 1, in Appendix), the identification of Hgb S by solubility (see Procedure 2), and paper electrophoresis studies (Procedure 3).

TREATMENT.—No treatment is required for those with the sickle cell trait. Among those with sickle cell anemia, the administration of oxygen is useful during a sickle cell crisis. However, whole-blood transfusions should be used only during an aplastic phase.

Allison, A. C.: Protection afforded by sickle-cell trait against subtertian malarial infection, Brit. M. J. 1:290, 1954.

Beet, E. A.: The genetics of the sickle-cell trait in a Bantu tribe, Ann. Eugenics 14:279, 1949.

*Chernoff, A. I.: The human hemoglobins in health and disease, New England J. Med. 253:322, 365, and 416, 1955.

Harris, J. W.: Studies on the destruction of red blood cells: VIII. Molecular orientation in sickle cell hemoglobin solutions, Proc. Soc. Exper. Biol. & Med. 75:197, 1950.

Ingram, V. M.: A specific chemical difference between the globins of normal human and sickle cell anemia hemoglobins, Nature 178:792, 1956.

————: How do genes act? Scient. Am. 198:68, 1958.

Neel, J. V.: The inheritance of sickle cell anemia, Science 110:64, 1949.

*————: The genetics of human haemoglobin differences: Problems and perspectives, Ann. Human Genet. 21:1, 1956.

Pauling, L.; Itano, H. A.; Singer, S. J.; and Wells, I. C.: Sickle cell anemia, a molecular disease, Science 110:543, 1949.

2. OTHER ABNORMAL HEMOGLOBIN VARIANTS

The differentiation of Hgb S from Hgb A was quickly followed by a series of reports on the identification of other abnormal hemoglobins. Each appeared to be inherited according to Mendelian laws and manifested itself, whether in the homozygous or heterozygous state, by specific changes in the hemoglobin pattern in the individual, much in the same way as does Hgb S (see Fig. 12). These hemoglobins do not differ significantly from each other. They have identical molecular weights, the isolated heme portions are alike, and the quantitative differences in the composition of the amino acids of the globulin portion of the molecule have not always been striking. There are some suggestions that the differences in their physical properties are due to alterations in amino acid arrangement, types of end-groups, or in the folding of the amino acid chains in the hemoglobin molecule.

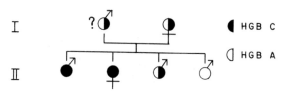

Fig. 12.—Other abnormal hemoglobin variants. (After Huisman *et al.*, 1955.)

Anderson and Griffith have suggested that abnormal hemoglobins may be complexes of normal hemoglobins with some other macromolecule which is constantly present and genetically inherited. In some instances the differences may so alter the solubility properties of the hemoglobin as to give rise to sickling. If this is the case, these complexes might be comparable to the polysaccharides responsible for the blood-group characteristics.

HEMOGLOBIN C

In 1950, Itano and Neel examined by electrophoresis the hemoglobin derived from members of two unusual families. In these families there occurred one or more children with the hematological picture of sickle cell anemia, but the disease was somewhat less severe than that usually encountered and the situation was peculiar in that the erythrocytes of only one parent in each case could be induced to sickle. Those of the other parent were apparently normal. Electrophoretically, it was found that the hemoglobin from two of these anemic children separated into two distinct components: one corresponding to that of Hgb S, and the other migrating as an even more positive ion than that of Hgb S. In another anemic child, both of these components were present as well as a small proportion of hemoglobin with a mobility corresponding to Hgb A. Studies of the parents in each case showed the findings typical of sickle cell trait in one parent while the other parent was found to have hemoglobins resolving into two types, Hgb A and the new component, which Itano and Neel designated as Hgb C.

Hemoglobin C (see Table 1) differs from the other hemoglobins in three respects: (1) it has an electrophoretic mobility faster than either Hgb S or Hgb A; (2) its solubility is greater than that of the reduced compounds of Hgbs F, S, and A; and (3) studies in molecular structure have revealed that in the same abnormal peptide the glutamic acid unit has been replaced by a lysine unit (Fig. 11).

Hemoglobin C trait ($h_1{}^C/h_1{}^A$) is present in about 2% of the American Negro population. In certain parts of western Central Africa, a prevalence up to 15% has been observed. Clinically, the hematological findings are entirely normal except for an increase in the number of target cells and a very mild hypochromia of the red cells. Sickling does not occur.

Homozygous Hgb C disease ($h_1{}^C/h_1{}^C$) is a rare condition, calculated as occurring once in every 6,000 Negroes in America. The condition is considerably more mild than the homozygous form of Hgb S (sickle cell anemia), with only vague intermittent arthralgia and occasional abdominal pain being present. Persons with this condition do not usually develop a true crisis, as in sickle cell anemia. Hemoglobin C disease is not incompatible with a normal life span.

Huisman, T. H. J.; Jonxis, J. H. P.; and Schaaf, P. C.: Amino acid composition of four different kinds of human hemoglobin, Nature 175:902, 1955.
————; Schaaf, P. C.; and Sar, A.: Some characteristic properties of hemoglobin C, Blood 10:1079, 1955.
Itano, H. A., and Neel, J. V.: A new inherited abnormality of human hemoglobin, Proc. Nat. Acad. Sc. 36:613, 1950.
Neel, J. V.; Kaplan, E.; and Zuelzer, W. W.: Further studies on hemoglobin C: I. A description of three additional families segregating for Hgb C and sickle cell hemoglobin, Blood 8:724, 1953.
Spaet, T. H.; Alway, R. H.; and Ward, G.: Homozygous Type C hemoglobin, Pediatrics 12:483, 1953.

HEMOGLOBIN D

In 1934, Cooke and Mack described a family, apparently of American ancestry, in which the father and two children all exhibited slow sickling of the red cells on reduction. In 1951, Itano re-examined the hemoglobin of these offspring and found that, electrophoretically, the hemoglobin in these children corresponded closely to that generally found in sickle cell anemia. However, in the mother and two siblings, none of whom showed the sickle cell trait, there were, nevertheless, two electrophoretically different components in their hemoglobin. Between 35 and 49% of their hemoglobin was found to migrate as Hgb S and the remainder as Hgb A. Thus, electrophoretically, these persons could be regarded as sickle cell heterozygotes even though they failed to show the sickling phenomenon.

The explanation of this anomalous result was found as a result of solubility studies. It was learned that Hgb D (Table 1) was much more soluble than Hgb S and that its solubility corresponded to that of reduced Hgb A. Thus, tactoids, the gelling phenomenon, and sickling cannot be elicited from the red cells of individuals with Hgb D trait. In its alkali resistance, Hgb D reacts in a manner similar to that of Hgbs A, S, and C.

Hemoglobin D trait (h^D/h^A) and *homozygous Hgb D disease* (h^D/h^D) have been observed in several parts of the world, including Caucasian families in America, Sikhs, Turks, and Negroes.

Bird, G. W. G., and Lehmann, H.: The finding of haemoglobin D disease in a Sikh, Man 55:1, 1956.
——; ——; and Mourant, A. E.: A third example of hemoglobin D, Tr. Roy. Soc. Trop. Med. & Hyg. 49:399, 1955.
Cabannes, R.; Sendra, L.; and Dalaut: Hemoglobin D, a hereditary hemoglobin abnormality in an Algerian Moslem: Observations of two families, Algéria méd. 59:387, 1955.
Cooke, J. V., and Mack, J. K.: Sickle cell anemia in a white family, J. Pediat. 5:601, 1934.
Itano, H. A.: A third abnormal hemoglobin associated with hereditary hemolytic anemia, Proc. Nat. Acad. Sc. 37:775, 1951.
Sturgeon, P.; Itano, H. A.; and Bergren, W. R.: Clinical manifestations of inherited and abnormal hemoglobins: I. The interaction of Hgb S and D, Blood 10:389, 1955.

Hemoglobin E

In 1954, Itano, Bergren, and Sturgeon identified a fourth abnormal hemoglobin, which they designated as Hgb E (Table 1), in a child with an atypical anemia. At approximately the same time, Chernoff, Minnich, and Chongchareonsuk detected the same pigment in a group of patients in Thailand, who, although having a clinical picture resembling Mediterranean anemia, failed to fulfill the genetic criteria postulated for that disease.

Hemoglobin E can be differentiated from the other hemoglobins by its electrophoretic pattern. In ultraviolet and visual absorption spectra, solubility, amino acid composition, and resistance to alkali denaturation it is similar to Hgb A.

Hemoglobin E trait (h^E/h^A) has been observed in about 13% of the Thai population. It has also been found among the Burmese, Malayans, the Veddas of Ceylon and in about 6% of the Indonesians in Djakarta. The condition, however, has not been reported from other parts of the world. From the anthropological viewpoint, the condition is of interest because, although it is seen among peoples of similar racial background, many of whom are believed to have originated in northern China and to have been driven southward by successive invasions, the trait has not been seen among some 200 pure Chinese living in Thailand.

Homozygous Hgb E disease (h^E/h^E) may be expected to occur in approximately 1 out of 250 Thais. At present, 6 instances of this syndrome have been encountered in patients ranging from 19 to 40 years of age. All are in good to fair health, although a history of easy fatigability and mild arthralgia can be elicited.

Chernoff, A. I.; Minnich, V.; and Chongchareonsuk, S.: Hemoglobin E, a hereditary abnormality of human hemoglobin, Science 120:605, 1954.
————; ————; Na-Nakorn, S.; Tuchinda, S.; Kashemsant, C.; and Chernoff, R. R.: Studies on hemoglobin E: I. The clinical, hematologic, and genetic characteristics of the hemoglobin E syndromes, J. Lab. & Clin. Med. 47:455, 1956.
Itano, H. A.; Bergren, W. R.; and Sturgeon, P.: Identification of a fourth abnormal hemoglobin, J. Am. Chem. Soc. 76:2278, 1954.
Jonxis, J. H. P.; Huisman, T. H. J.; van der Schaaf, P. C.; and Prins, H. K.: Amino acid composition of Hgb E, Nature 177:627, 1956.
Lehmann, H.; Story, P.; and Thein, H.: Haemoglobin E in Burmese, Brit. M. J. 1:544, 1956.
Na-Nakorn, S.; Minnich, V.; and Chernoff, A. I.: Studies on hemoglobin E: II. The incidence of hemoglobin E in Thailand, J. Lab. & Clin. Med. 47:490, 1956.

HEMOGLOBIN G

In the course of a survey among Gold Coast Africans, Edington and Lehmann described an individual who had both normal hemoglobin and a form hitherto not known, which they designated as Hgb G (Table 1). Family studies revealed that he was the offspring of a mother who had only normal hemoglobin (h_2^A/h_2^A) and a father who had only this abnormal hemoglobin (h_2^G/h_2^G). All except one of the siblings were heterozygotes (h_2^G/h_2^A). The homozygote was not anemic, and it was not possible to detect fetal hemoglobin in his blood. Sickling was not observed either in the individuals with Hgb G trait or in the one with homozygous hemoglobin G disease. A second example of Hgb G trait has been described by Schwartz and Spaet in a white family.

Hemoglobin G differs from all other known hemoglobins in its mobility by paper electrophoresis at pH 8.6. This hemoglobin can be differentiated from Hgb F (which has a similar mobility) by its not being resistant to denaturation by alkaline reagents, and from Hgb S by the failure of the cells to sickle. The solubility of Hgb G is consistently higher than that of Hgb S but is lower or similar to that of Hgb A.

Edington, G. M., and Lehmann, H.: Hemoglobin G: New hemoglobin found in West Africa, Lancet 2:173, 1954.
————; ————; and Schneider, R. G: Characterization and genetics of Haemoglobin G, Nature 175:850, 1955.
Schwartz, H., and Spaet, T. H.: Hemoglobin G: Fifth abnormal hemoglobin, Clin. Res. Proc. 3:51, 1955.

HEMOGLOBIN H

In 1955, Rigas, Koler, and Osgood described three members of a Chinese family with a hypochromic, microcytic anemia with blood smears resembling thalassemia. The electrophoretic pattern, however, revealed an abnormal hemoglobin migrating more rapidly than normal hemoglobin. Other features included refractoriness to iron therapy, reticulocytosis, poikilocytosis, intraerythrocytic inclusion bodies, and changes in erythrocytic fragility. The abnormal hemoglobin accounted for 35-40% of the total hemoglobin, the fetal hemoglobin was slightly increased, and the remainder was normal hemoglobin.

Family studies on the inheritance of Hgb H have failed to demonstrate the abnormal pigment in the parents of known cases. Instead, one of the parents and several other members of the family have the thalassemia trait without Hgb H. Since small population surveys have failed to reveal any carriers of the Hgb H trait, Motulsky has suggested that heterozygotes either do not exist or have poor penetrance.

Eng, L. I. L.; Hin, P. S.; Keng, K. L.; and Endenburg, D. M.: Chronic hypochromic microcytic anaemia associated with haemoglobin H, Acta haemat. 18:156, 1957.

Motulsky, A. G.: Genetic and haematological significance of haemoglobin H, Nature 178:1055, 1956.

Rigas, D. A.; Koler, R. D.; and Osgood, E. A.: New hemoglobin possessing a higher electrophoretic mobility than normal adult hemoglobin, Science 121:372, 1955.

——; ——; and ——: Hemoglobin H, J. Lab. & Clin. Med. 47:51, 1956.

HEMOGLOBIN I

Also in 1955, Rucknagel, Page, and Jensen reported a similar hemoglobin in three generations of a single family possessing a mobility on paper electrophoresis at pH 8.6 which was similar to that of Hgb H. There was, however, a marked dissimilarity at pH 7.0. Furthermore, the Hgb H of Rigas precipitates on standing, whereas that of Rucknagel and his co-workers does not. This hemoglobin appears, therefore, to represent a new type, which has now been designated as Hgb I.

The Hgb I trait has only been demonstrated in this one family. No homozygote for Hgb I has been described.

Rucknagel, D. L.; Page, E. B.; and Jensen, W. N.: Hemoglobin I: An inherited hemoglobin anomaly, Blood 10:999, 1955.

Hemoglobin J

In 1956, Thorup, Itano, Wheby, and Leavell described another new abnormal hemoglobin in a young Negro female with bilateral cystosarcoma phylloides. The same abnormality was found in 7 out of 13 other members of the family examined; but so far, no case of *homozygous Hgb J disease* (h^J/h^J) has been found. In the cases of *Hgb J trait* (h^J/h^A), there is more Hgb J than Hgb A in all of the individuals examined, which is different from the proportions in all the other abnormal hemoglobins.

By using boundary electrophoresis, Hgb J has a mobility between that of Hgb A and that of Hgb I. The solubility of Hgb J is higher than Hgb A, and sickling has not been observed in the cases studied.

Ager, J. A. M.; Lehmann, H.; and Vella, F.: Haemoglobin "Norfolk": A new haemoglobin found in an English family, Brit. M. J. 2:539, 1958.

Eng, L. I. L.: Haemoglobin J in an Indonesian family, Acta haemat. 19:126, 1958.

Huisman, T. H. J.; Noordhoek, K.; and da Costa, G. J.: A case of haemoglobin J in an Indonesian family, Nature 179:322, 1957.

Robinson, A. R.; Zuelzer, W. W.; Neel, J. V.; Livingstone, F. B.; and Miller, M. J.: Two "fast" hemoglobin components in Liberian blood samples, Blood 11:902, 1956.

Thorup, O. A.; Itano, H. A.; Wheby, M.; and Leavell, B. S.: Hemoglobin J, Science 123:889, 1956.

Hemoglobin K

In 1956, Cabannes described a new, fast-moving abnormal hemoglobin which he designated as Hgb K. This has since been described in three Berber families in North Africa, among Liberian natives, and East Indians.

Ager, J. A. M., and Lehmann, H.: Haemoglobin K in an East Indian and his family, Brit. M. J. 1:1449, 1957.

Cabannes, R.; Buhr, J. L.; and Sendra, L.: Hemoglobin J: A new hereditary hemoglobinopathy described in certain Kabyle families of Algeria, Blood 11:591, 1957.

Robinson, A. R.; Zuelzer, W. W.; Neel, J. V.; Livingstone, F. B.; and Miller, M. J.: Two "fast" hemoglobin components in Liberian blood samples, Blood 11:902, 1956.

Vella, F.: Haemoglobin K in Singapore, Brit. M. J. 1:755, 1958.

Unclassified Abnormal Hemoglobins

In addition to the above, a number of new abnormal hemoglobins have recently been described under the terms: Hopkins-1, Hopkins-2, IV (Barts), O (Buginese X), (Galveston type), and Q. The proper classification of these new entities will have to await more agreement on nomenclature.

Ager, J. A. M., and Lehmann, H.: Observations on some "fast" haemoglobins: K, J, N and "Bacts," Brit. M. J. 1:929, 1958.

Eng, L. I. L., and Sadona: Haemoglobin O (Buginese X) in Sulawesi, Brit. M. J. 1:1461, 1958.

Schneider, R. G., and Haggard, M. E.: Haemoglobin P (the Galveston type), Nature 182:322, 1958.

Smith, E. W., and Torbert, J. V.: Study of two abnormal hemoglobins with evidence for a new genetic locus for hemoglobin formation, Bull. Johns Hopkins Hosp. 101:38, 1958.

Vella, F.; Wells, R. H. C.; Ager, J. A. M.; and Lehmann, H.: A haemoglobinopathy involving haemoglobin H and a new (Q) haemoglobin, Brit. M. J. 1:752, 1958.

3. MIXED HETEROZYGOUS HEMOGLOBIN DISEASES

Four hemolytic diseases are now recognized as falling into the group of mixed hemoglobin disturbances: S–C disease; S–D disease; S–E disease; and S–G disease.

SICKLE CELL–HEMOGLOBIN C DISEASE

In this disease, the genes are either alleles or closely linked at the same locus. One of the parents is heterozygous for Hgb S (h_1^S/h_1^A);

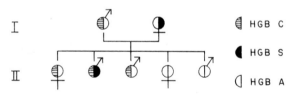

Fig. 13.—Mixed heterozygous hemoglobin diseases. (After Neel, Kaplan, and Zuelzer, 1953.)

the other is heterozygous for Hgb C (h_1^C/h_1^A); and the patient is heterozygous for both (h_1^S/h_1^C), as shown in Figure 13.

The disease was first suspected in patients with atypical sickle cell anemia who did not fulfill all the criteria for that diagnosis. Among the atypical features were: (1) only one parent showed sickling; (2) the spleen was usually easily palpable; and (3) the anemia was often mild, requiring few, if any, transfusions. In retrospect, about 15-20% of the cases previously classified as sickle cell anemia must be considered as having sickle cell–Hgb C disease.

Neel, J. V.; Kaplan, E.; and Zuelzer, W. W.: Further studies on hemoglobin

C: I. A description of three additional families segregating for Hgb C and sickle cell hemoglobin, Blood 8:724, 1953.

Schneider, R. G.: Incidence of hemoglobin C trait in 505 normal Negroes; family with homozygous hemoglobin C and sickle cell trait union, J. Lab. & Clin. Med. 44:133, 1954.

Smith, E. W., and Conley, C. L.: Filter paper electrophoresis of human hemoglobins with special reference to the incidence and clinical significance of Hgb C, Bull. Johns Hopkins Hosp. 93:94, 1953.

SICKLE CELL–HEMOGLOBIN D DISEASE

In 1956 Stewart and MacIver reported on a mulatto woman with sickle cell–Hgb D disease ($h_1{}^S/h_1{}^D$). She had inherited one abnormality from her mother, who was heterozygous for Hgb D ($h_1{}^D/h_1{}^A$). The father, a West African Negro, was dead and is assumed to have supplied the gene for the Hgb S. One of the patient's brothers had also inherited the abnormal Hgb D.

Stewart, J. W., and MacIver, J. E.: Sickle cell/haemoglobin D disease in a mulatto girl, Lancet 1:23, 1957.

SICKLE CELL–HEMOGLOBIN E DISEASE

The combination of sickle cell and Hgb E in the same patient ($h_1{}^S/h_1{}^E$) has been reported once.

Avisoy, M., and Lehmann, H.: The first observation of sickle cell–haemoglobin E disease, Nature 179:1248, 1957.

SICKLE CELL–HEMOGLOBIN G DISEASE

In 1957, Schwartz and his co-workers reported on a 28-year-old white male who had frequently been transfused because of persistent anemia. Laboratory studies revealed that not only was he a carrier of Hgbs S and G but also that he had thalassemia minor ($h_1{}^S/h_1{}^A$; $h_2{}^G/h_2{}^A$; $h_t{}^T/h_t{}^A$). His wife had always been healthy; and all laboratory studies, including sickling preparation, were negative ($h_1{}^A/h_1{}^A$; $h_2{}^A/h_2{}^A$; $h_t{}^A/h_t{}^A$). His son showed no abnormal hemoglobins but had signs of thalassemia minor ($h_1{}^A/h_1{}^A$; $h_2{}^A/h_2{}^A$; $h_t{}^T/h_t{}^A$). Further investigation revealed that the propositus had inherited the Hgb S abnormality from his father's side of the family and the Hgb G and thalassemia traits from his mother's side, as shown in Figure 14.

This family is of considerable importance because from it the following conclusions can be drawn: (1) The genes responsible for hemoglobins G and S cannot be alleles. If they were, the son would have inherited one or the other abnormality from the father. (2) The genes responsible for hemoglobin G and thalassemia cannot be alleles. The propositus could not have inherited both of these genes from his mother. (3) Since

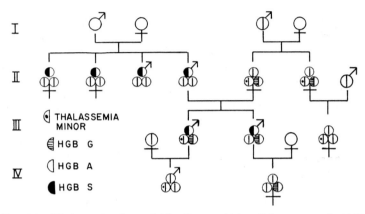

FIG. 14.—Thalassemia—hemoglobin disease. (After Schwartz *et al.*, 1957.)

it has previously been shown that the genes responsible for Hgb S and thalassemia are not allelic, one must conclude that there are at least three different loci in hemoglobin production.

Schwartz, H., and Spaet, T. H.: Hemoglobin G: A fifth abnormal hemoglobin, Clin. Res. Proc. 3:51, 1955.

*———; ———; Zuelzer, W. W.; Neel, J. V.; Robinson, A. R.; and Kaufman, S. F.: Combinations of hemoglobin G, hemoglobin S, and thalassemia occurring in one family, Blood 12:238, 1957.

4. THE THALASSEMIA SYNDROME

Patients with this syndrome inherit the thalassemia gene from one of the parents and a gene for one of the abnormal hemoglobins from the other parent, as shown in Figure 14. Since the gene for thalassemia and the genes for the abnormal hemoglobins are located at different loci, they have to be expressed separately.

THALASSEMIA—HEMOGLOBIN S

This mixed condition ($h_1{}^S/h_1{}^A$; $h_t{}^T/h_t{}^A$) was first described by Silvestroni and Bianco in Italy and is now being recognized with increasing frequency in other parts of Europe and in the United States.

Clinically, the symptoms start before the age of 10. In addition to the symptoms usually encountered in severe hemolytic anemias, patients complain of bone and joint pains, occasional abdominal discomfort, and rare clinical crises. Jaundice is usually mild. The hematological findings closely resemble those of thalassemia major, with moderately severe anemia and the presence of target cells and normoblasts on smear. Also, sickling can be found in the peripheral blood. Hemoglobin studies reveal a complex mixture of pigments, with Hgbs S, F, and A all being present.

Neel, J. V.; Itano, H. A.; and Lawrence, J. S.: Two cases of sickle cell disease presumably due to the combination of the genes for thalassemia and sickle cell hemoglobin, Blood 8:434, 1953.

Silvestroni, E., and Bianco, I.: Microcytemia, constitutional microcytic anemia, and Cooley's anemia, Am. J. Human Genet. 1:83, 1949.

———— and ————: Genetic aspects of sickle cell anemia and microdrepanocytic disease, Blood 7:429, 1952.

THALASSEMIA—HEMOGLOBIN C

This condition ($h_1{}^C/h_1{}^A$; $h_t{}^T/h_t{}^A$) has been diagnosed in only three patients. The combination sometimes causes a severe chronic microcytic anemia.

Singer, K.; Kraus, A. P.; Singer, L.; Rubinstein, H. M.; and Goldberg, S. R.: Studies on abnormal hemoglobins: X. A new syndrome: hemoglobin C–thalassemia disease, Blood 9:1032, 1954.

Zuelzer, W. W., and Kaplan, E.: Thalassemia–hemoglobin C disease, Blood 9:1047, 1954.

THALASSEMIA—HEMOGLOBIN E

This is a severe hemolytic syndrome which closely mimics Cooley's anemia in its manifestations. In all of the cases studied, one parent was found to have Hgb E ($h_1{}^E/h_1{}^A$) and the other had what appears to be, at best, a very mild thalassemia ($h_t{}^T/h_t{}^A$). Whether the parents without Hgb E really have thalassemia minor and whether this syndrome is correctly named remains to be proved.

Chernoff, A. I.; Minnich, V.; Na-Nakorn, S.; Tuchinda, S.; Kashemsant, C.; and Chernoff, R. R.: Studies on hemoglobin E: I. The clinical, hematologic, and genetic characteristics of the hemoglobin E syndromes, J. Lab. & Clin. Med. 47:455, 1956.

Lie-Injo, L. E.: Haemoglobin E in Indonesia, Nature 176:468, 1955.

Nagaratuam, N.; Wickremasinghe, R. L.; Jayawickreme, R. L.; and Maheson, V. S.: Haemoglobin E syndromes in a Ceylonese family, Brit. M. J. 1:866, 1958.

Punt, N., and Van Goal, J.: Thalassemia–haemoglobin E disease in Indo-European boys, Acta haemat. 17:305, 1957.

THALASSEMIA—HEMOGLOBIN G

Two patients with what is believed to be thalassemia–Hgb G disease were observed by Schwartz and his associates. The details are discussed in the previous section.

Schwartz, H. C.; Spaet, T. H.; Zuelzer, W. W.; Neel, J. V.; Robinson, A. R.; and Kaufman, S. F.: Combinations of hemoglobin G, hemoglobin S, and thalassemia occurring in one family, Blood 12:238, 1957.

5. OTHER MIXED DISTURBANCES

A similar combination of abnormal hemoglobins with hereditary spherocytosis and hereditary elliptocytosis has been reported. Again, the genes for spherocytosis, elliptocytosis, and the abnormal hemoglobins are undoubtedly located at separate loci.

SPHEROCYTOSIS-HEMOGLOBIN DISEASE

De Torregrosa and his co-workers have reported both the sickle cell trait and spherocytosis in the same patient. Family studies show that the

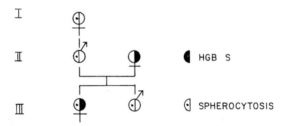

FIG. 15.—Spherocytosis-hemoglobin disease. (After de Torregrosa, 1956.)

spherocytosis trait was inherited from the father's side of the family and the sickle cell trait from the mother's side (Fig. 15). In this condition the patient suffered more from the effects of spherocytosis than from those of sickle cell trait. Splenectomy was of considerable value in treating the anemia.

De Torregrosa, M. V.; Ortiz, A.; and Vargas, D.: Sickle cell–spherocytosis associated with hemolytic anemia, Blood 11:260, 1956.
Smith, E. W., and Conley, C. L.: Genetic variants of sickle cell disease, Bull. Johns Hopkins Hosp. 94:289, 1954.

ELLIPTOCYTOSIS-HEMOGLOBIN DISEASE

At least three cases of elliptocytosis-hemoglobin disease have been recorded. In 1949, Fadem described hereditary elliptocytosis in association with the sickle cell trait in a 25-year-old Negro male. More recently, Avery has reported on two patients who manifested both hereditary elliptocytosis and the Hgb C trait. Genetic studies in the latter two cases clearly show how the two abnormal genes are transmitted through different members of the family to the affected individuals (Fig. 16).

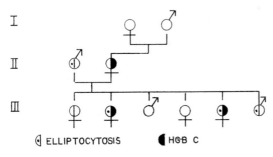

FIG. 16.—Elliptocytosis-hemoglobin disease. (After Avery, 1956.)

It is interesting to note that elliptocytosis and Hgb C trait in association do not produce a summation of effect. In fact, these patients show no clinical stigmata that can be attributed to their hematologic abnormalities. It appears that the two separate genetic effects can be manifested in the same cell, since some of the elliptical cells appear to contain abnormal hemoglobin.

Avery, M. E.: Hereditary elliptocytosis and hemoglobin C trait: A report of two cases, Bull. Johns Hopkins Hosp. 98:184, 1956.
Fadem, R. S.: Ovalocytosis associated with the sickle cell trait, Blood 4:505, 1949.

3

Other "Structural" Disturbances

WE NOW TURN to other conditions which may represent examples of disturbances in the structure of the stroma, or cell walls. These include: (1) *thalassemia,* (2) *hereditary elliptocytosis,* (3) *acanthrocytosis,* (4) *erythropoietic porphyria,* and (5) the *Pelger-Huet anomaly of the leukocytes.*

*Ponder, E.: Analytic review: Present concepts of the structure of the mammalian red cell, Blood 9:227, 1954.

I. THALASSEMIA (Cooley's, or Mediterranean, anemia)

Thalassemia is characterized by chronic hemolytic anemia associated with a hereditary defect in the synthesis of hemoglobin. The defect leads to the production of cells which are abnormal in shape, deficient in hemoglobin, and destroyed at an excessive rate. The condition was first described by Cooley in Detroit; and for some time it seemed to be limited exclusively to persons whose familial origins were in certain countries bordering the northern Mediterranean coast, particularly Italy, Greece, and Sicily.

CLINICAL FEATURES.—The onset of the condition is indicated by severe and progressive anemia early in infancy. Anemia is not present at birth but seems to develop in relation to the gradual decrease in production of fetal hemoglobin, which is normally expected. Pallor is usually marked, and there is often mild icterus. Splenomegaly is found early in the course of the disease and is progressive, and the spleen attains enormous proportions within a few years. If no supportive transfusion therapy is given, the anemia becomes progressive and leads to cardiorespiratory distress and eventual death.

With transfusions, hemosiderosis develops as a result of iron stores, causing the skin to become a muddy bronze color. The liver also becomes markedly enlarged because of extramedullary hematopoiesis. The skeletal changes associated with chronic hemolytic anemia become strikingly evident and exceed by far the changes found in other hemolytic anemias. Thickening of the membrane bones of the face and skull (Fig. 17) leads to a mongoloid facies, with a tendency toward protrusion of the

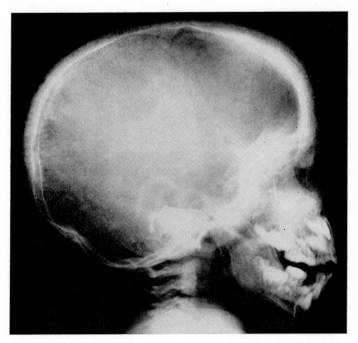

FIG. 17.—Lateral view of skull of a patient with thalassemia major. Marked thickening of the calvarium with multiple striations at right angles with the skull results in the "hair-on-end" appearance.

teeth. The hands become heavy and broad in appearance, owing to alterations in the metacarpal bones (Fig. 18).

The peripheral blood picture is typical and persists throughout life. There is severe anemia with a profound hypochromia. The erythrocyte count is below the normal range, and the hemoglobin is reduced to an even greater extent. The erythrocytes show marked anisocytosis and poikilocytosis. There are many microcytes, with a minority of contrasting large hypochromic cells 12-18 μ in diameter. The hemoglobin in these large cells is irregularly distributed, creating bizarre shapes. The presence

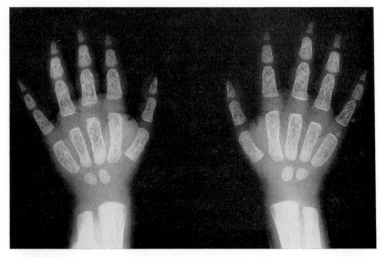

Fig. 18.—Anteroposterior view of hands in thalassemia major, showing marked coarsening of the trabecular pattern of metacarpals and phalanges. Owing to the pressure effects of the hyperplastic bone marrow, the trabecular pattern has coalesced and become coarse and heavy, producing the characteristic "bamboo" appearance.

of a small central mass of hemoglobin may give these cells a target-cell appearance. The rapid turnover of erythrocytes is shown by a moderate increase of reticulocytes and stippled cells. The indirect bilirubin is also increased.

HEREDITY.—The gene for thalassemia is expressed in two forms: (1) The homozygotes (those with a double dose of the abnormal gene) show the full clinical picture, which is known as *thalassemia major*. (2) The heterozygotes (those with only a single dose of the abnormal gene) show only minimal disturbances in hemoglobin synthesis, and this condition is known as *thalassemia minor*. The latter is characterized by mild anemia with moderate hypochromia, anisocytosis, and poikilocytosis. In most of the affected families, both parents are heterozygotes and, assuming a normal distribution, one offspring has thalassemia major, two have thalassemia minor, and a fourth is completely normal. The condition is seldom transmitted by homozygotes, since it is usually lethal before the age of reproduction.

A few years ago, Silvestroni and Bianco showed that certain persons may inherit one sickle cell gene from one parent and one thalassemia gene from the other, resulting in a clinical condition which is not very different from thalassemia major. (The condition is described in more detail in the section on sickle cell hemoglobins [p. 52].) If such a person should reproduce, either or both traits can be passed on to his (or her) children, since the genes for thalassemia and sickle cell hemoglobin are located on different chromosomes.

In a study of a predominantly Italian population in Rochester, New York, Neel and Valentine have estimated that thalassemia major occurs once in each 2,568 births (an incidence of 0.042%) and thalassemia minor once in each 25 births (an incidence of 4.1%). The incidence is probably higher in Mediterranean countries, since Banton showed that 20% of the total population in a remote part of Sicily carried the thalassemia trait. Although most of the cases of thalassemia originate in the Mediterranean area, cases have been reported in almost every part of the world.

PATHOGENESIS.—The exact nature of the defect in Cooley's anemia remains uncertain. The mutant gene may prevent some step necessary in the production of adult hemoglobin, or it may prevent the synthesis of normal adult stromal material, or in some other way impair normal red-cell production. There are several pieces of evidence to suggest this.

First, Smith and his co-workers have shown that patients with thalassemia major have a high serum iron content and an absent iron-binding capacity (Fig. 19). In normal adults or children, serum iron comprises one third of the total iron-binding capacity. In thalassemia major patients, the two values are about equal, suggesting that the iron-binding capacity is fully saturated and quantitatively lower than in normal children. The administration of fraction IV-7 of plasma results in a rise in serum iron values and an appearance of a latent capacity to further bind iron. This suggests that there is a release of iron from tissues to the blood when additional metal-combining globulin is supplied in this disease.

Second, the hemoglobin in thalassemia major consists of Hgb A and Hgb F. If it is generally assumed that Hgb A is the sole type of hemoglobin produced in the normal adult, there is little need to form Hgb F after early infancy. However, the latent ability to form fetal pigment is still present; and in a severe hematological disorder such as thalassemia major, Hgb F is produced to compensate for the lack of Hgb A production. Recently, Kunkel and Wallenius have shown that there is an increase of the slow component of Hgb A in patients with thalassemia minor. There seems to be no correlation between fetal hemoglobin levels and the clinical and hematological severity of the disease process.

Finally, Hoffman and his associates have studied the plasma membranes of erythrocytes by electron microscopy and have found that the surface texture of ghost cells from all of the thalassemia major bloods are distinctly different from ghost cells from thalassemia minor and normal bloods. These differences are observable whether the specimens for comparison are prepared at the same time or on different days. They conclude that these morphological changes in thalassemia major ghost cells constitute an expression of an alteration in the molecular structure of the plasma membranes of the cells.

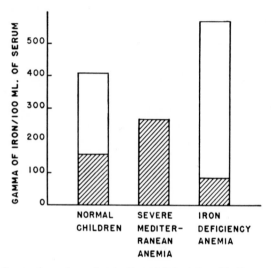

Fig. 19.—Serum iron (*crosshatched*) and latent iron-binding capacity (*clear area*). (After Smith, C. H.; Sisson, T. R. C.; Floyd, W. H., Jr.; and Siegal, S.: Serum iron and iron-binding capacity of the serum in children with severe Mediterranean [Cooley's] anemia, Pediatrics 5:799, 1950.)

Until recently, it has always been assumed that the defect in thalassemia is purely in the blood corpuscle itself and that splenectomy would not be helpful in such patients. However, Lichtman and his co-workers have shown that, if normal erythrocytes are transfused to patients with thalassemia major, the life span of the erythrocytes is shortened; and that if splenectomy is performed, the survival of the transfused cells becomes normal. It is difficult to interpret this new finding, except that it contributes partially to the increased destruction of erythrocytes in thalassemia.

If one postulates that thalassemia represents a basic defect in the proper production of Hgb A with possibly a defect of the cell membrane, the clinical signs and symptoms can all be attributed to these defects, as shown in Chart 2. The increased hemolysis and red-cell

CHART 2

THALASSEMIA

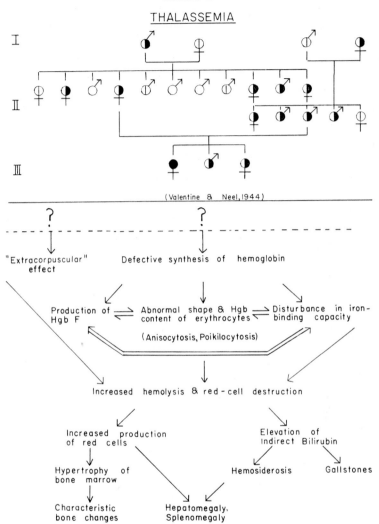

(Valentine & Neel, 1944)

? ?

"Extracorpuscular" effect   Defective synthesis of hemoglobin

Production of Hgb F ⇌ Abnormal shape & Hgb content of erythrocytes ⇌ Disturbance in iron-binding capacity

(Anisocytosis, Poikilocytosis)

Increased hemolysis & red-cell destruction

Increased production of red cells   Elevation of Indirect Bilirubin

Hypertrophy of bone marrow   Hemosiderosis   Gallstones

Characteristic bone changes   Hepatomegaly, Splenomegaly destruction causes an elevation of indirect bilirubin, which in turn causes the formation of gallstones and deposits of iron throughout the body. To compensate for this, the patient overproduces erythrocytes, and there are many sites of extramedullary hematopoiesis.

DIAGNOSIS.—Thalassemia major can be diagnosed by the characteristic hematological findings on a smear of the peripheral blood and by measurements of serum iron (see Procedure 4) and iron-binding capacity (see Procedure 5). The clinical picture for thalassemia minor is highly variable. In most instances, mild anemia and typical cell changes on a peripheral smear are sufficient to make the diagnosis.

TREATMENT.—Transfusions of whole blood to maintain an adequate hemoglobin concentration are essential. Despite this, most patients die from intercurrent infections before the age of puberty. Transfusion reactions can become serious problems, also. Splenectomy should only be performed for comfort when the spleen gets too large.

Cooley, T. B., and Lee, P.: A series of cases of anemia with splenomegaly and peculiar bone changes, Am. J. Dis. Child. 30:447, 1925.
Hoffman, J. F.; Wolman, I. J.; Millier, J.; and Parpart, A. K.: Ultra-structure of erythrocyte membranes in thalassemia major and minor, Blood 11:946, 1956.
Lichtman, H. C.; Watson, R. J.; Felman, F.; Ginzberg, V.; and Robinson, J.: Studies on thalassemia, J. Clin. Invest. 32:1229, 1953.
Silvestroni, E., and Bianco, I.: Microcytemia, constitutional microcytic anemia and Cooley's anemia, Am. J. Human Genet. 1:83, 1949.
Smith, C. H.: Detection of mild types of Mediterranean (Cooley's) anemia, Am. J. Dis. Child. 75:505, 1948.
——; Sisson, T. R. C.; Floyd, W. H., Jr.; and Siegal, S.: Serum iron and iron-binding capacity of the serum in children with severe Mediterranean (Cooley's) anemia, Pediatrics 5:799, 1950.
Sturgeon, P., and Finch, C. A.: Erythrokinetics in Cooley's anemia, Blood 12:64, 1957.
Valentine, W. N., and Neel, J. V.: Hematologic and genetic study of transmission of thalassemia, Arch. Int. Med. 74:185, 1944.

2. HEREDITARY ELLIPTOCYTOSIS

Oval or elliptically shaped erythrocytes (Fig. 20) normally occur in the camel and llama but are comparatively unusual as a hereditary trait in humans. Only about 400 cases of this anomaly have been reported.

CLINICAL FEATURES.—The patients with hereditary elliptocytosis may be divided into three groups: (1) those with no signs of hemolysis; (2) those with hemolysis but no anemia; and (3) those with hemolytic disease and anemia. In the first group, the condition is entirely benign and of no medical significance. Patients in the second group show reticulocytosis, mild icterus, and increased excretion of urobilinogen in the stools;

there is also a hyperplasia of the bone marrow and there may be changes in the osmotic fragility of the erythrocytes. Patients in the third group, in addition to having hemolytic disease, show a moderate to severe degree of anemia which may require transfusions. These patients show a

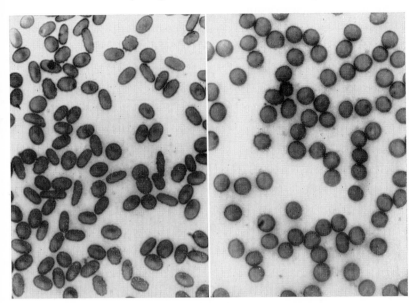

FIG. 20.—Smear from peripheral blood of a patient with elliptocytosis (*left*) compared with that of a normal person (*right*). (From Goodale, H. B.; Hendry, D. W. W.; and Lawler, S. D.: Data on linkage in man: Elliptocytosis and blood groups: II. Family three, Ann. Eugenics 17:272, 1952.)

shortened life span of erythrocytes as measured by the Ashby technique. Approximately 12% of all individuals with elliptocytosis belong in the last two groups.

HEREDITY.—The incidence of elliptocytosis in the general population has been estimated to be between 0.02 and 0.04%. The genetic mechanism responsible for this defect is similar to that present in thalassemia and sicklemia. Most of the affected individuals are heterozygous for the trait. When a gene for elliptocytosis is combined with another abnormal gene, a more severe hemolytic process occurs. Instances of elliptocytosis–Hgb S and elliptocytosis–Hgb C trait have been recorded. The homozygous form of hereditary elliptocytosis has only been recorded twice. This is not surprising, in view of the fact that known carriers are unlikely to mate other known carriers.

Recently, Lawler and her co-workers have shown that linkage exists between the locus for hereditary elliptocytosis and that for the cde (Rh) blood groups.

PATHOGENESIS.—Hereditary elliptocytosis represents an intrinsic defect of the erythrocyte itself. All attempts to show an extracorpuscular factor have been unsuccessful. Lipton has suggested that the microsphe-

CHART 3

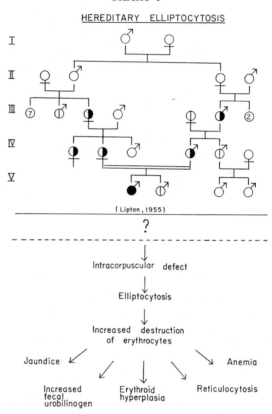

rocytes and microelliptocytes result in fragmentation of the erythrocytes. This increased destruction of red cells accounts for the shortened life span of elliptocytes, which in turn causes jaundice, increase of fecal urobilinogen, and compensatory hyperplasia of the bone marrow (Chart 3).

Splenectomy is usually successful in decreasing the degree of hemolysis. Although the reason for this is not known, some have suggested that this procedure results in the increased life span of the "fragmentation spherocytes" which had been selectively destroyed by the spleen.

DIAGNOSIS.—Elliptocytosis can easily be identified in the peripheral blood. Lipton has also outlined methods by which the cell eccentricity can be calculated by measuring the short and long diameter of each cell (see Procedure 6).

TREATMENT.—Splenectomy is the treatment of choice, especially when anemia or pancytopenia are serious problems.

Goodale, H. B.; Hendry, D. W. W.; and Lawler, S. D.: Data on linkage in man: Elliptocytosis and blood groups: II. Family three, Ann. Eugenics 17:272, 1952.

Lipton, E. L.: Elliptocytosis with hemolytic anemia: The effects of splenectomy, Pediatrics 15:67, 1955.

Motulsky, A. G.; Singer, K.; Crosby, W. H.; and Smith, V: The life span of the elliptocyte: Hereditary elliptocytosis and its relationship to other familial hemolytic disease, Blood 9:57, 1954.

Wyandt, H.; Bancroft, P. M.; and Winship, T. O.: Elliptic erythrocytes in man, Arch. Int. Med. 68:1043, 1941.

3. ACANTHROCYTOSIS

In 1950, Bassen and Kornzweig reported a hitherto undescribed malformation of the circulating erythrocytes. Since these misshapen cells have a thorny appearance, Singer coined the term "acanthrocytosis" to describe the condition.

CLINICAL FEATURES.—Acanthrocytosis seems to be characterized by a number of unrelated clinical features. The affected individuals show

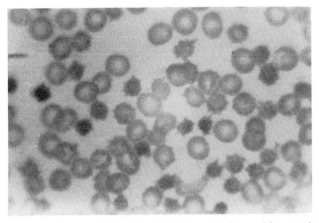

FIG. 21.—Smear from peripheral blood of a patient with acanthrocytosis. (From Singer, K.; Fisher, B.; and Perlstein, M. A.: Acanthrocytosis: A genetic erythrocyte malformation, Blood 7:577, 1952.)

evidence of celiac disease during early childhood. This state lasts for several years and then disappears. As they grow older, the patients develop a neurological picture which is not unlike Friedreich's ataxia: they walk on a broad base and waddle; there are extraneous athetoid movements of the head and arms, accompanied by tremor and poor co-ordination: there is impairment of vibratory and position sense; and the deep reflexes are absent.

CHART 4

ACANTHROCYTOSIS

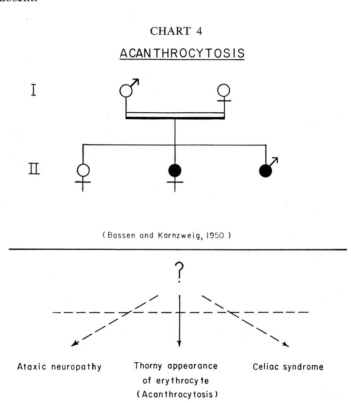

(Bassen and Kornzweig, 1950)

Ataxic neuropathy   Thorny appearance   Celiac syndrome
                         of erythrocyte
                         (Acanthrocytosis)

The erythrocyte anomaly represents an unusual type of crenation of the cells: The deformed cells show several irregularly spaced, large, and coarse projections and resemble spherocytes with pseudopods (Fig. 21). There are slight changes of osmotic, and more marked changes of mechanical, fragility but no evidence of increased hemolysis in vivo. Electrophoretic studies show that none of the abnormal hemoglobins are present.

HEREDITY.—Consanguinity was a factor in both of the two affected families that have been reported. This would suggest that acanthrocytosis is transmitted by a rare recessive gene. Presumably, the parents must be heterozygotes for the condition, but they have not been extensively studied.

The gene frequency of the condition is unknown. Both of the reported families are Jewish, but this may be a coincidence.

PATHOGENESIS.—Ponder has pointed out that there are two kinds of crenation. Type 1 represents an intermediary phase in the transformation of an erythrocyte from a disk to a sphere. In this type, the crenations tend to be fine and small, and they may be caused by extraneous lysis. Type 2 occurs when the cells undergo crenation spontaneously. Here the crenations are large and coarse and seem to be associated with gelation or crystallization of hemoglobin. Singer thinks that acanthrocytosis belongs to the second type, but he has not been able to identify any intra-erythrocyte factor which may be responsible for the alteration in the shape of the erythrocyte.

Thus far, it has not been possible to relate acanthrocytosis to the celiac syndrome and to ataxic neuropathy (Chart 4).

DIAGNOSIS.—Acanthrocytosis is diagnosed by the thorny appearance of the erythrocyte on a smear of peripheral blood.

TREATMENT.—None is required.

Bassen, F. A., and Kornzweig, A. L.: Malformation of the erythrocytes in a case of atypical retinitis pigmentosa, Blood 5:381, 1950.
Singer, K.; Fisher, B.; and Perlstein, M. A.: Acanthrocytosis: A genetic erythrocyte malformation, Blood 7:577, 1952.

4. ERYTHROPOIETIC PORPHYRIA (congenital or photosensitive porphyria)

Erythropoietic porphyria is an inborn error of metabolism characterized by photosensitivity, increased hemolysis and erythropoiesis, splenomegaly, and excessive and abnormal porphyrin formation in the bone marrow. The condition first came into prominence during the early decades of the present century, when Hans Fischer and his co-workers made most of the basic chemical observations on the porphyrins from studies on their celebrated patient, Petry, who suffered from this disorder.

CLINICAL FEATURES.—The signs and symptoms of erythropoietic porphyria appear very early in infancy. The first finding usually is red urine on the diaper. If the urine is examined under a Woods light, the characteristic red fluorescence of porphyria can be easily noted.

The skin photosensitivity is a striking feature of the disease. When exposed to sunlight, such infants form extensive bullous eruptions on the exposed surfaces (hydroa aestivale). Subsequently these eruptions break down and become infected, leaving shallow, slow-healing ulcers, and, ultimately, extensive scarring. It is believed that the photosensitivity is a reaction to the longer wavelengths of ultraviolet light (3,200-4,500 Å). Ordinary window glass offers no protection from the sun for such patients, a factor of considerable practical importance.

Other complications include: hypertrichosis (resembling that of Cushing's syndrome) along the hairline; and reddish brown staining of the deciduous teeth, caused by the deposition of porphyrins in the tooth substance. Sometimes splenomegaly is also seen.

A hemolytic process is nearly always present in patients with erythropoietic porphyria. This is shown by an increase of reticulocytes and circulating normoblasts, a short survival of erythrocytes (by the Ashby technique), an increase of urobilinogen in the stools, and a normoblastic hyperplasia of the bone marrow. Examination of the bone marrow under fluorescent light discloses the presence of porphyrins in the normoblasts.

In such patients, the urine contains large amounts of uroporphyrin I and smaller amounts of coproporphyrin I, while the reverse is found in the feces. Porphobilinogen is not encountered in erythropoietic porphyria, and the porphyrins in the excreta are in the free state, in contrast to their appearance as zinc complexes in hepatic porphyria.

HEREDITY.—Erythropoietic porphyria is an exceedingly rare disease, only about 40 cases having been reported. The condition has been seen among siblings in six families, but never among parents or offspring. Because of this, it is probably transmitted as an autosomal recessive. The heterozygous carriers of the abnormality have not been detected.

PATHOGENESIS.—Schmid and his associates have suggested that erythropoietic porphyria represents a constitutional fault in porphyrin synthesis in developing normoblasts in the bone marrow. They have shown that there exist two morphologically different varieties of normoblasts, which might be designated as normal and abnormal cells. The abnormal variety exhibits nuclear inclusion bodies, containing hemoglobin and red fluorescence. The fluorescence seems to originate predominantly from the normoblastic nucleus, while the cytoplasm around it shows only little fluorescence. Also, the polychromatophilic erythrocytes exhibit only weak fluorescence. These workers interpret these findings to indicate that there must coexist in the bone marrow two different lines of normoblasts. The nuclei of cells belonging to the abnormal line probably form excessive amounts of porphyrins and these are released into the plasma at a rela-

CHART 5

ERYTHROPOIETIC PORPHYRIA

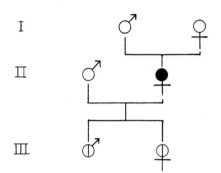

(Kench, Langley & Wilkinson, 1953)

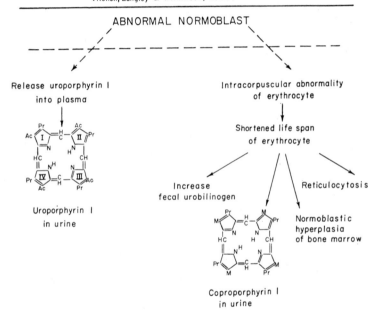

ABNORMAL NORMOBLAST

Release uroporphyrin I
into plasma

Intracorpuscular abnormality
of erythrocyte

Shortened life span
of erythrocyte

Uroporphyrin I
in urine

Increase
fecal urobilinogen

Reticulocytosis

Normoblastic
hyperplasia
of bone marrow

Coproporphyrin I
in urine

tively rapid rate as uroporphyrin I, which in turn is excreted in excess in the urine.

The abnormal normoblasts presumably are also responsible for producing erythrocytes with an intracorpuscular abnormality. This would result in the shortened life span of the erythrocytes in such patients and would result in increased hemolysis and erythropoiesis. The increase of coproporphyrin I in the urine is believed to be more of a reflection of the abnormally rapid hemoglobin synthesis stimulated by hemolysis than being related to the excess of uroporphyrin I (Chart 5).

DIAGNOSIS.—The diagnosis of erythropoietic porphyria is confirmed by (1) intense red fluorescence of normoblasts in the bone marrow by fluorescence microscopy (see Procedure 7); (2) marked increase of uroporphyrin I in the urine and erythrocytes (see Procedure 8); (3) increase of coproporphyrin I in the urine and erythrocytes (Procedure 9); and (4) absence of porphobilinogen in the urine (Procedure 10). The condition can also be differentiated from hepatic porphyria by the lack of involvement of the liver and central nervous system and the age of onset.

TREATMENT.—Management consists of (1) preventing the effects of photosensitivity and (2) controlling hemolysis. The former can be done by keeping the child in a shaded area, away from direct sunlight, and by putting protective clothing on him at all times. The hemolysis can be partially arrested by splenectomy, which also has a favorable effect on the photosensitivity. If the individual can be made to live with the disease, the ultimate outlook is good.

Aldrich, R. A.; Hawkinson, V.; Grinstein, M.; and Watson, C. J.: Photosensitivity or congenital porphyria with hemolytic anemia: I. Clinical and fundamental studies before and after splenectomy, Blood 6:685, 1951.

*————; Labbe, R. F.; and Talman, E. L.: A review of porphyrin metabolism with special reference to childhood, Am. J. M. Sc. 230:675, 1955.

Fischer, H.; Hilmer, H.; Linder, F.; and Putzer, B.: Zur Kenntnis der natürlichen Porphyrine XVIII: Mitteilung chemischer Befunde bei einem Fall von Porphyrinurise (Petry), Ztschr. physiol. Chem. 150:44, 1925.

Kench, J. D.; Langley, F. A.; and Wilkinson, J. F.: Biochemical and pathological studies of congenital porphyria, Quart. J. Med. 22:285, 1953.

*Schmid, R.; Schwartz, S.; and Sundberg, B.: Erythropoietic (congenital) porphyria: A rare abnormality of the normoblast, Blood 10:416, 1955.

5. PELGER-HUET ANOMALY OF THE LEUKOCYTES

This is a rare anomaly of the leukocytes characterized by an arrested segmentation of the granulocyte nucleus at the two-lobe level. The phenomenon was first noticed by Pelger, a Dutch physician, in 1928; and the familial nature of the condition was reported by Huet, another Dutch physician, 3 years later. Up to 1940 the anomaly had been noted in some 210 patients in 32 families from all over the world.

CLINICAL FEATURES.—Persons with this condition are completely

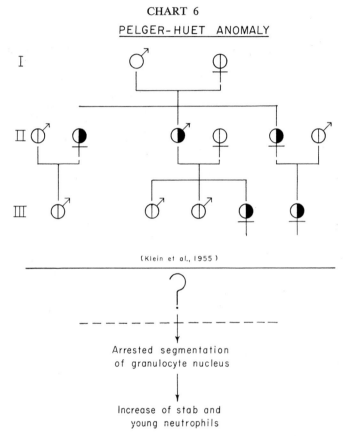

CHART 6

PELGER-HUET ANOMALY

(Klein et al., 1955)

Arrested segmentation
of granulocyte nucleus

Increase of stab and
young neutrophils

free of clinical symptoms and remain in good health throughout their lives.

Laboratory studies show that the total white blood count is normal. A diagnosis of Pelger-Huet anomaly is made by examining the granulocytes in the peripheral blood smear. In normal persons, there is found: non-segmentation in about 3-5% of the neutrophils, two segments in 15-20%, three or four segments in 70-75%, and more than four segments in about 5%. In persons with Pelger-Huet anomaly, an arrest of segmentation seems to have occurred at the two-lobe level. As a result, there is an increase of stab or younger neutrophils, and only an occasional three-segmented nucleus. The eosinophils and basophils are similarly affected.

Surprisingly, the Pelger-Huet anomaly does not cause a deficient defense mechanism against infection. The mature Pelger cells have essentially the same functional capacity as have normal mature white cells. However, there is some suggestion that the immature Pelger neutrophils may have less phagocytic activity than normal cells. Despite this, affected individuals do not suffer from infections or other illnesses any more than usual; and, when they do, their resistance is satisfactory.

HEREDITY.—The Pelger-Huet anomaly is transmitted as an autosomal dominant, with all of the affected individuals being heterozygotes.

Nachtsheim has mated heterozygous Pelger rabbits and shown that the Pelger anomaly is lethal in the homozygotes. Out of 39 rabbits, 27 died during parturition or shortly thereafter; and out of the 12 that survived, only 2 lived to maturity. The homozygous state has been seen in humans only once. This patient, a child, showed on peripheral smear that 92% of the neutrophils had round eccentric nuclei and 6% had indented stab forms, leaving only 2% with segmented forms.

It is estimated that the Pelger-Huet anomaly occurs about once in every 1,000 births.

PATHOGENESIS.—Essentially nothing is known about the etiology of this anomaly except that there seems to be an arrested segmentation of the granulocytic nuclei for some unknown reason (Chart 6).

DIAGNOSIS.—A careful differential count of the white-cell series will reveal the abnormality.

TREATMENT.—None is required.

Huet, G. J.: Familial anomaly of leukocytes, Nederl. tijdschr. geneesk. 75:5956, 1931.
*Klein, A.; Husson, A. E.; and Bornstein, S.: Pelger-Huet anomaly of the leukocytes, New England J. Med. 253:1057, 1955.
Nachtsheim, H.: Pelger-anomaly in man and rabbit: Mendelian character of nuclei of leukocytes, J. Hered. 41:131, 1950.
Pelger, K.: Demonstratie van een paar zeldzaam voorkumende typen van bloedlichaampjes en bespreking der patienten, Nederl. tijdschr. geneesk. 72:1178, 1928.

PART II

Disturbances in Molecular Synthesis (Protein Deficiencies)

SOME HEREDITARY DISEASES are the result of a quantitative deficiency or absence of one of the plasma proteins. Although the details have not been properly worked out, there is strong evidence suggesting that in these conditions the plasma protein in question is actually missing from the plasma. This defect is, therefore, a different type of defect from an alteration in the structure of the protein molecule, as has been described in Part I, and also from a functional change in the action of the protein, as will be described in Part III, on enzyme defects.

The disturbances in molecular synthesis may be divided into two groups: (1) the deficiencies of the plasma protein fractions, and (2) the deficiencies of clotting factors.

4

Deficiencies of
Plasma Protein Fractions

THE THREE congenital deficiencies of plasma proteins are: (1) *agammaglobulinemia,* (2) *ceruloplasmin deficiency* (Wilson's disease), and (3) *afibrinogenemia.*

I. CONGENITAL AGAMMAGLOBULINEMIA

In 1952, Colonel Ogden C. Bruton of the Walter Reed Army Medical Center described a new condition characterized by repeated episodes of infection during infancy and early childhood. Laboratory studies showed a failure to develop antibodies following antigenic stimulation and, by electrophoresis, the absence of gamma globulin in the plasma. Accordingly, the condition was named "agammaglobulinemia."

CLINICAL FEATURES.—All patients with this condition suffer from numerous severe bacterial infections, which may take any number of forms (Fig. 22). Some patients have repeated episodes of pneumonia or septicemia. Others have recurrent sinusitis and otitis media, which may eventually lead to meningitis. Although these infections respond satisfactorily to antibiotic therapy, sequelae frequently develop owing to the very frequency of attacks. Some of the children have irreversible bronchiectasis following numerous attacks of bronchopneumonia; others develop deafness, cerebral palsy, and mental retardation following meningitis. Some patients develop arthritis associated with tissue injury from repeated infections. On the other hand, all of these patients seem to respond normally to virus infections.

Patients with agammaglobulinemia fail to develop antibodies following antigenic stimulation. For example, repeated immunizations with

74

pertussis vaccine fail to produce the usual antibodies. Similarly, children with blood group O fail to develop anti-A and anti-B isohemagglutinins. Vaccination with vaccine virus results in a low antibody production even after three or four tries at different sites. However, revaccination 6 months later usually reveals an accelerated type of reaction, suggesting immunity.

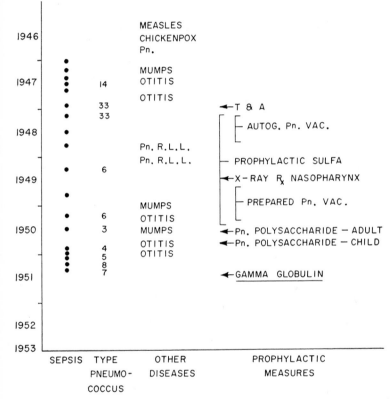

1946			MEASLES CHICKENPOX Pn.	
1947		14	MUMPS OTITIS	
			OTITIS	
		33		←T & A
		33		┌ AUTOG. Pn. VAC.
1948				
			Pn. R.L.L.	
			Pn. R.L.L.	├ PROPHYLACTIC SULFA
1949		6		←X-RAY Rₓ NASOPHARYNX
			MUMPS	┌ PREPARED Pn. VAC.
1950		6	OTITIS	
		3	MUMPS	←Pn. POLYSACCHARIDE — ADULT
		4	OTITIS	←Pn. POLYSACCHARIDE — CHILD
		5	OTITIS	
		8		
1951		7		←GAMMA GLOBULIN
1952				
1953				

SEPSIS | TYPE PNEUMO-COCCUS | OTHER DISEASES | PROPHYLACTIC MEASURES

FIG. 22.—The infections repeated, during a 5-year period, in a patient with congenital agammaglobulinemia. (After Bruton, O. C.: Agammaglobulinemia, Med. Ann. District of Columbia 22:648, 1953.)

HEREDITY.—Preliminary studies, based on a small number of families, suggest that the condition is probably transmitted by a sex-linked recessive gene. This form of transmission is suggested by the fact that in all the cases diagnosed up to the present, except for one instance, the patients have been boys. Frequently it has been found that other male members of the immediate family have died of presumably the same condition; and in three families, maternal uncles or maternal male cousins have been similarly affected. The appearance of a female with all the stigmata of the disease suggests that there may be a second mode of inheritance for the condition, about which we know little. The heterozygotes have not, as yet, been detectable by measurements of gamma globulin levels.

PATHOGENESIS.—The cause of this disease is poorly understood. The most striking abnormality is the marked deficiency of gamma globulin in the plasma. As a general rule, no gamma globulin can be detected by electrophoresis. However, by more sensitive immunochemical methods, amounts of less than 30 mg/100 ml have been found (normal, 600-1,200 mg/100 ml). Careful study by Gitlin and his associates has shown that this deficiency occurs because of a lack of production of gamma globulin; there is no evidence to suggest an increased rate of destruction in such patients.

Pathologically, the condition is characterized by an almost total absence of plasma cells in the body. Antigenic stimulation fails to produce specific antibodies in various parts of the body. Recently, Gitlin has demonstrated that there is a deficiency of at least two other beta globulins in the plasma of these patients. This clearly suggests that the deficiency of gamma globulin is not the primary defect in this condition. Rather, it appears that all the complications result from the absence of plasma cells and that this deficiency in turn results from an unknown, but probably more basic, process (Chart 7).

DIAGNOSIS.—The absence of isohemagglutinins is useful as a simple laboratory screening test for patients with blood groups O, A, or B. Very recently, Gitlin has developed a quantitative immunochemical procedure for measuring gamma globulin (see Procedure 11) which is more reliable and accurate than electrophoresis at very low concentrations.

Congenital agammaglobulinemia should be differentiated from adult agammaglobulinemia and from transient or physiological agammaglobulinemia, neither of which is hereditary or congenital.

TREATMENT.—The antibiotics, although useful in controlling an immediate infection in these children, have been only partially successful in prevention. On the other hand, gamma globulin administered intramuscularly in dosages of from 0.6 to 1.0 ml per kilogram body weight once a month has given considerable protection against infection.

Bruton, O. C.: Agammaglobulinemia, Pediatrics 9:722, 1952.
Gitlin, D.: Low resistance to infections: Relationship to abnormalities in gamma globulin, Bull. New York Acad. Med. 31:359, 1955.
———; Hitzig, W. H.; and Janeway, C. A.: Multiple serum protein defi-

CHART 7

CONGENITAL AGAMMAGLOBULINEMIA

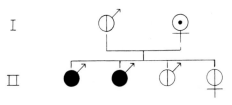

(Janeway & Gitlin, 1957)

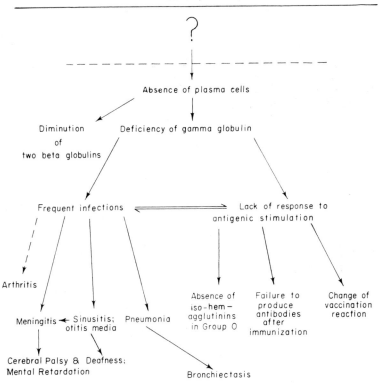

ciencies in congenital and acquired agammaglobulinemia, J. Clin. Invest 35:1199, 1956.

Good, R. A.: Studies on agammaglobulinemia: II. Failure of plasma cell formation in the bone marrow and lymph nodes of patients with agamma-globulinemia, J. Lab. & Clin. Med. 46:167, 1955.

*Janeway, C. A., and Gitlin, D.: The gamma globulins, Advances Pediat 9:65, 1957.

2. CERULOPLASMIN DEFICIENCY (Wilson's disease)

In 1912, Sir Kinnier Wilson, an English neurologist, described a new familial condition characterized by degeneration of the basal ganglia and cirrhosis of the liver (hepatolenticular degeneration). This condition has now been shown to be related to an abnormality of copper metabolism resulting from a deficiency of the plasma protein "ceruloplasmin" and should be included, therefore, among the inborn errors of metabolism.

CLINICAL FEATURES.—One can do no better than quote Wilson's original description of the disease:

> Progressive lenticular degeneration may be defined as a disease which oc curs in young people, often familial but not congenital or hereditary; it is essentially and chiefly a disease of the extrapyramidal motor system and is characterized by involuntary movements, usually in the nature of tremor, dysphagia, emaciation. With these may be associated emotionalism and certain symptoms of a mental nature. It is progressive, and after a longer or shorter period fatal. Pathologically, it is characterized predominantly by bilateral degeneration of the lenticular nucleus, and in addition cirrhosis of the liver [Fig. 23] is constantly found, the latter morbid condition rarely, if ever, giving rise to symptoms during the life of the patient.

Subsequently, pathologists noted a brown or grayish ring at the limbus of the cornea in these patients, which they named "Kayser-Fleischer rings."

HEREDITY.—Ceruloplasmin deficiency is transmitted by a single autosomal recessive gene. This is shown by a high incidence of consanguinity among the parents and by the frequent occurrence of the condition among siblings without the parents or other near relatives being affected. Detection of a heterozygote has so far been unsuccessful, although Bearn has noted a slight but definite decrease of ceruloplasmin synthesis in an asymptomatic sister of a patient with Wilson's disease.

Bearn has estimated that the gene frequency is roughly 1 in 2,000; and so the expected incidence of this condition would be about 1 in 4,-000,000 births. It is actually considerably higher in New York City, where there may be isolates with a high incidence of consanguinity. There is some suggestion that males are affected more frequently than females, although this may in part be due to variations in the age of the patient at the onset of symptoms.

PATHOGENESIS.—The etiology of this rather diffuse condition presents a fascinating story. Wilson originally thought that the disease might be due to an unidentified toxin which damaged the brain and liver only. Later, it was thought that the disease was due to copper intoxication. For a period, all of the signs were attributed to the aminoaciduria which is a complication of this disease. At present it is believed to be due to a deficiency of ceruloplasmin, a blue copper-containing protein in the serum.

Plasma copper occurs in two forms: In one form, a small fraction of the copper reacts with diethylthiocarbamate and is known as the "direct-

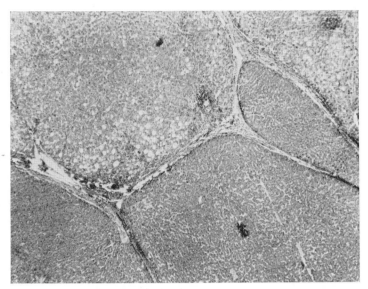

FIG. 23.—Photomicrograph of a section of liver from a patient with Wilson's disease. Prominent fibrous septa circumscribe irregular pseudolobules of liver tissue. The vacuolated hepatic cells indicate an associated fatty metamorphosis.

reacting" fraction (this has been shown to be bound to albumin). In the other form, the greater part of the copper does not react and is known as the "indirect-reacting" fraction (this corresponds to ceruloplasmin). In the normal individual, an intravenous injection of Cu^{64} results in a rapid fall in serum radioactivity, followed by a large increase some time later. In patients with Wilson's disease, there is a slightly slower fall and no secondary rise whatsoever. Since the latter rise is due to the Cu^{64} being incorporated into ceruloplasmin, the failure to rise indicates a deficiency of that protein. This reaction has also been demonstrated with immunochemical techniques by Scheinberg and Gitlin.

Ceruloplasmin deficiency results (see Chart 8) in a decrease or absence of the indirect-reacting fraction of copper. This causes two effects: (1) an increased absorption of copper through the gastrointestinal tract, and (2) an increase of the direct-reacting fraction of copper in plasma. The excess copper is deposited in the tissues of the body. Some of the copper is chelated with amino acids and excreted in the urine, and this explains both the increased absorption and the excretion of copper among patients with Wilson's disease. The deposition of copper in various organs is responsible for the signs and symptoms of the disease: in the brain, lenticular degeneration; in the liver, cirrhosis; and in the cornea, Kayser-Fleischer rings.

Finally, copper is deposited in the kidneys and appears to interfere with the enzyme systems responsible for the transport of a variety of substances across the tubular epithelium. This results in: (1) a generalized aminoacidura (described first by Dent in 1947). Although most of the amino acids are involved, the loss is particularly marked in threonine, cystine, serine, glycine, asparagine, valine, tyrosine, and lysine; (2) a glycosuria with considerable reduction in glucose T_m; (3) a phosphaturia which eventually causes bony irregularities and sclerosis; and (4) an increased loss of uric acid, resulting in hypouricemia in the serum. The relatively late onset of the clinical symptoms in Wilson's disease is in part due to the effect of the gradual increase in the amounts of copper in the tissues over a period of years. For example, at least one child has been described in whom aminoaciduria was not present early in life but became increasingly marked as the child grew older.

DIAGNOSIS.—Wilson's disease can be diagnosed by the deficiency of ceruloplasmin in plasma (see Procedure 12) and the proportion of the direct-reacting plasma copper fraction (see Procedure 13).

TREATMENT.—Replacement with injections of ceruloplasmin is impractical at the present time because of the very limited quantities of the protein available in pure form. However, BAL (British anti-lewisite) is effective in greatly increasing the urinary output of copper, and Denny-Brown feels that great improvement may ensue if such treatment is vigorously pursued. Also, favorable results have been reported with the use of penicillamine.

Bearn, A. G.: Genetic and biochemical aspects of Wilson's disease, Am. J. Med. 15:442, 1953.
*———: Wilson's disease, Am. J. Med. 22:747, 1957.
Cartwright, G. E.; Hodges, R. E.; Gubler, C. J.; Mahoney, J. P.; Daum, K.; and Wintrobe, M. M.: Studies on copper metabolism: XIII. Hepatolenticular degeneration, J. Clin. Invest. 33:1487, 1954.

CHART 8

CERULOPLASMIN DEFICIENCY (WILSON'S DISEASE)

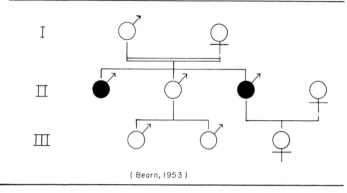

I

II

III

(Bearn, 1953)

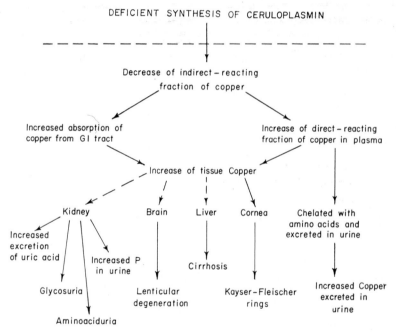

DEFICIENT SYNTHESIS OF CERULOPLASMIN

Decrease of indirect – reacting
fraction of copper

Increased absorption of
copper from GI tract

Increase of direct – reacting
fraction of copper in plasma

Increase of tissue Copper

Kidney   Brain   Liver   Cornea   Chelated with
amino acids and
excreted in urine

Increased
excretion
of uric acid

Increased P
in urine

Glycosuria

Aminoaciduria

Lenticular
degeneration

Cirrhosis

Kayser–Fleischer
rings

Increased Copper
excreted in
urine

Denny-Brown, D., and Porter, H.: The effect of BAL on hepatolenticular degeneration, New England J. Med. 245:917, 1951.

Holmberg, C. G., and Laurell, C. B.: Investigations in serum copper: II. Isolation of the copper containing protein and a description of some of its properties, Acta chem. scandinav. 2:550, 1948.

Scheinberg, I. H., and Gitlin, D.: Deficiency of ceruloplasmin in patients with hepatolenticular degeneration, Science 116:484, 1952.

Wilson, S. A. K.: Progressive lenticular degeneration, Brain 34:295, 1912.

3. CONGENITAL AFIBRINOGENEMIA

The congenital absence of fibrinogen is a rare condition which was first described in 1920 by Rabe and Salomon.

CLINICAL FEATURES.—Bleeding is the primary manifestation of congenital afibrinogenemia. It usually begins at an early age, frequently at birth; and it recurs in association with the eruption and shedding of teeth, with trauma, with infections, and after surgery. It is surprising, however, that, despite the complete incoagulability of the blood, patients with afibrinogenemia have, on the average, less difficulty with bruising and bleeding than have those with hemophilia. Also, despite the lack of a fibrin net, the healing of wounds is not usually retarded.

HEREDITY.—Congenital afibrinogenemia is probably transmitted by a rare recessive gene. This is suggested by the fact that one third of the cases come from cousin marriages, and the condition is seen frequently among siblings without the parents being affected. Up to the present, the sex distribution has been 21 males and 8 females, a difference which may be significant.

About half of the parents and many of the near relatives of known patients show a moderate decrease of plasma fibrinogen levels without clinical symptoms of bleeding. This would suggest that the heterozygotes are sometimes detectable, although there is considerable overlap with the normal range.

PATHOGENESIS.—The primary defect in this condition appears to be a marked deficiency of fibrinogen in the plasma. Using immunochemical methods, Gitlin and Borges have shown that there is no more than 1.2 mg/100 ml of fibrinogen or fibrinogen-like material present in such patients, as compared with 300-500 mg/100 ml in normal controls. It appears unlikely that the protein is present in another form, since one would have to account for a missing 5-8% component of the total plasma proteins. It has also been shown that the deficiency of fibrinogen is due to a lack of synthesis; there is no evidence of increased breakdown of this protein fraction when it is transfused to affected individuals.

The deficiency of fibrinogen is responsible for the bleeding tendency.

Normally, under the action of the active enzyme, thrombin, fibrinogen is polymerized to the larger molecule, fibrin, which forms the clot. When fibrin is deficient, this process no longer takes place and the patient bleeds (Chart 9).

DIAGNOSIS.—A deficiency of fibrinogen in the plasma can be shown by one of the following tests: (1) plasma coagulation (see Procedure

CHART 9

CONGENITAL AFIBRINOGENEMIA

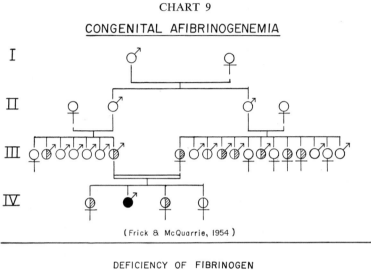

(Frick & McQuarrie, 1954)

DEFICIENCY OF FIBRINOGEN

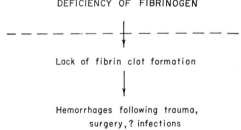

Lack of fibrin clot formation

Hemorrhages following trauma,
surgery, ? infections

14), (2) quantitative measurement of fibrinogen in the plasma (see Procedure 15), (3) electrophoresis, and (4) immunochemical techniques.

TREATMENT.—During periods of bleeding, patients with congenital afibrinogenemia can be greatly helped by intravenous transfusions of fibrinogen, plasma, or whole blood. This treatment is usually effective in promptly stopping the bleeding, and the effect lasts for 4-5 days.

Alexander, B., et al.: Congenital afibrinogenemia: A study of some basic aspects of coagulation, Blood 9:843, 1954.

Frick, P. G., and McQuarrie, I.: Congenital afibrinogenemia, Pediatrics 13:44, 1954.

Gitlin, D., and Borges, W. H.: Studies on the metabolism of fibrinogen in two patients with congenital afibrinogenemia, Blood 8:679, 1953.

Henderson, J. L.; Donaldson, G. M. M.; and Scarborough, H.: Congenital afibrinogenemia, Quart. J. Med. 14:101, 1945.

5

Deficiencies of Clotting Factors

DURING THE PAST half century the field of blood coagulation has become so complex that we might do well to start off by reviewing a few of the fundamental concepts involved. First, we should remember that these represent deficiencies of "trace proteins." Unlike gamma globulin or fibrinogen, the amounts of these proteins normally present are so small that they cannot be detected by chemical or electrophoretic methods. Most of the clotting factors have not been isolated, purified, or characterized in the chemical sense. Rather, their absence can only be implied by the failure of blood to clot. This is a functional demonstration of deficiency, much like the enzyme defects to be described in the next section. Second, the existence of these proteins can only be established by deductive reasoning. For example, when the plasma from an apparent case of hemophilia corrects the clotting defect in the plasma from a patient with known hemophilia, the diseases are assumed to be due to deficiencies of entirely different substances. When the exceptional plasma is found to correct the clotting defect in all other types of hemophilia-like deficient plasmas, it is generally agreed that this plasma is unique and the patient is considered to be suffering from a new, previously undescribed condition. Despite these limitations, the deficiency or absence of certain specific clotting factors appears to be quite definite. These factors can be distinguished by the genetic and biochemical characteristics, and they will be discussed in some detail.

At the present time, the exact role that each of the specific factors plays in the formation of the blood clot is not entirely settled. In order to avoid this highly controversial subject, I have chosen to adopt Graham's simplification of Marowitz's theory of blood coagulation, as illustrated in Figure 24. It is generally agreed that there are at least two essential steps in the formation of a clot: (1) prothrombin is converted to thrombin in the presence of Ca⁺⁺ and certain thromboplastic effects, and (2) fibrinogen is converted to fibrin in the presence of thrombin. All of the clotting factors have something to do with the first step and can be classi-

PLATELETS

+

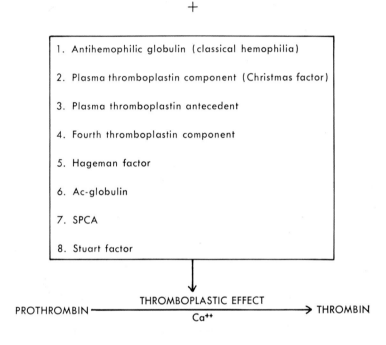

1. Antihemophilic globulin (classical hemophilia)

2. Plasma thromboplastin component (Christmas factor)

3. Plasma thromboplastin antecedent

4. Fourth thromboplastin component

5. Hageman factor

6. Ac-globulin

7. SPCA

8. Stuart factor

THROMBOPLASTIC EFFECT
PROTHROMBIN ——————————————————→ THROMBIN
Ca⁺⁺

THROMBIN
FIBRINOGEN ——————————————————→ FIBRIN

FIG. 24.—A modification of the Marowitz theory of blood coagulation. (Proposed by Graham, J. B.: The genetic biochemistry of human blood coagulation, Am. J. Human Genet. 8:63, 1956.)

fied under the over-all term of "thromboplastic effects" without specifying the specific role of each.

Eight congenital deficiencies of specific clotting factors have been described: (1) *deficiency of antihemophilic globulin* (classical hemophilia), (2) *deficiency of plasma thromboplastin component* (Christmas disease), (3) *deficiency of plasma thromboplastin antecedent,* (4) *deficiency of a fourth thromboplastin component,* (5) *Hageman trait,* (6) *deficiency of Ac-globulin,* (7) *SPCA deficiency,* and (8) *Stuart defect.* There is still considerable controversy as to whether idiopathic hypothrombinemia is a true inborn error of metabolism, or, for that matter, whether such a defect exists at all.

*Brinkhous, K. M.; Langdell, R. D.; Penick, G. D.; Graham, J. B.; and Wagner, R. H.: Newer approaches to the study of hemophilia and hemophiloid states, J.A.M.A. 154:481, 1954.

*Graham, J. B.: The genetic biochemistry of human blood coagulation, Am. J. Human Genet. 8:63, 1956.

Rosenthal, R. L.: Hemophilia and hemophilia-like diseases caused by deficiencies in plasma thromboplastin factors: Anti-hemophilic globulin (AHG), plasma thromboplastin component (PTC), and plasma thromboplastin antecedent (PTA), Am. J. Med. 17:57, 1954.

I. DEFICIENCY OF ANTIHEMOPHILIC GLOBULIN (AHG) (classical hemophilia; hemophilia A; deficiency of thromboplastinogen; alpha prothrombin deficiency)

Hemophilia is of particular interest because it is probably the oldest hereditary disease known. Both the Jews and Arabs knew of the condition in ancient times, and more recently its mode of transmission has been recorded among many of the royal houses of Europe (Chart 10).

CLINICAL FEATURES.—Hemophilia is usually diagnosed early in childhood by signs of a hemorrhagic tendency following circumcision, by easy bruising, and by difficulty in stopping bleeding after a cut. In older children, uncontrollable bleeding following the extraction of teeth or removal of tonsils may be the first serious sign of hemophilia. Bleeding may also affect the internal organs, and death may result from intracranial hemorrhage. Hemarthrosis is a characteristic lesion of hemophilia and, after repeated hemorrhages, the joints tend to become fixed.

HEREDITY.—In most instances the defect is transmitted as a sex-linked recessive character. This means that an affected male will transmit the defect to all of his daughters, who will become carriers. All of his sons, however, will escape the defect and be perfectly normal. If a woman is a carrier, one half of her male offspring will be active bleeders, while the other half will be normal. Similarly, one half of her female offspring will be carriers, while the other half will be normal. In this condition, most of the affected individuals will be males. A homozygous female is possible if an affected male mates with a female carrier. Only one or two instances of this situation have been noted, but this mode of transmission has been well worked out in hemophilic dogs.

The female carriers of hemophilia do not show any consistent clotting defect. Apparently, the overlap between normals and carriers is so great that no definite trend emerges from such a study.

At least two other types of antihemophilic globulin (AHG) deficiency have been reported. In 1953, Graham, McLendon, and Brink-hous described a pedigree in which the AHG was not completely absent but was reduced to about a quarter that of normal. Bleeding was much less severe among the affected individuals. The condition was transmitted as a sex-linked recessive. However, the heterozygous females showed some, definitely detectable, deficiency of AHG. In 1956, Schulman and his co-workers and Matter and his associates described families with "vascular hemophilia." In addition to a deficiency of AHG, the affected individuals showed vascular abnormalities characteristic of pseudohemophilia (von Willebrand's disease). The trait appears to be transmitted by an autosomal dominant gene with high penetrance and variable expressivity. At the present time, it is not clear whether these latter forms represent variants of the classical disease, are alleles in the same locus, or are separate entities, all showing a deficiency of AHG. It may be that the production of AHG requires both a normal sex-linked and another autosomal locus. If so, the forms studied by Graham are probably alleles of the former, and those described by Schulman and Matter represent a defect in the latter.

PATHOGENESIS.—Classical hemophilia is the direct result of a congenital deficiency of the AHG in the plasma (Chart 10). The absence of this factor reduces the thromboplastic effect and causes the failure of the blood to clot. Hemorrhagic diathesis is the direct result of prolonged clotting time. The AHG is carried in the fraction I of Cohn and can be precipitated by CO_2 saturation of diluted plasma. It is quite labile when stored under blood-bank conditions, and as much as 50% will disappear in 24 hours. However, if plasma is frozen or lyophilized, the anti-hemophilic activity is maintained for long periods of time.

DIAGNOSIS.—The diagnosis of classical hemophilia is based on certain negative findings, such as normal fibrinogen, prothrombin, clotting inhibitors, and platelet numbers, coupled with the positive findings suggesting delayed conversion of prothrombin to thrombin. For example, the findings may show (1) that the whole-blood clotting time (see Procedure 16) and plasma clotting time (see Procedure 17) are abnormal; (2) that the plasma clots relatively slowly, despite normal prothrombin levels as shown by the one-stage method (Procedure 18); (3) that there is slow disappearance of prothrombin from clotting blood, as shown by prothrombin utilization or consumption tests (Procedure 21); and (4) that the thromboplastin generation test (Procedure 23), where the patient's adsorbed plasma, normal serum, platelets, and calcium are incubated together, is delayed. Further localization of the clotting defect is dependent on special studies. In the main, these consist of determining

CHART 10

DEFICIENCY OF ANTIHEMOPHILIC GLOBULIN

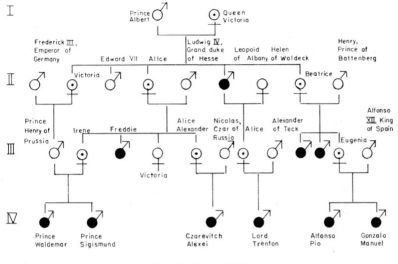

(After Brinkhous, 1954)

DEFICIENCY OF AHG

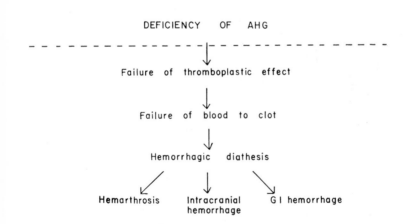

the effectiveness of normal plasma and serum fractions and of plasmas with known deficiencies on the clotting defect under study.

The principal findings in AHG deficiency are shown in Table 2. Fresh normal plasma and adsorbed fresh normal plasma will correct the defect. Aged plasma will not correct the defect because AHG is lost upon stand-

TABLE 2.—CLOTTING CHARACTERISTICS OF THE VARIOUS HEMOPHILIAS*

	EFFECT ON CLOTTING TIME OF PATIENT'S PLASMA BY ADDITION OF—			
DEFECT	Fresh Normal Plasma	Aged Normal Plasma	Adsorbed Normal Plasma	Normal Serum
AHG deficiency	+	0	+	0
PTC deficiency	+	+	0	+
PTA deficiency	+	(+)	(+)	+

*Symbols: +, correction; 0, no correction; (+), partial correction.

ing. Normal serum will not correct the clotting time because AHG is lost upon clotting. Finally, the antihemophilic factor (AHF) (see Procedure 20) is greatly decreased or absent in AHG deficiency.

Proper diagnostic proof requires that the clotting defect can be corrected by plasma from patients with every other type of known hemophilic disorder—namely, plasma thromboplastin component (PTC) deficiency, plasma thromboplastin antecedent (PTA) deficiency, fourth plasma thromboplastin component deficiency, etc.

TREATMENT.—In the management of the hemophiliac, it should be recognized that bleeding occurs when the vascular system is injured or when capillaries become hyperpermeable. While the basic defect is the lack of thromboplastic effect, which remains constant throughout life, the immediate cause of bleeding is always vascular, and this is variable. The immediate approach to controlling hemorrhage is local. Cold and pressure are the key guides to staunching. When bleeding cannot be controlled by local measures, systemic treatment is mandatory. The only form of treatment which has stood the test of time is transfusion of fresh whole blood, or fresh frozen or lyophilized plasma.

*Brinkhous, K. M.; Langdell, R. D.; Penick, G. D.; Graham, J. B.; and Wagner, R. H.: Newer approaches to the study of hemophilia and hemophiloid states, J.A.M.A. 154:481, 1954.

Graham, J. B.; McLendon, W. W.; and Brinkhous, K. M.: Mild hemophilia: An allelic form of the disease, Am. J. M. Sc. 225:46, 1953.

Margolius, A., Jr., and Ratnoff, O. D.: A laboratory study of the carrier state in classic hemophilia, J. Clin. Invest. 35:1316, 1956.

Matter, M.; Newcomb, T. F.; Melly, A.; and Finch, C. A.: Vascular hemophilia: The association of a vascular defect with a deficiency of antihemophilic globulin, Am. J. M. Sc. 232:421, 1956.

Merskey, C.: The occurrence of haemophilia in the human, Quart. J. Med. 20:299, 1951.

Schulman, I.; Smith, C. H.; Erlandson, M.; Fort, E.; and Lee, R. E.: Vascular hemophilia: A familial hemorrhagic disease in males and females characterized by combined antihemophilic globulin deficiency and vascular abnormality, Pediatrics 18:347, 1956.

Taylor, F. H. L.; Davidson, C. S.; Tagnon, H. J.; Adams, M. A.; MacDonald, A. H.; and Minot, G. R.: Studies in blood coagulation: The coagulation properties of certain globulin fractions of normal plasma in vitro, J. Clin. Invest. 24:698, 1945.

2. DEFICIENCY OF PLASMA THROMBOPLASTIN COMPONENT (PTC) (Christmas disease; hemophilia B; deficiency of beta prothromboplastin)

This disease was probably discovered, and was reported with the wrong interpretation, by Pavlovsky in 1947. He suggested that not all cases of hemophilia were "uniform in nature," because the blood of certain hemophiliacs improved the clotting time of others. Five years later, workers in England and America reported, almost simultaneously, on certain hemophilic families whose blood would correct the clotting defect of other known hemophiliacs, and vice versa. The English family was named Christmas, and the report appeared during Christmas week; hence, the name "Christmas disease" has become permanently attached to the nomenclature of hemophilia.

CLINICAL FEATURES.—Clinically, the hemorrhagic diathesis cannot be distinguished from classical hemophilia except that some of the cases are rather mild.

HEREDITY.—Like classical hemophilia, Christmas disease is transmitted as a sex-linked recessive character. However, a decrease of the PTC factor can be found in about half of the mothers of known cases, indicating that the heterozygote may be detected.

It is estimated that 1 out of every 6 so-called "hemophiliacs" has Christmas disease.

PATHOGENESIS.—The congenital deficiency of PTC factor in the plasma is responsible for the hemorrhagic diathesis (Chart 11). The PTC factor is precipitated by 45-50% saturation of normal plasma with ammonium sulfate. It is also adsorbed by $BaSO_4$, which distinguishes it from the other hemophilic factors.

DIAGNOSIS.—As in AHG deficiency, the diagnosis is suggested by a delay in the generation of thromboplastin. The condition is also suggested by abnormalities in the partial thromboplastin time (see Procedure 22), the thromboplastin generation test (Procedure 23), and the prothrombin utilization test (Procedure 21). The AHG (Procedure 20) is normal in the patient with PTC deficiency.

The principal findings in PTC deficiency are shown in Table 2. Fresh normal plasma, aged normal plasma, and normal serum will correct the defect. This is because PTC is not destroyed by aging or clot forma-

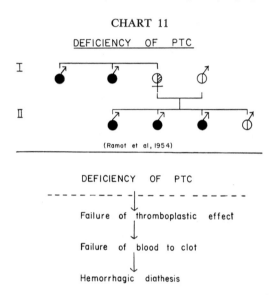

CHART 11

DEFICIENCY OF PTC

(Ramot et al, 1954)

DEFICIENCY OF PTC

Failure of thromboplastic effect

Failure of blood to clot

Hemorrhagic diathesis

tion. However, the PTC is adsorbed by $BaSO_4$, and therefore adsorbed normal plasma will not correct the defect.

Final diagnostic proof requires that the clotting defect be corrected by plasma from patients with every other type of known hemophilic disorder.

TREATMENT.—The condition can be effectively controlled by transfusions of fresh plasma or whole blood, but fraction I of Cohn is of no therapeutic value.

Aggeler, P. M.; White, S. G.; Glending, M. B.; Page, E. W.; Leake, T. B.; and Bates, G.: Plasma thromboplastin component (PTC), a new disease resembling hemophilia, Proc. Soc. Exper. Biol. & Med. 79:692, 1952.

Biggs, P.; Douglas, A. S.; MacFarlane, R. G.; Dacie, J. V.; Pitney, W. R.; Merskey, C.; and O'Brien, J. R.: Christmas disease, a condition previously mistaken for hemophilia, Brit. M. J. 2:1378, 1952.

Pavlovsky, A.: Contribution to the pathogenesis of hemophilia, Blood 2:185, 1947.

Ramot, B.; Angelopoulos, B.; and Singer, K.: Variable manifestations of plasma thromboplastin deficiency, J. Lab. & Clin. Med. 46:80, 1955.

Soulier, J. P., and Larrieu, M. J.: Differentiation of hemophilia into two groups: A study of 33 cases, New England J. Med. 249:547, 1953.

3. DEFICIENCY OF PLASMA THROMBOPLASTIN ANTECEDENT (PTA) (hemophilia C)

In 1953, Rosenthal, Dreskin, and Rosenthal described still another hemophilia-like condition, which appears to be due to the deficiency of a third thromboplastic factor, which they named "plasma thromboplastin antecedent" (PTA). The coagulation disorder in these patients is cor-

CHART 12

DEFICIENCY OF PTA

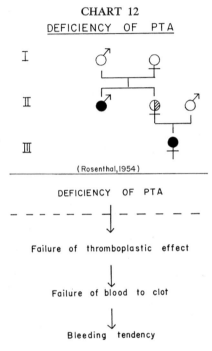

(Rosenthal, 1954)

DEFICIENCY OF PTA

Failure of thromboplastic effect

Failure of blood to clot

Bleeding tendency

rected by both AHG- and PTC-deficient plasma as well as by normal plasma or serum.

CLINICAL FEATURES.—Clinically, the bleeding tendency is very slight, occurring usually after the extraction of teeth or tonsillectomy. Purpura and joint involvement rarely occur.

HEREDITY.—Rosenthal has suggested that the condition is transmitted as a simple autosomal dominant and affects both males and females about equally. The condition can also occur to a lesser degree in individuals without bleeding tendencies. For instance, he reports a PTA carrier who is the mother of one patient and the sister of another. The mother showed an abnormal utilization of prothrombin, and her plasma failed to correct the clotting defect in her daughter.

PATHOGENESIS.—This bleeding tendency is due to the deficiency of the PTA factor in the plasma (Chart 12). The PTA can be partially purified by ammonium sulfate fractionation (it is present in the 25-35% fraction). It is stable on storage at temperatures ranging from —20° C to 28° C, is chiefly present in Cohn's fraction IV-1, and is localized in the beta$_2$ globulin fraction of serum separated by paper electrophoresis. Seitz filtration and BaSO$_4$ treatment of normal plasma and serum irregularly remove slight amounts of PTA, which can then be eluted by NaCl and sodium citrate.

DIAGNOSIS.—The condition is suggested by a delay in the generation of thromboplastin and also by a prolongation of the partial thromboplastin time (see Procedure 22).

The principal findings in PTA deficiency are shown in Table 2. All of the plasmas and normal serum will partially correct the defect. This is because aging and clotting only partially destroy the PTA factor and because only a portion of PTA is adsorbed by BaSO$_4$ treatment.

Final diagnostic proof requires that the clotting defect be corrected by plasma from patients with every other type of known hemophilic disorder.

TREATMENT.—The administration of stored, refrigerated plasma has been found to correct the clotting defect and is effective in controlling hemorrhage or as a prophylactic measure prior to surgery.

Rosenthal, R. L.: Hemophilia and hemophilia-like diseases caused by deficiencies in plasma thromboplastin factors: Anti-hemophilic globulin (AHG), plasma thromboplastin component (PTC), and plasma thromboplastin antecedent (PTA), Am. J. Med. 17:57, 1954.

———; Dreskin, O. H.; and Rosenthal, N.: New hemophilia-like disease caused by deficiency of a third thromboplastin factor, Proc. Soc. Exper. Biol. & Med. 82:171, 1953.

——— and Gendelman, E.: Properties of plasma thromboplastin antecedent (PTA) in relation to blood coagulation, J. Lab. & Clin. Med. 45:123, 1955.

4. DEFICIENCY OF A FOURTH PLASMA THROMBOPLASTIN COMPONENT (PTF-D)

CLINICAL FEATURES.—In 1954, Spaet, Aggeler, and Kinsell reported on a patient with a persistent tendency to bleed following injury, surgery, and dental extractions. Clotting studies revealed a prolonged prothrombin utilization and retarded generation of plasma thromboplastin. No anticoagulant was demonstrable, and all previously described coagulation factors were normally present. As a result, the condition was described as due to a deficiency of a fourth plasma thromboplastin component.

HEREDITY.—The bleeding tendency has been present in both male and female bleeders in the patient's family for three generations. It is presumed, therefore, to be transmitted as an autosomal dominant, with the affected individuals being heterozygous for the condition.

PATHOGENESIS.—The hemorrhagic diathesis is presumably due to a deficiency of the fourth thromboplastin component (Chart 13). The fac-

CHART 13

DEFICIENCY OF 4th PLASMA THROMBOPLASTIN COMPONENT

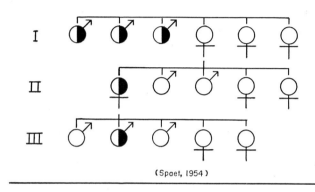

(Spaet, 1954)

DEFICIENCY OF 4th PLASMA THROMBOPLASTIN COMPONENT

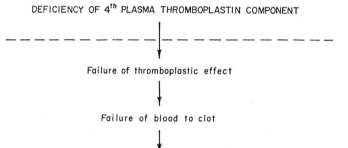

Failure of thromboplastic effect

Failure of blood to clot

Bleeding tendency

tor is found in Cohn's fractions III and IV and in the 50% ammonium sulfate precipitation of normal plasma. The activity is heat labile and storage stable; and the factor is not adsorbed on $BaSO_4$ but is removed only by high-concentration asbestos Seitz filters.

DIAGNOSIS.—This condition is suggested by prolonged prothrombin utilization (see Procedure 21) and the thromboplastin generation test (Procedure 23). The defect can be corrected by the plasmas from patients with AHG, PTC, and PTA deficiencies.

TREATMENT.—Transfusion with whole blood or its fractions does not improve the clotting condition in the patient.

Spaet, T. H.; Aggeler, P. M.; and Kinsell, B. C.: A possible fourth thromboplastin component, J. Clin. Invest. 33:1095, 1954.

5. HAGEMAN TRAIT

CLINICAL FEATURES.—In 1956, Margolius and Ratnoff described three patients with a new clotting defect. The patients were remarkable in being totally free from bleeding difficulties, and there was no evidence

CHART 14

HAGEMAN TRAIT

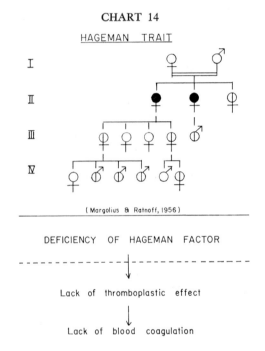

(Margolius & Ratnoff, 1956)

DEFICIENCY OF HAGEMAN FACTOR

Lack of thromboplastic effect

Lack of blood coagulation

of hemorrhagic diathesis despite operations and dental extractions. The clotting defect was uncovered only in routine preoperative studies.

HEREDITY.—The condition occurs in both males and females. It is probably familial, since two of the patients were sisters. However, none of some 15 relatives in four generations tested showed any clotting abnormalities.

PATHOGENESIS.—The clotting abnormality is presumably due to a deficiency of the Hageman factor in the serum (Chart 14). The fraction can be purified by precipitating the $BaSO_4$-treated aged serum with

30-40% ammonium sulfate; it can then be adsorbed onto kaolin and eluted with some selectivity, resulting in apparent concentration (about 500-fold, compared with the original serum). However, the globulin will still not be homogeneous electrophoretically. Small amounts of this purified substance will shorten the prolonged recalcified clotting time and restore the thromboplastic effect to normal.

DIAGNOSIS.—The defect can be shown by the thromboplastin generation test (see Procedure 23) and by prothrombin activity of the serum. Hageman factor can be differentiated from some of the other factors in that it is not destroyed by aging of the serum (which excludes fibrinogen, prothrombin, Ac-globulin, and AHF), adsorption with BaSO₄ (which excludes PTC and SPCA), and heating at 56° C for 30 minutes (which excludes the fourth thromboplastin component).

The final diagnosis of the clotting defect depends on the plasma being corrected by plasma from patients with deficiencies of AHF, PTC, PTA, and fourth thromboplastin component.

TREATMENT.—None is required. A small transfusion of 50 ml of 20-day-old blood will normalize clotting tests.

Margolius, A., Jr., and Ratnoff, O. D.: Observations on the hereditary nature of Hageman trait, Blood 11:565, 1956.

Ramot, B.; Singer, K.; Hiller, P.; and Zimmerman, H. J.: Hageman factor (HF) deficiency, Blood 11:745, 1956.

Ratnoff, O. D., and Colopy, J. E.: A familial hemorrhagic trait associated with a deficiency of a clot promoting fraction of plasma, J. Clin. Invest. 34:602, 1955.

6. DEFICIENCY OF AC-GLOBULIN (parahemophilia; deficiencies of factor V; prothrombin A; prothrombin accelerator; labile factor; plasma accelerator globulin; plasma prothrombin conversion factor; and proaccelerin)

CLINICAL FEATURES.—In 1944, Owren described the case of a 29-year-old woman who gave a history of abnormal bleeding time since the age of 3½ years. Investigation of the patient disclosed prolongation of the whole-blood clotting time as well as a prolonged "prothrombin time," both of which could be corrected by the addition of prothrombin-free fresh normal plasma. This represented a new coagulation defect, which was called "parahemophilia."

Clinically, such patients have mucous membrane bleeding, and epistaxis and menorrhagia are common features. The latter can be very severe; two affected women have bled to death at the first menstrual period.

HEREDITY.—The condition appears to be transmitted by an autosomal recessive gene. Consanguinity has been reported in a large pedigree from South Africa. The heterozygous carriers of the abnormal gene can be detected by a partial deficiency of Ac-globulin although they show no hemorrhagic tendencies.

The incidence of the condition in the population is not known.

PATHOGENESIS.—The hemorrhagic diathesis is caused by a congenital absence of Ac-globulin factor in the plasma (Chart 15). This

CHART 15

AC-GLOBULIN DEFICIENCY

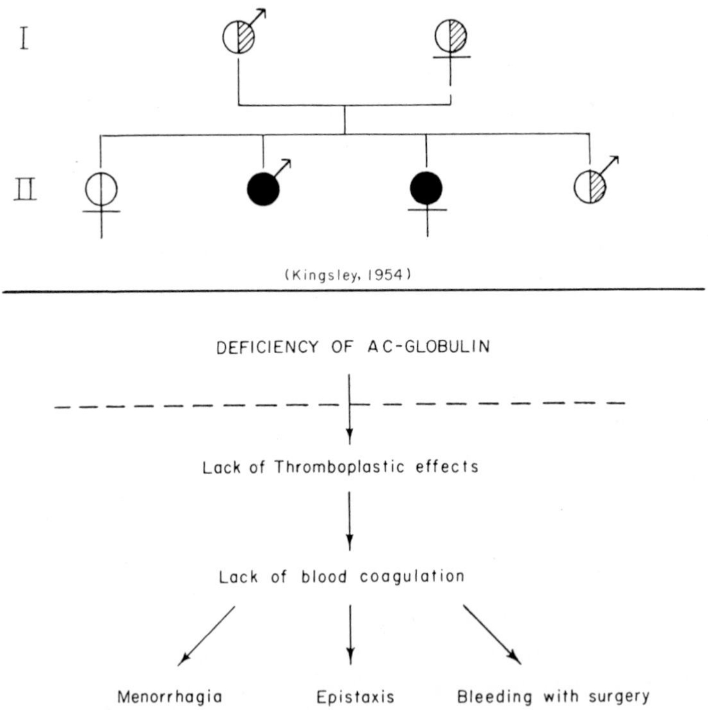

(Kingsley, 1954)

DEFICIENCY OF AC-GLOBULIN

Lack of Thromboplastic effects

Lack of blood coagulation

Menorrhagia   Epistaxis   Bleeding with surgery

factor precipitates from plasma with the globulins at pH 5.3 and is found preponderantly in fractions II and III of plasma. It is not adsorbed by $BaSO_4$, and only slightly by $Mg(OH)_2$ and Seitz filters. The distinguishing characteristic of Ac-globulin is that it is relatively labile, deteriorating rapidly in plasma. It tends to deteriorate more rapidly in the absence of calcium and is more labile in oxalated than in citrated plasma.

DIAGNOSIS.—The coagulation time (see Procedure 16) and one

stage prothrombin time (Procedure 18) are prolonged. The presence of Ac-globulin can quickly be detected by its ability to reduce the prothrombin time of stored human plasma (Procedure 24).

TREATMENT.—Transfusions with fresh whole blood or plasma will correct the deficiency to a clinically significant degree for about a day. The administration of vitamin K has been uniformly unsuccessful.

Kingsley, C. S.: Familial factor V deficiency: The pattern of heredity, Quart. J. Med. 23:323, 1954.
Owren, P. A.: Parahemophilia: Hemorrhagic diathesis due to absence of a previously unknown clotting factor, Lancet 1:446, 1947.
Ware, A. G., and Seegers, W. H.: Plasma accelerator globulin: Partial purification, quantitative determination, and properties, J. Biol. Chem. 172:699, 1948.

7. DEFICIENCY OF SERUM PROTHROMBIN CONVERSION ACCELERATOR (SPCA) (deficiencies of cothromboplastin; prothrombin conversion factor; prothrombinogen; proconvertin-convertin; and factor VII)

CLINICAL FEATURES.—After the discovery of the Ac-globulin factor, it was soon realized that some other factor was also important for the conversion of prothrombin into thrombin. Studies with Dicumarol® suggested that the compound caused a decrease not only of prothrombin but of an additional factor as well. In 1949, Alexander and his associates made the first complete observations on a patient lacking this factor and named the factor the "serum prothrombin conversion accelerator" (SPCA).

Congenital lack of SPCA constitutes a clinical entity which is difficult to distinguish from true congenital hypoprothrombinemia. In fact, several cases of true SPCA deficiency were previously misdiagnosed as being due to hypoprothrombinemia. Patients with SPCA deficiency show an excessive tendency to bleed early in life. In fact, infants will frequently bleed to death at delivery from this defect. Later in life, patients suffer from recurrent epistaxis, excessive bruising, subarachnoid hemorrhage, and melena.

HEREDITY.—The condition is probably transmitted by an autosomal recessive gene, although very few complete families have been described. Parents and some siblings of known patients have been shown to have a normal concentration of prothrombin but a moderate delay of prothrombin conversion by the modified two-stage method for determining prothrombin (see Procedure 19). This defect can be corrected by the addition of small amounts of partially purified SPCA.

PATHOGENESIS.—The congenital deficiency of SPCA is responsible for the bleeding difficulties (Chart 16). The SPCA factor has been partially purified from human serum. Its main characteristics are: (1) it can be quantitatively adsorbed from serum by $BaSO_4$; (2) it is nondialyzable; (3) it is not precipitated from dilute serum at pH 5.8; (4) it is destroyed at 56° C in 2 minutes; and (5) it is stable at 4°-5° C for at

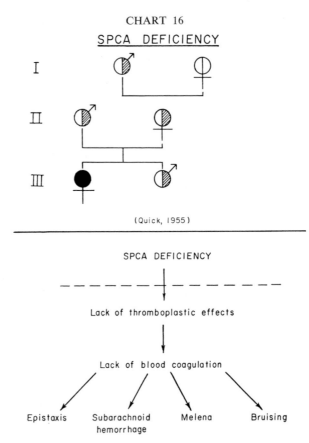

CHART 16

SPCA DEFICIENCY

(Quick, 1955)

SPCA DEFICIENCY

Lack of thromboplastic effects

Lack of blood coagulation

Epistaxis   Subarachnoid   Melena   Bruising
             hemorrhage

least 3 days in serum and 9 days in purified fractions. Also, the coagulation of hemophilic or heparinized blood is accelerated by SPCA.

DIAGNOSIS.—The SPCA deficiency is characterized by a prolongation of the one-stage prothrombin time (see Procedure 18) and by the modified two-stage prothrombin determination (Procedure 19). The defect can be readily corrected by the addition of partially purified SPCA. The deficiency can also be detected by adding normal serum and observing the enhancement of prothrombin activity (Procedure 25).

TREATMENT.—The transfusion of serum appears to be the treatment of choice during periods of bleeding.

Alexander, B.; Goldstein, R.; and Landwehr, G.: The prothrombin conversion accelerator of serum (SPCA): Its partial purification and its properties compared with serum Ac globulin, J. Clin. Invest. 29:881, 1950.

———; ———; ———; and Cook, C. D.: Congenital SPCA deficiency: A hitherto unrecognized coagulation defect with hemorrhage rectified by serum and fractions, J. Clin. Invest. 30:596, 1951.

DeVries, A.; Alexander, B.; and Goldstein, A.: A factor in serum which accelerates the conversion of prothrombin to thrombin: I. Its determination and some physiologic and biochemical properties, Blood 4:247, 1949.

Frick, P. G., and Hagen, P. S.: Congenital familial deficiency of the stable prothrombin conversion factor: Restudy of case originally reported as "idiopathic hypoprothrombinemia," J. Lab. & Clin. Med. 42:212, 1953.

Quick, A. J.; Pisciotta, A. V.; and Hussey, C. V.: Congenital hypoprothombinemic states, Arch. Int. Med. 95:2, 1955.

8. STUART CLOTTING DEFECT

In 1957, Houghie, Barrow, and Graham restudied a patient who had previously been diagnosed as having SPCA deficiency. They showed by cross-matching techniques that the bleeding tendency was due to a lack, not of SPCA, but of a hitherto undescribed clotting factor. They named this the "Stuart factor," after the patient's surname.

CLINICAL FEATURES.—The patient with this deficiency appeared clinically to be identical with patients having SPCA deficiency. He gave a history of frequent episodes of epistaxis and hematomata, and on one occasion developed a severe hemarthrosis with severe anemia.

HEREDITY.—The Stuart factor appears to be transmitted as a highly penetrant, but incompletely recessive, autosomal characteristic (Chart 7). In the family studied by Graham, consanguinity was present. The heterozygotes are only mildly affected clinically but show 1½- to 3-second prolongations of the prothrombin time and the thromboplastin generation test.

Graham has suggested that about 2 in 1,000 individuals are heterozygous carriers of this abnormality.

PATHOGENESIS.—Stuart factor, like SPCA, can be adsorbed from serum by $BaSO_4$; it is stable at pH 6-9 and will remain so when heated up to 56° C. It is essential for the formation of blood thromboplastin at an early stage and is required for the optimal activity of brain, lung, and platelet thromboplastin and of cephalin and Stypven®.

Stuart factor will correct the clotting defect in SPCA deficiency in the prothrombin time test. Similarly, SPCA will correct the clotting defect in Stuart factor deficiency. A mixture of equal parts of plasmas of patients with SPCA and Stuart factor deficiency will give 50% proconvertin activity in the Owren assay.

DIAGNOSIS.—Stuart factor deficiency is characterized by an abnormal thromboplastin generation test (see Procedure 23). The defect can readily be corrected by normal serum or by serum from a patient with

CHART 17

STUART DEFECT

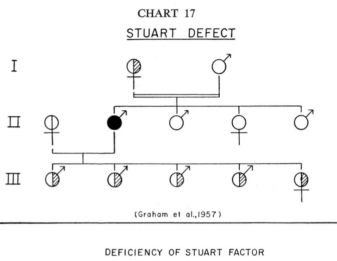

(Graham et al.,1957)

DEFICIENCY OF STUART FACTOR

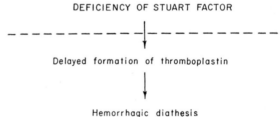

Delayed formation of thromboplastin

Hemorrhagic diathesis

SPCA deficiency. The deficiency can also be detected by adding Dicumarol® plasma to oxalated plasma from a patient with Stuart defect and observing the enhancement of prothrombin activity (see Procedure 25).

TREATMENT.—The transfusion of serum appears to be the treatment of choice in correcting the bleeding.

Graham, J. B.; Barrow, E. M.; and Houghie, C.: Stuart clotting defect: II Genetic aspects of a "new" hemorrhagic state, J. Clin. Invest. 36:497, 1957.
Houghie, C.; Barrow, E. M.; and Graham, J. B.: Stuart clotting defect: I. Segregation of an hereditary hemorrhagic state from the heterogeneous group heretofore called "stable factor" (SPCA, proconvertin, factor VII) deficiency J. Clin. Invest. 36:485, 1957.

9. OTHER DEFICIENCIES

The conditions described above probably do not represent all of the known congenital defects in blood coagulation. For example, the existence of two other defects is still questionable. The Swiss have reported the deficiency of an unknown plasma factor which they have called "factor X," but its existence requires confirmation. Also, there probably exists a true congenital deficiency of prothrombin; however, except for the cases reported by Quick, no cases have appeared.

In addition, combined coagulation defects have been reported in the literature. Two examples of AHG and PTC deficiency occurring in the same patient have been suggested by the failure of the patients' plasmas to correct the defect of either type of hemophilia. And instances of combined AHG and Ac-globulin deficiency and of combined PTC and SPCA deficiency have also been found.

It is apparent that in regard to coagulation we should retain an open mind about these inborn errors of metabolism until we have had more success in chemically isolating and identifying the missing factors.

Bell, W. N., and Alton, H. G.: Christmas disease associated with factor VII deficiency, Brit. M. J. 1:330, 1955.

Duckert, F.; Flückiger, P.; Matter, M.; and Koller, F.: Clotting factor X: physiologic and physicochemical properties, Proc. Soc. Exper. Biol. & Med. 90:17, 1955.

Flückiger, P.; Duckert, F.; and Koller, F.: Die Bedeutung des Factor X für die Antikoagulantientherapie, Schweiz. med. Wchnschr. 84:1127, 1954.

Hill, J. M., and Speer, R. J.: Combined hemophilia and PTC deficiency, Blood 10:357, 1955.

Iversen, T., and Bastrup-Madsen, P.: Congenital familial deficiency of factor V (parahemophilia) combined with deficiency of antihemophilic globulin, Brit. J. Haemat. 2:265, 1956.

Quick, A. J.; Pisciotta, A. V.; and Hussey, C. V.: Congenital hypoprothrombinemic states, Arch. Int. Med. 95:2, 1955.

Soulier, J. P., and Larrieu, M. J.: Differentiation of hemophilia into two groups: A study of 33 cases, New England J. Med. 249:547, 1953.

PART III

Disturbances in Molecular Function (Enzyme Defects)

IT WAS Sir Archibald Garrod who first postulated that all hereditary diseases were due to metabolic blocks which occurred because of the absence of specific "enzymes." In looking back, it appears probable that he had only a vague idea as to what the term meant, and certainly he could not have conceived of the complex protein molecules which we call enzymes. In the intervening years, some of the hereditary conditions have, in fact, been shown to be due to enzyme deficiencies. Alkaptonuria and albinism, two of the original diseases described by Garrod, are almost certainly in that group. Others, including cystinuria, do not appear to represent primary enzyme defects at the present time. It would be better, therefore, to regard the deficiency of an enzyme as one of several mechanisms responsible for inborn errors of metabolism in man.

It should be noted that, when we refer to an "enzyme defect," we mean that we can demonstrate the defect only indirectly. None of the enzymes to be described herein have been crystallized, and there are no physical means of showing whether they are absent or present. All we can say is that a specific enzyme, such as the one responsible for the conversion of phenylalanine to tyrosine, does not appear to be working properly. The enzyme could be absent, and hence unable to do its work. It could be present but have a slight structural abnormality, such as having one more or one less of the amino acids, making it incapable of performing its function properly. It might differ from the normal enzyme much in the same way that sickle cell hemoglobin differs from normal hemoglobin. Finally, it is possible that the enzyme could be both present and structurally normal but unable to function in the environment because of alterations in the host or within the cell.

The hereditary diseases which probably are caused by enzyme defects may be divided into five groups: disturbances in amino acid metabolism, disturbances in carbohydrate metabolism, disturbances in endocrine metabolism, disturbances in pigment metabolism, and miscellaneous disturbances.

6

Disturbances in
Amino Acid Metabolism

AROMATIC AMINO ACID DISTURBANCES

During the past few years rapid strides in biochemistry have permitted a proper understanding of the normal pathway for the degradation of phenylalanine and tyrosine in man. This occurs in a series of separate steps, each of which is catalyzed by an enzyme system (Fig. 25):

Phenylalanine is first converted to tyrosine in the presence of the enzyme system "phenylalanine hydroxylase." The absence of this enzyme is responsible for the clinical condition *phenylketonuria*.

Tyrosine is next converted to *p*-hydroxyphenylpyruvic acid in the presence of the enzyme "tyrosine transaminase."

The *p*-hydroxyphenylpyruvate is converted to homogentisic acid in one step in the presence of the enzyme "*p*-hydroxyphenylpyruvic oxidase." An absence of this enzyme is apparently responsible for the condition known as *tyrosinosis*.

Homogentisic acid is then converted to maleylacetoacetate in the presence of the enzyme "homogentisic oxidase." An absence of this enzyme is responsible for the third metabolic defect, known as *alkaptonuria*.

Maleylacetoacetate is then converted, by two additional steps, to acetoacetate and fumarate by enzymes which will be discussed later.

As another pathway of metabolism, tyrosine is also converted to 3,4-dihydroxyphenylalanine (dopa) and eventually to melanin by the action of the enzyme "tyrosinase." The absence of this enzyme is responsible for the hereditary defect *total albinism* and probably is responsible for *partial albinism*.

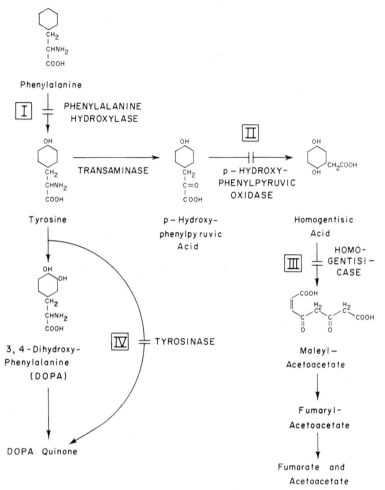

Fig. 25.—The normal pathway for the degradation of phenylalanine and tyrosine in man. The known metabolic defects are I, phenylketonuria; II, tyrosinosis; III, alkaptonuria; and IV, albinism.

1. PHENYLKETONURIA (phenylpyruvic oligophrenia)

Phenylketonuria is a hereditary condition characterized by mental retardation and the presence of phenylpyruvic acid in the urine. Nearly 400 cases have been reported from all parts of the world since the first cases were described by Folling, a Norwegian biochemist, in 1934.

CLINICAL FEATURES.—Though patients seem to be ordinary imbeciles, they are noted for their unusually attractive features in early childhood. Unlike other mental defectives, they show only a slight reduction in stature and head size, as compared with the normal average of same age and sex. Many of the children have blond hair, blue eyes, and fair skin. A few show a tendency toward developing dermatitis or eczema.

Neurologically, phenylketonurics show no paralysis and no changes in muscle tone. However, there is usually a marked accentuation of both the superficial and deep tendon reflexes. The majority of patients have an I.Q. of 30 or less. However, a few high-grade cases with near normal intelligence have been described recently; it is believed that these atypical cases represent less than 1% of all cases of phenylketonuria.

HEREDITY.—It is estimated that phenylketonuria accounts for about 1% of all mental defectives in institutions. The condition arises once in every 40,000 births in the United States and is transmitted by a rare recessive gene. In any given family with one affected child, the chances of another case occurring in a subsequent pregnancy is 1 in 4, or 25%. The heterozygous carriers of the phenylketonuric gene can be identified by means of phenylalanine tolerance tests.

PATHOGENESIS.—Phenylalanine is converted to tyrosine by the enzyme system "phenylalanine hydroxylase." Mitoma and his co-workers have shown that two protein fractions are involved in this reaction: a labile fraction I, which is present only in the liver; and a more stable fraction II, found also in the kidney and heart. The system requires DPNH and Fe^{++}, and the over-all reaction appears to occur in one step, with no intermediates. Recent studies have shown that in phenylketonurics, fraction II is present in the tissues in normal amounts and that the disease occurs because of a deficiency of fraction I in this enzyme system.

The deficiency of phenylalanine hydroxylase causes an excessive accumulation of l-phenylalanine in the blood and spinal fluid. This in turn causes three kinds of effects (Chart 18). (1) The excessive phenylalanine is converted, by its transaminase, to phenylpyruvic acid. This in turn is converted to phenyllactic acid, phenylacetic acid, and phenylacetylglutamine and excreted in the urine. For reasons which are still obscure, o-hydroxyphenylacetic acid, m-hydroxyphenylacetic acid, and indole products derived from tyrosine and tryptophane are also found in the urine of such patients. (2) The excessive phenylalanine also inhibits the normal pathways of tyrosine metabolism. There is a decreased production of melanin, and this is responsible for the light pigment in the skin and hair of such patients. There is also a disturbance in adrenalin production, since phenylketonurics have unusually low blood adrenalin levels. (3) The excessive phenylalanine or one of its products probably causes some, as yet unexplained, damage to the central nervous system; this is

CHART 18

PHENYLKETONURIA

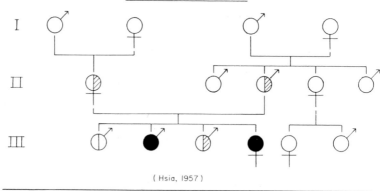

(Hsia, 1957)

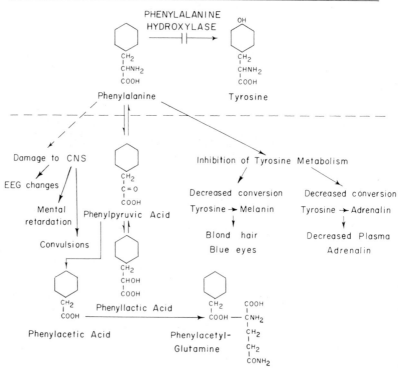

characterized by mental retardation, epileptic seizures, and abnormal electroencephalogram changes.

DIAGNOSIS.—A diagnosis of phenylketonuria can be established by (1) the presence of phenylpyruvic acid in the urine (see Procedure 26) and (2) an increase of *l*-phenylalanine level in the plasma (see Procedure 27).

TREATMENT.—Young infants should be treated by a special diet low in phenylalanine content. This consists of (1) low phenylalanine protein

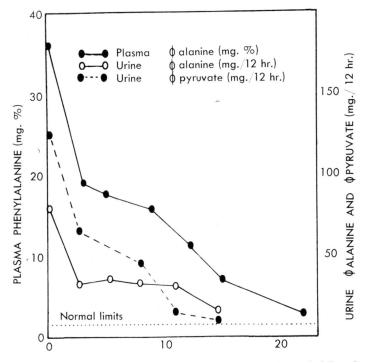

FIG. 26.—Reduction of plasma phenylalanine levels after administration of low-phenylalanine diet in patient with phenylketonuria. The reduction in urine phenylpyruvate and urine phenylalanine excretion also parallels that of the plasma phenylalanine. (From Hsia, D. Y. Y.: Recent developments in the study of hereditary diseases in children, Postgrad. Med. 22:203, 1957.)

hydrolysate manufactured by Mead Johnson and Merck & Company, Inc., (2) 1% protein fruits and vegetables, (3) gluten-free bread, (4) sugar, (5) butter or lipomal, and (6) vitamins and minerals. This diet is effective in reducing plasma phenylalanine levels down to the normal range (Fig. 26). At present, it is felt that this diet is effective in bringing about normal development if started shortly after birth; it has less value in older infants, and appears to have no effect upon phenylketonuric children after the age of 6 years.

Armstrong, M. D., and Robinson, K. S.: On the excretion of indole derivatives in phenylketonuria, Arch. Biochem. 52:287, 1954.

Bickel, H.; Gerrard, J.; and Hickmans, E. M.: Influence of phenylalanine intake on phenylketonuria, Lancet 2:812, 1953.

Dancis, J., and Balis, M. E.: A possible mechanism for disturbance in tyrosine metabolism in phenylpyruvic oligophrenia, Pediatrics 15:63, 1955.

Hsia, D. Y. Y.: Recent developments in the study of hereditary diseases in children, Postgrad. Med. 22:203, 1957.

———; Driscoll, K. W.; Troll, W.; and Knox, W. E.: Detection of the heterozygous carrier for phenylketonuria by phenylalanine tolerance tests, Nature 178:1239, 1956.

———; Knox, W. E.; and Paine, R. S.: A case of phenylketonuria with borderline intelligence, A.M.A. J. Dis. Child. 1957.

——— et al.: A one year controlled study on the effect of a low-phenylalanine diet on phenylketonuria, Pediatrics 21:178, 1958.

*Jervis, G. A.: Phenylpyruvic oligophrenia, Nerv. & Ment. Dis. 33:259, 1954.

*Knox, W. E., and Hsia, D. Y. Y.: Pathogenetic problems in phenylketonuria, Am. J. Med. 22:687, 1957.

Mitoma, C.; Auld, R. M.; and Udenfriend, S.: On the nature of enzymatic defect in phenylpyruvic oligophrenia, Proc. Soc. Exper. Biol. & Med. 94:634, 1957.

2. TYROSINOSIS

In 1932, Medes described the first authentic case of tyrosinosis. In this patient there was a continuous excretion of large quantities of p-hydroxyphenylpyruvic acid but no other clinical symptoms. Recently, Felix and his co-workers have made similar observations on two patients with liver disease. It would appear that tyrosinosis should be included among the conditions defined as inborn errors of metabolism.

HEREDITY.—The mode of transmission of tyrosinosis is completely unknown. The condition certainly appears to occur very rarely. Blatherwick has examined the urine of 26,000 persons and could not find a single individual showing a positive reaction to the Millon test.

PATHOGENESIS.—Tyrosinosis appears to occur as the result of a metabolic block at the conversion of p-hydroxyphenylpyruvic acid to homogentisic acid, as shown in Chart 19. This reaction is catalyzed by the liver enzyme, p-hydroxyphenylpyruvic acid oxidase and requires glutathione and either ascorbic acid or dichlorophenolendophenol as cofactors.

If the protein intake is increased, or if tyrosine itself is fed to these patients, the amount of p-hydroxyphenylpyruvate in the urine is increased. The following substances will also appear in the urine, in this order: tyrosine, p-hydroxyphenyllactic acid, and 3,4-dihydroxyphenyl-

CHART 19

TYROSINOSIS

UNKNOWN

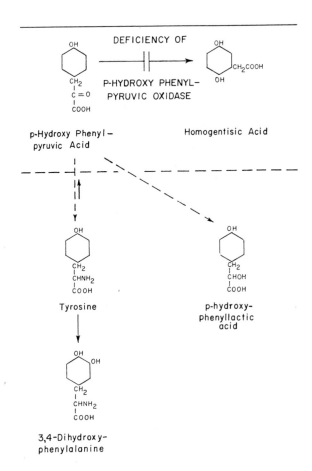

DEFICIENCY OF

P-HYDROXY PHENYL-
PYRUVIC OXIDASE

p-Hydroxy Phenyl-
pyruvic Acid

Homogentisic Acid

Tyrosine

p-hydroxy-
phenyllactic
acid

3,4-Dihydroxy-
phenylalanine

alanine. On the other hand, if homogentisic acid is fed to the patient, p-hydroxyphenylpyruvate does not appear in the urine, and it exerts no influence upon the excretion of any of the other compounds.

DIAGNOSIS.—The presence of p-hydroxyphenylpyruvic acid in the urine (see Procedure 28) is suggested by a positive reaction to the Millon test but needs to be confirmed by its conversion to the enol form.

TREATMENT.—None is required.

Blatherwick, N. R.: Tyrosinosis: A search for additional cases, J.A.M.A. 103: 1933, 1934.

Edwards, S.; Hsia, D. Y. Y.; and Knox, W. E.: The first oxidative enzyme of tyrosine metabolism, p-hydroxyphenylpyruvate oxidase, Fed. Proc. 14:206, 1955.

Felix, L.; Leonhardi, G.; and Glaseivapp, I.: Über Tyrosinosis, Ztschr. physiol. Chem. 287:141, 1951.

Medes, G.: A new error of tyrosine metabolism: Tyrosinosis, Biochem. J. 26:917, 1932.

3. ALKAPTONURIA

Alkaptonuria is an inborn error of aromatic amino acid metabolism characterized by the excretion of homogentisic acid in the urine.

CLINICAL FEATURES.—The condition is compatible with long life. Except for the discoloration of the urine, there are no clinical manifestations until the second or third decade, when ochronosis begins to appear. This consists of deposits of ocher-like pigments in various parts of the body. The deposits are particularly prominent in the scleras on either side of the corneal limbus, in the ear and nasal cartilages, and in the superficial tendons of the hand.

By the time alkaptonurics reach middle age, they generally complain of pain and stiffness in the large joints, owing to a deforming arthritis. The spine becomes rigid; there is kyphosis in the dorsal region; and motion of the hip, knee, or shoulder joints becomes limited and painful. On x-ray examination, the presence of thin, densely calcified intervertebral disks is characteristic.

HEREDITY.—Alkaptonuria can be transmitted by two means. In the majority of cases, the condition is transmitted by a single recessive gene; in such families, the expectation will be that 1 out of 4 children will be affected. So far, no method has been worked out for detecting the heterozygotes for this condition, but the occurrence of a very high incidence of parental consanguinity makes such a conclusion almost certain.

In a few families the condition appears to be transmitted as a simple dominant. In these pedigrees, individuals in a series of successive generations are affected, and there are no indications of any cousin marriages.

CHART 20

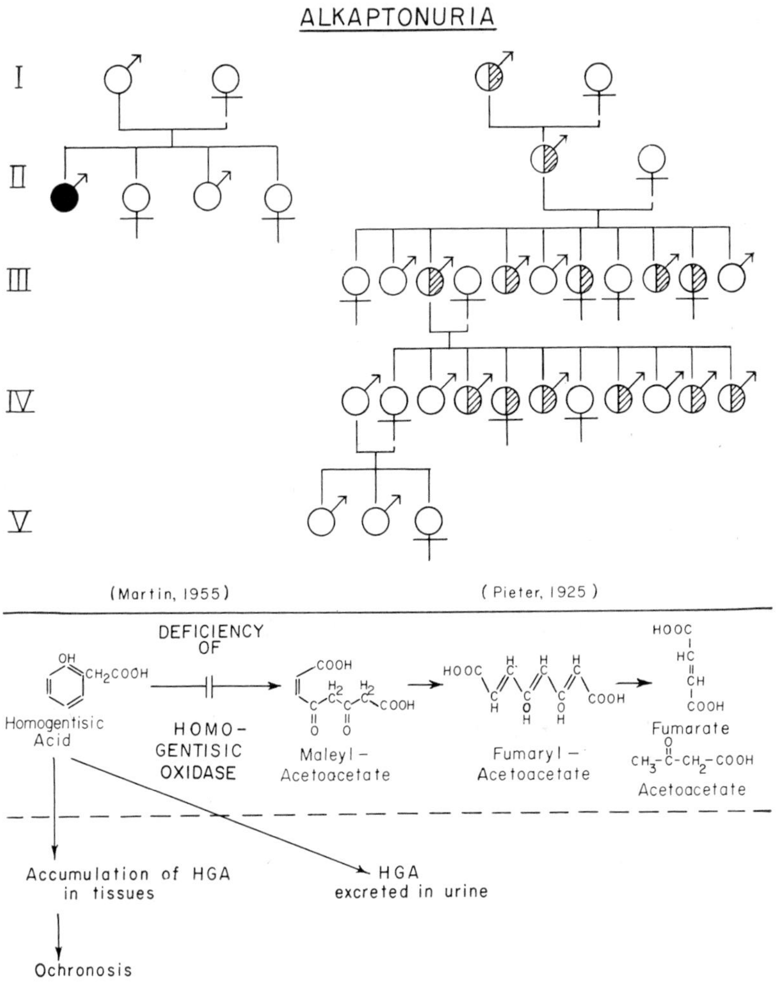

ALKAPTONURIA

(Martin, 1955)   (Pieter, 1925)

Homogentisic Acid — DEFICIENCY OF HOMOGENTISIC OXIDASE → Maleyl-Acetoacetate → Fumaryl-Acetoacetate → Fumarate, Acetoacetate

Accumulation of HGA in tissues

HGA excreted in urine

Ochronosis

Here the affected individuals must be regarded as heterozygous for al-kaptonuria, since it is highly unlikely that their mates in each generation were all heterozygous for alkaptonuria.

It would appear that there are two separate types of alkaptonuria, which are not related to each other. At the present time, it is not known whether the two types are alleles or are at different loci on the chromosomes.

PATHOGENESIS.—Since the feeding of homogentisic acid to alkapto-

CHART 21

TOTAL ALBINISM

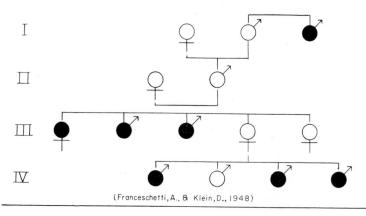

(Franceschetti, A., & Klein, D., 1948)

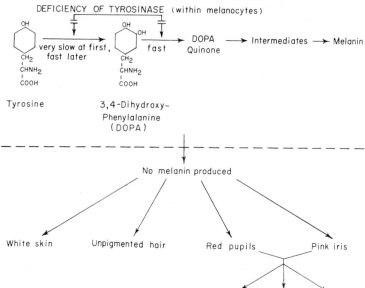

118

normal numbers in such patients but that the enzyme is not present within the cells and hence melanin is not produced.

The action of tyrosinase is shown in Chart 21. Tyrosinase is oxidized to 3,4-dihydroxyphenylalanine (dopa) in the presence of molecular oxygen and tyrosinase. Dopa is then further changed to dopa quinone in the presence of tyrosinase. Ultimately, dopa quinone is converted to melanin without tyrosinase. However, it should be noted that in the absence of dopa, tyrosinase cannot act on tyrosine. Even when dopa is present, there is a lag period in the action of the first step. No such lag is noted in the second step of the reaction.

These findings seem to support the concept that total albinism arises as a result of the absence of a single enzyme and a block in the normal pathway of metabolism; and, therefore, albinism can be included among the conditions known as the inborn errors of metabolism.

DIAGNOSIS.—The diagnosis can usually be made on clinical grounds alone.

TREATMENT.—Prevention of exposure to sunlight and proper protection of the eyes by dark glasses.

Fitzpatrick, T. B.: Human melanogenesis: The tyrosinase reaction in pigment cell neoplasma, with particular reference to malignant melanoma: Preliminary report, A.M.A. Arch. Dermat. 65:379, 1952.

———— and Lerner, A. B.: Pigment and pigment tumors: Biochemical basis of human melanin pigmentation, A.M.A. Arch. Dermat. 69:133, 1954.

Franceschetti, A., and Klein, D.: Rétinite dominante avec surdité, Confinia neurol. 8:339, 1948.

*Lerner, A. B., and Fitzpatrick, T. B.: Biochemistry of melanin formation, Physiol. Rev. 30:91, 1950.

5. PARTIAL ALBINISM

Partial albinism is characterized by a congenital absence of pigment in specific parts of the body. The areas affected are of irregular distribution but sometimes follow the course of cutaneous nerves. There are many varieties of partial albinism, each of which probably arose from a different mutation.

CLINICAL FEATURES AND HEREDITY.—At least three well-defined types have been described: piebald albinism; white forelock and spotting of the skin; and albinism of the eye alone.

1. *Piebald albinism.*—This form was first described in 1934 by Keeler, who interpreted it as a dominant mutation. It was found in 25 out of 85 individuals in four generations of one family. Members of this family have exhibited themselves in sideshows since the nineteenth cen-

tury. The condition appears to be transmitted as a dominant; no normal individuals within the family have ever transmitted the condition to their offspring, while the affected ones have transmitted it to about half of their children.

2. *White forelock and spotting of the skin.*—In the majority of instances, the affected persons in these families have the white forelock and also moderately well-distributed white spotting of the skin. The condition is again believed to be transmitted as a simple dominant, since in a recent study it was found that more than half of some 769 children born of parents with this trait also inherited it, while only 15 out of 474 born of unaffected normal parents in these same families inherited the trait.

3. *Albinism of the eye alone.*—This form is characterized by albinism in the fundus, hypoplasia of the macula, head nodding, nystagmus, and amblyopia. Unlike the other types of partial albinism, this condition is transmitted as a sex-linked recessive, where only male offspring of mothers who are carriers are affected. The heterozygous carriers of the abnormal gene show a permeability of the iris to light on transillumination of the scleras, and macular retinal pigmentation which is stippled, cocoa brown in color, and very sparse.

PATHOGENESIS.—The pathogenesis is not known.

DIAGNOSIS.—This can usually be established on clinical grounds.

TREATMENT.—None is required except for proper protection of the eyes.

Cooke, J. V.: Familial white skin spotting with white forelock, J. Pediat. 41:1, 1952.
Falls, H. F.: Sex-linked ocular albinism displaying typical fundus changes in the female heterozygote, Am. J. Ophth. 34:41, 1951.

OTHER AMINO ACID DISTURBANCES

6. MAPLE SUGAR URINE DISEASE (progressive familial cerebral dysfunction associated with an unusual urinary substance)

In 1954, Menkes, Hurst, and Craig described a new syndrome characterized by cerebral symptoms and the passage of urine with an odor strikingly similar to that of maple sugar. This has recently been shown to represent a defect in the branched chain amino acids.

CLINICAL FEATURES.—All of the affected infants begin to show clinical symptoms between the third and fifth days of life. There is difficulty in feeding, an absence of the Moro reflex, and the development of irregular, jerky respirations. This is followed by signs of spasticity and opisthotonos, and the infants go rapidly downhill and die within a few

CHART 22

MAPLE SUGAR URINE DISEASE

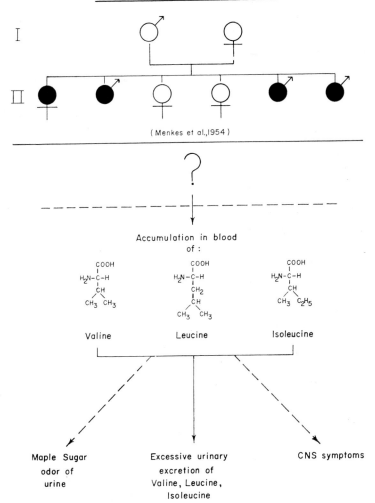

(Menkes et al.,1954)

Accumulation in blood
of :

| Valine | Leucine | Isoleucine |

Maple Sugar
odor of
urine

Excessive urinary
excretion of
Valine, Leucine,
Isoleucine

CNS symptoms

121

weeks or months. Surprisingly, convulsions and paralyses are not usually noted in this disease.

In all instances, the odor of the urine resembles that of maple sugar. This seems to become more striking as the disease progresses. At post-mortem, none of the findings are specific or unusual; rather, they are consistent with those of very acute diseases or with those occurring during the agonal period of any systemic condition.

HEREDITY.—The mode of transmission of maple sugar urine disease is yet to be worked out. Out of the six children in the original family studied by Menkes and his co-workers, four had a maple sugar odor in the urine, developed cerebral signs, and died. There were three boys and one girl in the affected group. The two remaining siblings and their parents did not have maple sugar odor in the urine and were perfectly healthy.

PATHOGENESIS.—Westall and his associates have studied the urine and blood of a patient with this condition. Using a Dowex 50 column, for separation, they showed that the three branched chain amino acids—valine, leucine, and isoleucine—were greatly increased in both the blood and urine. On the other hand, threonine, serine, and alanine showed exceptionally low figures. A single enzymatic defect involving the branched chain amino acids could explain these changes.

At present, the material in the urine giving rise to the maple sugar odor has not been identified. Similarly, the relationship between the central nervous system symptoms and the amino acid abnormalities has not been clarified (Chart 22).

DIAGNOSIS.—The diagnosis can be established by the typical neurological signs and by demonstrating excessive amounts of the branched chain amino acids in the blood and urine by means of paper chromatography (see Procedure 30).

TREATMENT.—None is of any avail.

Menkes, J. H.; Hurst, P. L.; and Craig, J. M.: A new syndrome: Progressive familial infantile cerebral dysfunction associated with an unusual urinary substance, Pediatrics 14:462, 1954.
Westall, R. G.; Dancis, J.; and Miller, S.: Maple sugar urine disease—a new molecular disease, A.M.A. J. Dis. Child. 94:571, 1957.

7. H DISEASE (hereditary pellagra-like skin rash with temporary cerebellar ataxia, constant renal aminoaciduria, and other bizarre biochemical features)

In 1956, Baron, Dent, Harris, Hart and Jepson described a new clinical syndrome characterized by a pellagra-like skin rash, neurological changes resembling cerebellar ataxia, a constant aminoaciduria, and other biochemical changes suggesting a disturbance of nicotinic acid utilization. They named the condition "H disease," after the surname of the affected family.

CLINICAL FEATURES.—The first patient who was studied showed skin changes similar to those in pellagra. There was a rash over the exposed surfaces of the face, neck, hands, and legs. After being exposed to the sun, the skin became very red, raw, and started to ooze. Neurologically, the patient presented a varied picture. At times he had only a mild ataxia. On other occasions he showed a coarse nystagmus, ptosis, an increase of deep reflexes, and poor performance of fine movements. There was a tremor of the outstretched hands, and his hands and tongue showed spontaneous involuntary movements. With the passage of time, he became more irritable and hard to handle. Psychological tests indicated that he was mentally retarded, and there was some suggestion of increased mental deterioration.

The most consistent laboratory finding was a gross generalized aminoaciduria. Except for proline, all of the amino acids in the urine were increased. The aminoaciduria was renal in origin, since the plasma α-aminonitrogen was within normal limits.

There was also an increase in the urinary excretion of indole compounds. In addition to an increase in indican, there was an excess of tryptophane, indole-acetic acid, and an unidentified indolic material, U.I. However, tryptamine, serotonin, 5-hydroxyindole-acetic acid, and indole-lactic acid were not detectable.

The patients in the H family have been followed over a period of years. The skin changes persist and are accentuated by sunlight. The neurological signs come and go, but they tend to get worse when the rash is marked and also following infections without rash. The youngest sibling shows only aminoaciduria, without skin rash or neurological signs. It is not clear whether these symptoms will develop as he grows older.

HEREDITY.—Among the eight children in this family, three males and one female are affected. Also, the parents are first cousins. This suggests that the condition is transmitted as an autosomal recessive. The heterozygous carriers for H disease have not, so far, been detected either clinically or in the laboratory.

Although only one family has so far appeared in the literature, several other families with what appears to be the same condition are known to exist.

PATHOGENESIS.—Baron and his co-workers have suggested that H

disease represents a disorder of tryptophane metabolism whereby a metabolic block exists somewhere along the pathway from tryptophane to
nicotinic acid. If one also postulates that some enzyme systems in the
body require nicotinic acid or nicotinamide as prosthetic groups and that

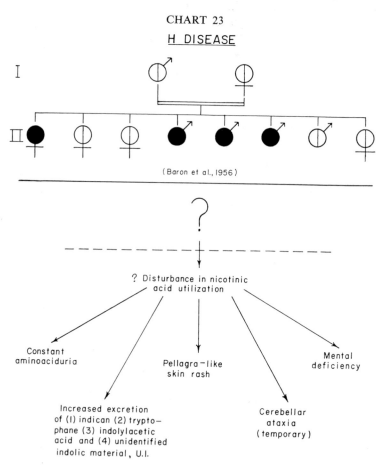

CHART 23

H DISEASE

(Baron et al., 1956)

? Disturbance in nicotinic
acid utilization

Constant
aminoaciduria

Pellagra–like
skin rash

Mental
deficiency

Increased excretion
of (I) indican (2) trypto–
phane (3) indolylacetic
acid and (4) unidentified
indolic material, U.I.

Cerebellar
ataxia
(temporary)

they can only get these from tryptophane, this could explain the pellagra-
like lesions and disturbances in indole metabolism (Chart 23).

The aminoaciduria, cerebellar ataxia, and mental deficiency would
be more difficult to interpret. The only possible explanation for these is
that the former is a consequence, on the level of cellular metabolism, of
an apparent nicotinamide deficiency and that the latter may in some way

be similar to the disturbances in indole metabolism in phenylketonuria, which is another cause for mental deficiency.

DIAGNOSIS.—A gross aminoaciduria (see Procedure 30) plus the characteristic skin and nervous system changes would strongly suggest this condition.

TREATMENT.—Nicotinamide has been used as a form of therapy, but there is considerable skepticism as to whether it is really of any value.

Baron, D. N.; Dent, C. E.; Harris, H.; Hart, E. W.; and Jepson, J. B.: Hereditary pellagra-like skin rash with temporary cerebellar ataxia, constant renal amino-aciduria, and other bizarre biochemical features, Lancet 2:421, 1956.

7

Disturbances in Carbohydrate Metabolism

UP TO THE PRESENT, the disturbances in carbohydrate metabolism have been divided into four groups: (1) an inborn error of metabolism involving a five-carbon sugar, which results in the clinical condition *pentosuria, or l-xyloketosuria;* (2) inborn errors of metabolism involving two six-carbon sugars, which result in the clinical conditions *fructosuria* and *galactosemia;* (3) disturbances in glycogen metabolism, which result in four clinical conditions: Type I, *glycogen storage disease of the liver and kidneys* (von Gierke's disease); Type II, *glycogen storage disease of the heart;* Type III, *diffuse glycogenosis with hepatic cirrhosis;* Types IVa and IVb, *glycogen storage of liver and muscle;* and (4) disturbances in the glycolysis of red cells which appear to be responsible for *hereditary spherocytosis* and *hereditary nonspherocytic hemolytic anemia.* These disturbances will now be described.

METABOLIC DISTURBANCE INVOLVING A FIVE-CARBON SUGAR

I. PENTOSURIA (*l*-xyloketosuria)

The presence of pentose in the urine was first described by Salkowski and Jastrowitz in 1892. The condition is of historic interest because it is one of the four inborn errors of metabolism described by Garrod in the Croonian Lectures of 1908.

CLINICAL FEATURES.—The condition appears to be harmless to health and well-being. Patients excreting this substance show no symptoms, the diagnosis usually being made by examiners for life insurance

CHART 24

L-XYLOKETOSURIA

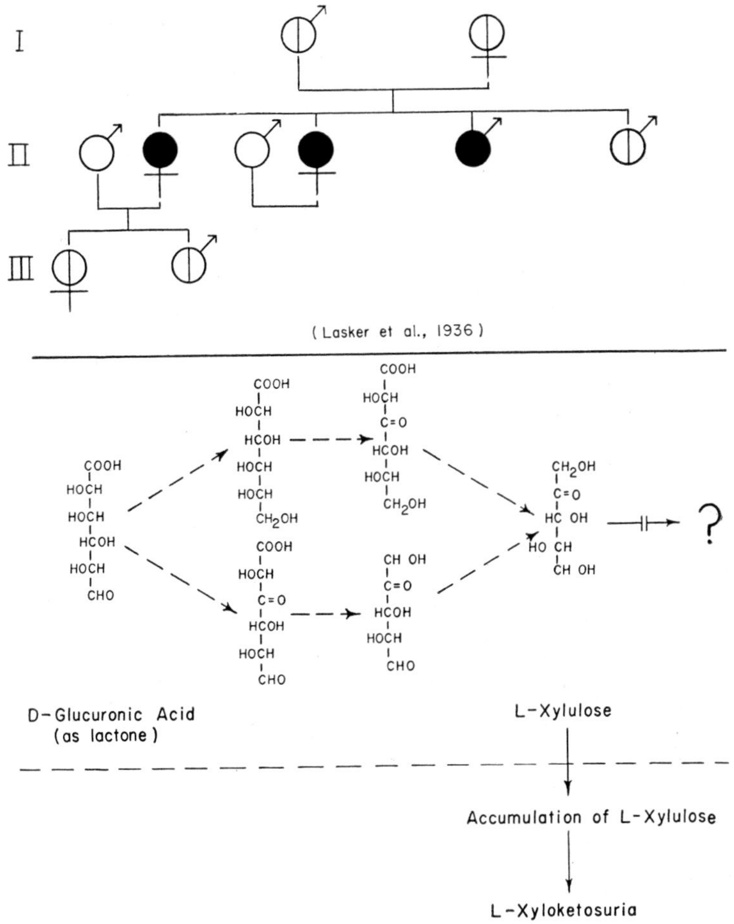

(Lasker et al., 1936)

D-Glucuronic Acid
(as lactone)

L-Xylulose

Accumulation of L-Xylulose

L-Xyloketosuria

companies. It should be remembered, however, that pentosuria can occur in normal people after they have eaten large amounts of fruits and berries, and it is also sometimes seen in patients with muscular dystrophy.

HEREDITY.—The incidence of essential pentosuria is estimated to be 1 in 50,000; the condition is found almost exclusively in people of Jewish ancestry from a certain part of Russia, but recently a few cases have been reported among non-Hebrews. Lasker and her co-workers believe that pentosuria is transmitted by a recessive gene. The condition has been found more often in males than females, but this may merely reflect the fact that more males than females apply for life insurance. The heterozygotes for this condition have not been identified.

PATHOGENESIS.—Touster and his associates have suggested that glucuronic acid is metabolized by a series of steps, as shown in Chart 24: (1) Glucuronic acid is first converted to *l*-xylulose by one or more intermediate steps which are as yet poorly defined. There is good evidence that *l*-xylulose is the end-product of this series of reactions, since it has been isolated in the urine of normal subjects and guinea pigs fed glucuoronolactone. (2) Then *l*-xylulose is degraded to *l*-xylitol by an enzyme present in the mitochondrial fraction of guinea pig liver homogenate. This enzyme requires MgCl, *l*-glutamate, and atmospheric oxygen. The reaction occurs without the accumulation of any known intermediates or xylulose phosphate; and the product, *l*-xylitol, has been identified by its pentose acetate.

In 1936, Enklewitz and Lasker showed that there is a direct relationship between the amount of glucuronic acid administered and the extra amount of xylulose excreted. Since feeding glucuronic acid to normal individuals does not produce this effect, they postulated that there was a defect in the system that decarboxylates glucuronic acid to xylulose. Now that *l*-xylulose has been identified as an intermediate in the normal pathway of glucuronic acid metabolism, it is believed the defect must occur at the stage immediately following *l*-xylulose. Pentosuria must, therefore, represent a deficiency of the enzyme described by Touster; however, this remains to be demonstrated in a patient with known pentosuria.

DIAGNOSIS.—The diagnosis of pentosuria is established by identifying *l*-xylulose in the urine (see Procedure 31). Up until the present, no authentic case of *l*-arabinosuria, the isomer of *l*-xylulose, has been reported.

TREATMENT.—None is required.

Barnes, H. D., and Bloomberg, B. M.: Paper chromatography of the urinary sugar in essential pentosuria, South African J. M. Sc. 18:93, 1953.

Enklewitz, M., and Lasker, M.: The origin of *l*-xyloketosuria, J. Biol. Chem. 110:443, 1935.

Lasker, M.; Enklewitz, M.; and Lasker, G. W.: The inheritance of *l*-xyloketosuria, Human Biol. 8:243, 1936.

Touster, O.; Hutcheson, R. M.; and Rice, L.: The influence of *d*-glucuoronolactone and the excretion of *l*-xylulose by humans and guinea pigs, J. Biol. Chem. 215:677, 1955.

———; Reynolds, V. H.; Hutcheson, R. M.; and Hollmann, S.: Reduction of *l*-xylulose to xylitol by an enzyme of guinea pig liver mitochondria, Fed. Proc. 15:372, 1956.

METABOLIC DISTURBANCE INVOLVING SIX-CARBON SUGARS

2. FRUCTOSURIA

Essential fructosuria is an extremely rare error of metabolism characterized by a congenital inability to utilize fructose completely. The first cases were probably described by Zumier and Czapek in 1876.

CLINICAL FEATURES.—Individuals who excrete fructose in their urine show no clinical symptoms, and the condition is completely harmless. It is only important as a differential for diabetes mellitus, and most cases are discovered by life insurance examiners.

HEREDITY.—Fructosuria is transmitted by an autosomal recessive gene. The condition usually occurs among siblings and is not found in parents or other relatives. The heterozygous carrier for the abnormality has not yet been detected. Lasker has estimated that fructosuria occurs only once in every 120,000 births.

PATHOGENESIS.—The exact pathogenesis of fructosuria is not known at the present time. Hers has recently outlined the major metabolic pathway for fructose in the liver, as shown in Figure 28: (1) Fructose is converted to fructose-1-PO_4 by the action of ATP in the presence of the enzyme "fructokinase." (2) Fructose-1-PO_4 cleaves to form two three-carbon fragments—glyceraldehyde phosphate and dihydroxyacetone phosphate—in the presence of the enzyme "aldolase." (3) Glyceraldehyde is phosphorylated by ATP in the presence of the enzyme "triokinase." (4) Glyceraldehyde phosphate and dihydroxyacetone phosphate are also interconvertible in the presence of the enzyme "triosephosphate isomerase." (5) The glyceraldehyde phosphate is subsequently converted to 1,3-diphosphoglyceric acid by the enzyme "phosphoglyceraldehyde dehydrogenase" and is subsequently converted to pyruvic and lactic acid in the usual way. (6) The two isomeric triose phosphates, dihydroxyacetone phosphate and glyceraldehyde phosphate, can be reconverted to fructose-1,6-diphosphate in the presence of aldolase. (7) Fructose-1,6-diphosphate is converted to fructose-6-PO_4 and ATP in the presence of the enzyme "hexose diphosphatase." (8) Finally, fructose-6-PO_4 is converted to glucose-6-PO_4 by the enzyme "phosphohexose isomerase."

In addition to the above pathway, fructose is undoubtedly utilized in two other ways: (*a*) in the brain and muscle, fructose is converted directly to fructose-6-PO_4 in the presence of hexokinase and ATP, and (*b*) fructose-1-PO_4 can also be phosphorylated in position 6 to fructose-1,6-diphosphate.

In the normal individual, when fructose is ingested there is a rapid

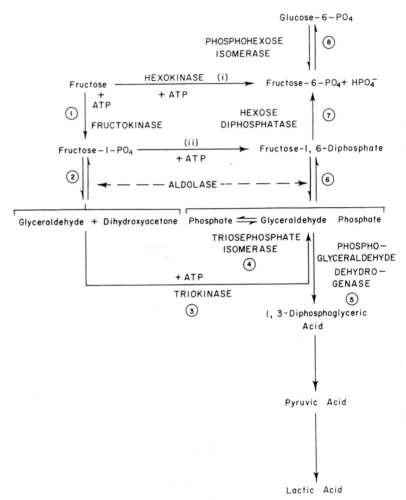

FIG. 28.—Postulated metabolic pathway for fructose.

rise of the respiratory quotient and an elevation of lactic acid in the blood. Patients with fructosuria do not show this characteristic response (Chart 25), which would suggest that the metabolic defect in the liver in fructosuria must occur in the first three steps of fructose metabolism, since a block beyond glyceraldehyde phosphate would not result in a disturbance of lactic acid metabolism.

Recently, Froesch and his associates have reported on a family of fructosurics presenting an, as yet unknown, inborn error of fructose metabolism, distinguished from the so-called "essential fructosuria" by the occurrence of severe symptoms upon ingestion of fructose. The mode of inheritance of this disorder seems to be of the autosomal recessive type. The administration of fructose leads to an excessive and prolonged rise of

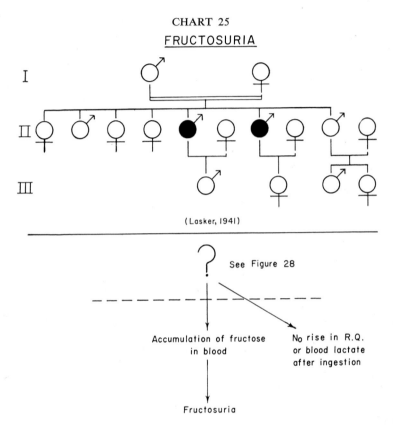

CHART 25

FRUCTOSURIA

(Lasker, 1941)

? See Figure 28

Accumulation of fructose in blood

No rise in R.Q. or blood lactate after ingestion

Fructosuria

the fructose concentration in the blood; 10% of the ingested fructose is excreted in the urine, and, simultaneously with the rise in blood fructose, the blood glucose falls to levels as low as 10 mg/100 ml. This severe hypoglycemia lasts for several hours and is accompanied by nausea, hemorrhagic vomiting, trembling, profuse sweating, and somnolence. After cessation of the acute symptoms a slight and transient icterus, albuminuria, and aminoaciduria are observed. An allergy toward fructose can be excluded as a cause of this disorder, which seems likely to be due to a congenital lack of an enzyme responsible for one of the steps of fructose metabolism by the fructose-1-PO_4-triose pathway. The red cells of these patients respire normally with fructose as a substrate, meaning that the hexokinase system functions normally. Instead, it is believed that the accumulation of fructose-1-PO_4 leads to a block of gluconeogenesis by inhibiting the aldolase which splits fructose-1,6-phosphate.

DIAGNOSIS.—Fructosuria can be diagnosed by the presence of fructose in the urine (see Procedure 32) and a delayed fructose tolerance test (see Procedure 33).

TREATMENT.—None is required.

Froesch, E. R.; Prader, A.; Labhart, A.; Stuber, H. W.; and Wolf, H. P.: Die hereditäre Fructose-Intoleranz, eine bisher nicht bekannte kongenitale Stoffwechselstörung, Schweiz. Med. (in press).

Hers, H. G.: The conversion of fructose-1-C^{14} and sorbitol-1-C^{14} to liver and muscle glycogen in the rat, J. Biol. Chem. 214:373, 1955.

Lasker, M.: Essential fructosuria, Human Biol. 13:51, 1941.

Renold, A. E., and Thorn, G. W.: Editorial: Clinical usefulness of fructose, Am. J. Med. 19:163, 1955.

3. GALACTOSEMIA

Galactosemia is a hereditary condition characterized by an inability to convert galactose to glucose in a normal manner. The disease was first described by von Reuss, a German physician, in 1908.

CLINICAL FEATURES.—Infants with this condition appear to be normal at birth; but after a few days of milk feeding, they begin to vomit, become lethargic, fail to gain weight, and show enlargement of the liver. Prolonged jaundice during the neonatal period is a common finding. Ascites and edema may develop (Fig. 29); and in severe cases death occurs, owing to malnutrition and wasting. Those who survive are usually malnourished and dwarfed at 2 or 3 months of age, and mental retardation and cataracts may be discerned. Others may develop cirrhosis of the liver months or years after the acute phase of the disease. In all instances, the signs and symptoms regress after the deletion of milk and milk products from the diet. Laboratory studies reveal the constant presence of a reducing substance in the urine which is not glucose. An excessive excretion of amino acids in the urine is also a common finding.

HEREDITY.—Galactosemia is transmitted as an autosomal recessive. The defect has been noted among siblings in about half of the families reported, and it would be expected to occur in 1 out of 4 births in such families in a normal distribution. The heterozygous carrier of the abnormal gene can be detected by means of galactose tolerance tests. Recently, we have also found a decrease of P-gal-uridyl-transferase among parents of such children.

The incidence of the condition in the population is not known. Galactosemia is probably quite rare; only about 75 cases have been reported from all over the world.

PATHOGENESIS.—LeLoir and his co-workers have shown that galactose is converted to glucose in a series of four separate steps, as shown in Figure 30A. Each step is catalyzed by a specific enzyme (in capital letters in the chart).

The site of the metabolic defect in galactosemia was found by two ingenious experiments. In 1955, Schwarz and his associates in Manches-

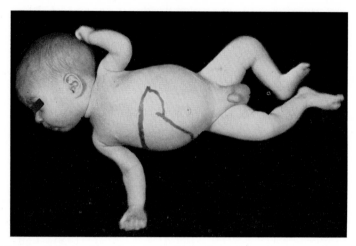

FIG. 29.—Infant with galactosemia. Note the massive hepatomegaly and abdominal distention.

ter, England, showed that when milk was given to a galactosemic child there was an abnormal accumulation of galactose-1-PO_4 in the red cells, while this metabolite was not found in normal children. This meant that the block must have occurred somewhere beyond galactose-1-PO_4 and that galactokinase, the enzyme needed for the first reaction, was present in adequate amounts. In 1956, Isselbacher and his co-workers in the United States demonstrated that uridine diphosphogalactose-4-epimerase and uridine diphosphoglucose pyrophosphorylase, the enzymes needed for the third and fourth steps, were present in normal amounts in the erythrocytes of galactosemic children. However, P-gal-uridyl-transferase, the enzyme needed for the second step, was barely detectable in 10 such children. They therefore concluded that galactosemia occurs as a result of an enzyme deficiency which causes a metabolic block in step 2 and that all other pathways of metabolism in such patients are normal and intact.

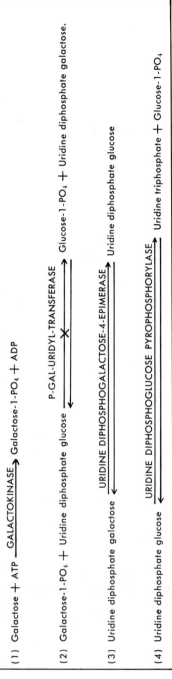

(1) Galactose + ATP $\xrightarrow{\text{GALACTOKINASE}}$ Galactose-1-PO$_4$ + ADP

(2) Galactose-1-PO$_4$ + Uridine diphosphate glucose $\underset{\times}{\overset{\text{P-GAL-URIDYL-TRANSFERASE}}{\rightleftharpoons}}$ Glucose-1-PO$_4$ + Uridine diphosphate galactose.

(3) Uridine diphosphate galactose $\underset{\text{URIDINE DIPHOSPHOGALACTOSE-4-EPIMERASE}}{\longrightarrow}$ Uridine diphosphate glucose

(4) Uridine diphosphate glucose $\underset{\text{URIDINE DIPHOSPHOGLUCOSE PYROPHOSPHORYLASE}}{\longrightarrow}$ Uridine triphosphate + Glucose-1-PO$_4$

Fig. 30A.—Normal pathway of galactose metabolism in erythrocytes. The enzymes for each step are denoted by capital letters. The metabolic block in galactosemia is marked by an $\times$.

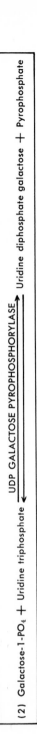

(2) Galactose-1-PO$_4$ + Uridine triphosphate $\underset{\text{UDP GALACTOSE PYROPHOSPHORYLASE}}{\longrightarrow}$ Uridine diphosphate galactose + Pyrophosphate

Fig. 30B.—Alternate pathway of galactose metabolism in the liver.

CHART 26

GALACTOSEMIA

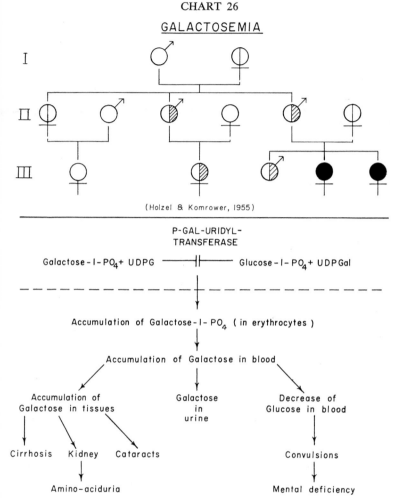

(Holzel & Komrower, 1955)

P-GAL-URIDYL-
TRANSFERASE

$$Galactose-1-PO_4 + UDPG \longrightarrow\!\!\!\!\parallel\!\!\!\!\longrightarrow Glucose-1-PO_4 + UDPGal$$

Accumulation of Galactose-1-PO_4 (in erythrocytes)

Accumulation of Galactose in blood

| Accumulation of Galactose in tissues | Galactose in urine | Decrease of Glucose in blood |

Cirrhosis   Kidney   Cataracts   Convulsions

Amino-aciduria   Mental deficiency

The pedigree of causes of galactosemia is shown in Chart 26. The decrease or absence of P-gal-uridyl-transferase results in the accumulation of galactose-1-PO_4 in the red cells, and this in turn is responsible for the accumulation of galactose in the blood. The excessive galactose can have three types of effects: (1) Galactose and galactose-1-PO_4 can accumulate in the tissues, and over a period of time are probably responsible for cirrhosis of the liver, cataracts, and renal changes which are also responsible for aminoaciduria. (2) Galactose can be excreted in the urine (easily detectable as a reducing substance). (3) Galactose depresses the blood glucose level, and this in turn may cause convulsions and mental retardation.

DIAGNOSIS.—Galactosemia can be diagnosed by the presence of galactose in the urine (see Procedure 34) and by the excessively high galactose levels in the blood (Fig. 31) (see Procedure 35).

TREATMENT.—Withholding all milk and milk products will clear up all acute symptoms, and no long-term effects will result if the lactose or

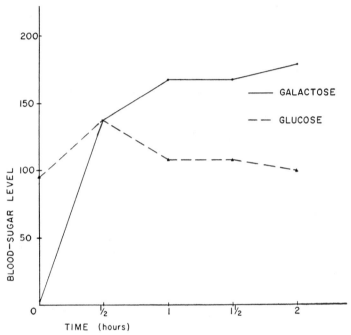

FIG. 31.—Galactose tolerance curve of patient with galactosemia. The continued elevation of the galactose levels is characteristic. (From Hsia, Hsia, Green, Kay, and Gellis, 1954.)

galactose is withdrawn from the diet in the first few weeks of life. Nutramigen® or protein hydrolysates can be used as a substitute for milk.

As the child gets older, small amounts of milk products can be tolerated without any ill effects. Presumably, this occurs because an accessory pathway of galactose metabolism is present in the liver which can convert small amounts of galactose to glucose (Fig. 30B).

Holzel, A., and Komrower, G. M.: A study of the genetics of galactosemia, Arch. Dis. Childhood 30:155, 1955.

Hsia, D. Y. Y.; Hsia, H. H.; Green, S.; Kay, M.; and Gellis, S. S.: Aminoaciduria in galactosemia, A.M.A. Am. J. Dis. Child. 88:458, 1954.

Hsia, D. Y. Y.; Huang, I.; and Driscoll, S. G.: The heterozygous carrier in galactosemia, Nature 16:1389, 1958.

Isselbacher, K. J.: Evidence for an accessory pathway of galactose metabolism in man, J. Clin. Invest. 36:902, 1957.

————; Anderson, E. P.; Kurahashi, K.; and Kalckar, H. M.: Congenital galactosemia, a single enzymatic block in galactose metabolism, Science 123:635, 1956.

*Komrower, G. M.; Schwarz, V.; Holzel, A.; and Golberg, L.: A clinical and biochemical study of galactosemia, Arch. Dis. Childhood 31:254, 1956.

LeLoir, L. F.: The metabolism of hexose phosphates, in McElroy, W. D., and Glass, H. B. (eds.): *Phosphorus Metabolism* (Baltimore: Johns Hopkins Press, 1951), p. 67.

Schwarz, V.; Golberg, L.; Komrower, G. M.; and Holzel, A.: Some disturbances of erythrocyte metabolism in galactosemia, Biochem. J. 62:34, 1956.

GLYCOGEN STORAGE DISEASE

"Glycogen storage disease" is an over-all term applied to a group of congenital and familial disorders characterized by the deposition of abnormally large quantities of glycogen in the tissues. At least three of the several types of the disease represent metabolic blocks in the normal pathway of glycogen metabolism (see Fig. 32). Glucose is converted to glycogen by three separate steps: (1) Glucose reacts with ATP to form glucose-6-PO_4 and ADP. This reaction is catalyzed by the enzyme "hexokinase." (2) Glucose-6-PO_4 is then converted to glucose-1-PO_4 in the presence of the enzyme "phosphoglucomutase." (3) Glucose-1-PO_4 is then converted to glycogen by the action of two separate enzymes. Phosphorylase acts to remove the phosphate group from glucose-1-PO_4 and attaches the bared first carbon atom to the fourth carbon atom of a glucose residue on the glycogen nidus. This addition occurs on the nonreducing end of the molecule. In this way, successively longer 1,4-glucose chains are added. When the chain has been lengthened to a critical level of eight glucose residues, the molecule becomes the substrate for the second enzyme, brancher enzyme amylo-(1,4- to 1,6)-transglucosidase. The enzyme transfers the α-1,4-linkage to an α-1,6-linkage, thus establishing a branch point of the molecule. The absence of this branching enzyme appears to be responsible for the glycogen storage disease characterized by *diffuse glycogenosis with hepatic cirrhosis* (Type III).

Glycogen is also converted back to glucose by three separate steps: (4) Glycogen is converted to glucose-1-PO_4 by the action of two enzymes. Phosphorylase first acts to remove the 1,4-linked glucose residues from the outermost tier and converts these to glucose-1-PO_4 and bares the 1,6-links. The debrancher enzyme (amylo-1,6-glucosidase) causes hydrolytic cleavage of the 1,6-linkage and liberates glucose. The absence of this debrancher enzyme appears to be responsible for *glycogen storage disease of the liver and muscle* (Type IV). (5) The glucose-1-PO$_4$ is then converted to glucose-6-PO$_4$ by the enzyme action of phosphoglucomutase. (6) Finally, the glucose-6-PO$_4$ is transformed to glucose by the enzyme glucose-6-phosphatase. An absence of this enzyme

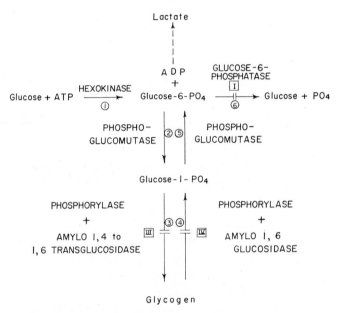

Fig. 32.—Normal pathway of glycogen formation and breakdown. A block at site I results in von Gierke's disease; at site III in diffuse glycogenosis with hepatic cirrhosis; and at site IV in glycogen storage disease of liver and muscle.

is responsible for *von Gierke's disease* (Type I, glycogen storage disease of the liver and kidneys).

*Cori, G. T.: Glycogen structure and enzyme deficiencies in glycogen storage disease, Harvey Lect. 48:145, 1953.

*Recant, L.: Recent developments in the field of glycogen metabolism and the diseases of glycogen storage, Am. J. Med. 19:610, 1955.

4. TYPE I, GLYCOGEN STORAGE DISEASE OF THE LIVER AND KIDNEYS (von Gierke's disease)

In 1928, van Crevald and von Gierke independently reported on a condition characterized by excessive enlargement of the liver and other organs during early infancy, owing to the accumulation of glycogen. This has since been found to be a hereditary disease resulting from an inborn error of glycogen metabolism.

CLINICAL FEATURES.—The condition is usually diagnosed during the first year of life because of asymptomatic liver enlargement. Initially, the infant appears to be completely well; but it may develop anorexia, weight loss, and vomiting, and in the later stages hypoglycemia, convulsions, and coma. Since it is essential to differentiate this form of glycogen storage disease from the other types, Holt has recommended that, to establish the diagnosis, these five criteria be met: (1) marked enlargement of the liver; (2) rapid development of hypoglycemia and ketosis when food is

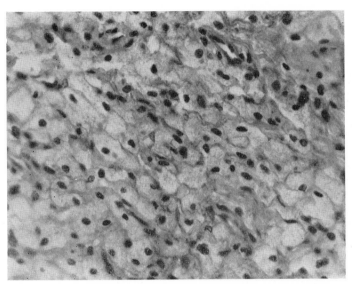

FIG. 33.—Photomicrograph of section from liver of a patient with glycogen storage disease of liver and kidney (Type I). The hepatic cells show clear cytoplasm and small nuclei; there is also a suggestion of fine cytoplasmic granules. These cells contain abundant stored glycogen, which is unstained, producing the clear, swollen appearance.

withheld; (3) subnormal or absent response of the blood sugar to an injection of epinephrine; (4) glycogen content of the liver representing 12-16% of the wet weight and no marked increase in fat (Fig. 33); and (5) an abnormal stability of the liver glycogen both in vitro and after death.

It is interesting to note that, despite the low blood-sugar levels and failure to respond to epinephrine, infants with this disease seldom show symptoms of hypoglycemia. However, they do show a low resistance to infection, and some retardation of growth and development is a frequent finding. In most cases, death ensues in the first two years of life, but an occasional patient may reach adult life and do moderately well.

HEREDITY.—The incidence of glycogen storage disease of the liver in the population is not known. The condition appears to be transmitted as a simple autosomal recessive. Many of the reported cases are among siblings, and consanguinity is not an unusual finding. The heterozygous carrier of the abnormal gene can be detected by elevated glucose-6-PO_4 and fructose-6-PO_4 levels in the red cells.

PATHOGENESIS.—Since the condition represents an inborn error of converting glycogen back to glucose, it appears improbable that the defect represents a block in steps 1, 2, and 3 (see p. 137). Also, step 5 can be excluded because it is merely a reverse reaction of step 2. In 1952, Cori and Cori showed that von Gierke's disease represents a block in step 6. First they showed that the structure of glycogen in the liver of these patients did not differ from that of normal individuals. Then they demonstrated that glucose-6-phosphatase either was absent or was present in greatly reduced amounts in every sample of liver from patients tested. Recently this has also been indirectly confirmed by the studies of Schwartz and his co-workers. They found that, although such infants show a normal response to intravenous galactose tolerance tests, the galactose is not converted to glucose, as in the normal infant, but is excreted as lactic acid, indicating an inability to convert glucose-6-PO_4 to glucose.

The pedigree of causes for glycogen storage disease of the liver is shown in Chart 27. The absence of glucose-6-phosphatase is responsible for at least three major effects. By depriving the patient of readily accessible sources of glucose, hypoglycemia is likely to ensue. This in turn causes ketosis, convulsions, increased gluconeogenesis from proteins, starvation diabetes, and a poor response to glucose tolerance tests. The absence of glucose-6-phosphatase also deprives the patient of a proper response to epinephrine injections. Finally, the absence of this enzyme causes the body organs to be loaded with glycogen. This in turn is responsible for obesity, impaired liver function, and poor resistance to infection.

DIAGNOSIS.—Von Gierke's disease should be seriously considered when a patient shows a poor response to epinephrine (see Procedure 36) and a flat glucose tolerance curve. The final diagnosis can only be established by the absence of glucose-6-phosphatase in the liver (see Procedure 37), obtained either by biopsy or at autopsy.

TREATMENT.—Frequent feedings and a high-protein diet are believed to be useful in reducing the rate of glycogen deposition, but the results of such therapy have not been impressive. ACTH or cortisone

CHART 27

GLYCOGEN STORAGE DISEASE OF LIVER & KIDNEYS
(TYPE I)

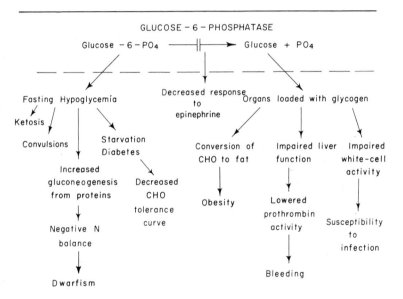

GLUCOSE – 6 – PHOSPHATASE

$$\text{Glucose} - 6 - PO_4 \longrightarrow\!|\!|\longrightarrow \text{Glucose} + PO_4$$

Fasting Hypoglycemia

Ketosis

Convulsions

Starvation
Diabetes

Increased
gluconeogenesis
from proteins

Negative N
balance

Dwarfism

Decreased response
to
epinephrine

Decreased
CHO
tolerance
curve

Organs loaded with glycogen

Conversion of
CHO to fat

Obesity

Impaired liver
function

Lowered
prothrombin
activity

Bleeding

Impaired
white-cell
activity

Susceptibility
to
infection

may be of value in controlling the hypoglycemia episodes. Sodium lactate is given for the acidosis, which can be quite marked.

Bridge, E. M., and Holt, L. E., Jr.: Glycogen storage disease: Observations on pathologic physiology of two cases of hepatic form of disease, J. Pediat. 27: 299, 1945.

Cori, G. T., and Cori, C. F.: Glucose-6-phosphatase of the liver in glycogen storage disease, J. Biol. Chem. 199:661, 1952.

Hsia, D. Y. Y., and Gawranska, E.: Detection of the heterozygous carrier in von Gierke's disease (to be published).

Illstrom, R. A.; Ziegler, M.; Doeden, D.; and McQuarrie, I. J.: Metabolic and

clinical effects of ACTH on essential glycogenesis, Metabolism 1:197, 1952.
Mason, H. H., and Andersen, D. H.: Glycogen disease, Am. J. Dis. Child. 61:795, 1941.
Schwartz, R.; Ashmore, J.; and Renold, A. E.: Galactose tolerance in glycogen storage disease, Pediatrics 19:585, 1957.

5. TYPE II, GLYCOGEN STORAGE DISEASE OF THE HEART

In 1950, di Sant'Agnese and his associates showed that glycogen storage disease of the heart should be regarded as a clinical entity separate from other forms of glycogen storage disease.

CLINICAL FEATURES.—The condition becomes manifest in early infancy. The infants feed poorly, become listless, and fail to gain weight

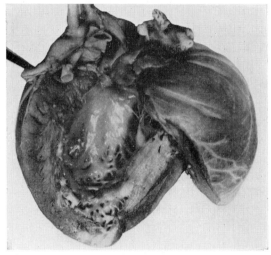

FIG. 34.—Glycogen storage disease of the heart. The weight of the organ is six times the normal weight, owing to marked myocardial glycogen deposition.

properly. This is followed by episodes of intermittent cyanosis, especially during feeding, and attacks of dyspnea without specific cause. Many parents report "excessively rapid breathing" as the reason for their bringing the baby to the doctor. All infants suffering from this disease die of heart failure, and in some instances bronchopneumonia, during the first 2 years of life.

The heart is usually enlarged, and systolic murmurs are sometimes heard. An x-ray examination shows the cardiac silhouette to be globular; and an electrocardiogram reveals inverted T waves, left-axis deviation, and ST depression with a normal PR interval. At autopsy the heart is found to weigh from 2 to 5.6 times the normal weight for the age (Fig. 34). Histologically, there is noted massive infiltration of the cardiac fibers by glycogen; and microscopically, a distinctive lacework appearance of the myocardium. Similar depositions are noted in the skeletal muscle, smooth muscle, and other organs of the body.

HEREDITY.—The condition is probably transmitted as a rare recessive. The condition is known to occur among siblings, and in one instance

CHART 28

GLYCOGEN STORAGE DISEASE OF HEART (TYPE II)

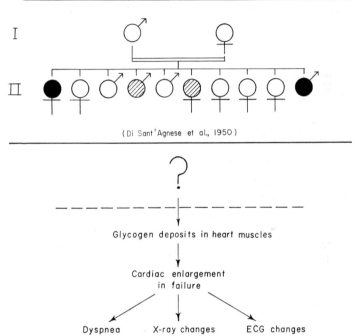

(Di Sant'Agnese et al., 1950)

the parents were first cousins. The heterozygous carrier for this abnormality has not been detected.

PATHOGENESIS.—The etiology of this condition is completely unknown (Chart 28). The Coris have found that both the structure of the glycogen and the glucose-6-phosphatase activity of the liver and kidney are within normal limits. However, the possibility of a metabolic block in some other stage of glucose metabolism has not been completely ruled out. For instance, a reduction of phosphohexoisomerase or phosphofructokinase content might lead to a moderate decrease in the rate of glycogen breakdown. With a normal rate of glycogen synthesis, this could lead to storage of glycogen. The predilection of glycogen for the heart and muscles also remains to be explained.

DIAGNOSIS.—Glycogen storage disease of the heart is suggested by cardiac enlargement or electrocardiographic changes during life. At postmortem the deposition of glycogen in the muscle fibers of the heart is found to be typical.

TREATMENT.—None is available.

Cori, G. T.: Glycogen structure and enzyme deficiencies in glycogen storage disease, Harvey Lect. 48:145, 1953.
*Di Sant'Agnese, P. A.; Andersen, D. H.; Mason, H. H.; and Bauman, W. A.: Glycogen storage disease of the heart: I. Report of 2 cases in siblings with chemical and pathologic studies, Pediatrics 6:402, 1950.
———; ———; and ———: Glycogen storage disease of the heart: II. Critical review of the literature, Pediatrics 6:607, 1950.

6. TYPE III, DIFFUSE GLYCOGENOSIS WITH HEPATIC CIRRHOSIS

In 1952, Andersen reported on a 17-month-old white male infant whose liver showed glycogen which on analysis was less branched and had longer inner and outer branches than normal.

CLINICAL FEATURES.—This form of glycogen storage disease becomes manifest in late infancy or early childhood. The complaints are primarily hepatic, with such features as edema, ascites, and occasional bleeding tendencies being prominent. Liver function tests are usually abnormal, but blood sugar is normal and no acidosis is present. When the glucose tolerance test is performed a moderate rise and a slow fall of the blood sugar is observed. The response to epinephrine is moderate, but less than in normal individuals. The clinical course appears to be highly variable, and children with this condition may survive up to 10 years of age.

At postmortem, the liver is found to have a finely nodular surface. Microscopic examination shows a diffuse, finely nodular cirrhosis with large amounts of glycogen in the liver cells. In the spleen there are accumulations of what appear to be reticulum cells loaded with glycogen. Phagocytic cells loaded with glycogen are also found in the lymph nodes and lymph follicles and in the intestinal mucosa. No glycogen appears to be present in the kidneys. The glycogen has been observed to be different in physical characteristics from that of von Gierke's disease, being sticky, hard to handle, and slow to precipitate.

HEREDITY.—Although the sibling of the first described case also died of glycogen storage disease, the diagnosis of Type III diffuse glycogenosis was not confirmed biochemically.

PATHOGENESIS.—Illingworth and Cori have studied the character of glycogen in the liver from a patient with this condition. End-group analysis showed branch points of 4.7% (normal, 7.1-8.4%), and the average chain length was 21.2 (normal, 11.9-14.1). The average outer

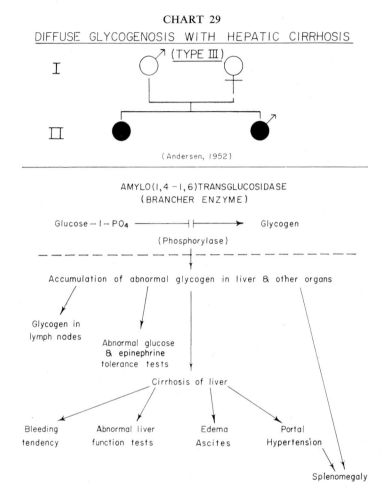

CHART 29

DIFFUSE GLYCOGENOSIS WITH HEPATIC CIRRHOSIS

(TYPE III)

(Andersen, 1952)

AMYLO(1,4 — 1,6)TRANSGLUCOSIDASE
(BRANCHER ENZYME)

Glucose — 1 — PO₄ $\longrightarrow$ Glycogen

(Phosphorylase)

Accumulation of abnormal glycogen in liver & other organs

Glycogen in lymph nodes

Abnormal glucose & epinephrine tolerance tests

Cirrhosis of liver

Bleeding tendency

Abnormal liver function tests

Edema Ascites

Portal Hypertension

Splenomegaly

chain length had 14.7 residues (normal, 7.1-8.9), and the inner chain length had 6.5 residues (normal, 3.0-5.6). Thus there were fewer branch points and significantly longer chains. It would appear that this form of glycogen storage disease is caused by a deficiency of brancher enzyme "amylo-(1,4 to 1,6)-transglucosidase."

The pedigree of causes for this condition is given in Chart 29. The deficiency of the brancher enzyme causes an accumulation of glycogen in the liver. Over a length of time the glycogen behaves as a foreign body, to which there is a tissue reaction. This causes cirrhosis of the liver, and all the ultimate complications of this disease can be attributed to liver damage.

DIAGNOSIS.—Demonstration of the glycogen abnormality (see Procedure 38) by liver biopsy will confirm the diagnosis.

TREATMENT.—None is available.

*Andersen, D. H.: Studies on glycogen disease with a report of a case in which the glycogen was abnormal, in Najjar, V. A. (ed.): *Symposium on the Clinical and Biochemical Aspects of Carbohydrate Utilization in Health and Disease* (Baltimore: Johns Hopkins Press, 1952).

————: Familial cirrhosis of the liver with storage of abnormal glycogen, Lab. Invest. 5:11, 1956.

Illingworth, B., and Cori, G. T.: Structure of glycogens and amylopectins: III. Normal and abnormal human glycogens, J. Biol. Chem. 199:653, 1952.

7. TYPE IV, GLYCOGEN STORAGE DISEASE OF LIVER AND MUSCLE

In 1953, Forbes reported on a fourth type of glycogen storage disease of the liver which was apparently caused by a deficiency of debrancher enzyme. In the same year, Krivit and his co-workers described a similar deficiency but with glycogen storage primarily in the skeletal muscle. It would appear that these two conditions represent different manifestations of the same basic defect and that they should be considered together.

TYPE IV*a*, GLYCOGEN STORAGE DISEASE OF LIVER

CLINICAL FEATURES.—The child described by Forbes was essentially well until age 12, when she was noted to have progressive hepatomegaly. Liver function tests showed a positive cephalin flocculation test and bromsulfalein retention. There was slightly less response to epinephrine than normal. A moderate amount of acetone was detected in the urine. Otherwise, the child was perfectly well, and she did not appear to be incapacitated by the defect.

Liver biopsy showed the parenchymal cells to be packed with glycogen, and a slight increase of connective tissue was noted in the periportal spaces. Both muscle and liver biopsies, however, showed increased amounts of glycogen.

HEREDITY.—The mode of transmission of this condition is not known. None of the siblings or near relatives of this patient were affected.

PATHOGENESIS.—Illingworth and Cori characterized the glycogen in this patient (see Procedure 38). End-group analysis revealed branch points of 10.8% for liver and 13.1% for muscle (normal, 7.1-8.4%), and the over-all chain length was 9.3 for liver and 7.6 for muscle (normal, 7.1-8.4). Degradation by phosphorylase was 12.2% for liver and 2.6% for muscle (normal, 25-41%). The average outer chain length had 5.1

CHART 30

GLYCOGEN STORAGE IN LIVER (TYPE IV A)

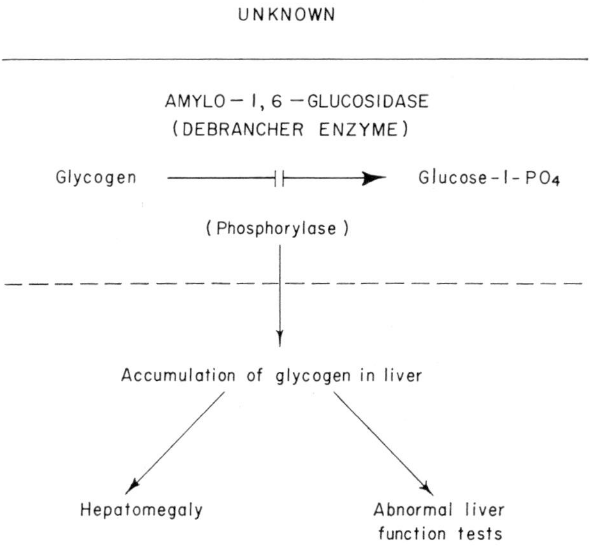

UNKNOWN

AMYLO – 1, 6 – GLUCOSIDASE
(DEBRANCHER ENZYME)

Glycogen ————————⊣⊢————➤ Glucose-1-PO$_4$

(Phosphorylase)

Accumulation of glycogen in liver

Hepatomegaly   Abnormal liver
function tests

residues for liver and 4.0 for muscle (normal, 7.1-8.9); and the inner chain length, 4.2 for liver and 3.6 for muscle (normal, 3.0-5.6). This indicates that the glycogen had an enormous number of branches and very short outer chains and suggests that there is a deficiency of the debrancher enzyme (see Procedure 38) (amylo-1,6-glucosidase) in step 4 of the glycogen pathway (Chart 30).

TYPE IV*b*, GLYCOGEN STORAGE DISEASE OF SKELETAL MUSCLE

CLINICAL FEATURES.—A number of cases of glycogen storage disease of skeletal muscle have been reported. The condition resembles Werdnig-Hoffmann disease clinically, with progressive weakness, difficulty in swallowing, and regurgitation of food. Also, there is macroglossia, cardiomegalia, and hepatomegalia. Laboratory studies show a normal response to glucose tolerance tests and to epinephrine. However, histochemically the muscles are found to be loaded with glycogen. Autoglycogenesis occurs to a degree but is less than in normal tissues.

HEREDITY.—The condition appears to be genetically determined.

CHART 31

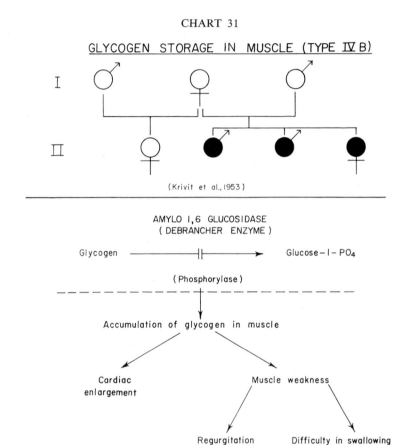

GLYCOGEN STORAGE IN MUSCLE (TYPE IV B)

(Krivit et al., 1953)

AMYLO I,6 GLUCOSIDASE
(DEBRANCHER ENZYME)

Glycogen ⟶ $Glucose-I-PO_4$

(Phosphorylase)

Accumulation of glycogen in muscle

Cardiac enlargement

Muscle weakness

Regurgitation   Difficulty in swallowing

Consanguinity has been found in one instance, and several siblings in other families have been found to have the same disease. This suggests that the disease is inherited as a rare recessive.

PATHOGENESIS.—The molecular structure of the glycogen in muscle has been studied in one case. An excessive number of branched linkages were found in the glycogen molecule, with a shorter-than-average chain length. Since this is similar to the changes in glycogen storage of the liver (Type IV*a*), it would appear that this condition should be regarded as a variant of the deficiency of the debrancher enzyme (Chart 31).

Forbes, G. B.: Glycogen storage disease, J. Pediat. 42:645, 1953.

Illingworth, B., and Cori, G. T.: Structures of glycogen and amylopectins: III. Normal and abnormal human glycogen, J. Biol. Chem. 199:653, 1952.

Krivit, W.; Polglase, W. J.; Gunn, F. D.; and Tyler, F. H.: Studies in disorders of muscle: IX. Glycogen storage disease primarily affecting skeletal muscle and clinically resembling amyotonia congenita, Pediatrics 12:165, 1953.

OTHER CARBOHYDRATE DISTURBANCES

8. HEREDITARY SPHEROCYTOSIS

Hereditary spherocytosis is a congenital hemolytic disorder characterized by the presence of spherocytes in the peripheral blood. The condition was first accurately described by Valair and Masius in 1871, but the merit of their observations was not appreciated until recent times. The disorder is believed to be due to a derangement in the energy-yielding reactions of glycolysis within the membranes of the erythrocytes.

CLINICAL FEATURES.—Patients with hereditary spherocytosis have a mild degree of anemia. The degree varies from patient to patient, but the anemia is rarely severe. This is because a balance seems to occur between the rate of red-cell production and destruction; the hemoglobin and hematocrit values show little variation. The slight increase of red-cell breakdown is characterized by an increase of indirect bilirubin in the serum, increased excretion of urobilinogen in the stools, and mild to moderate reticulocytosis. Cholecystitis and cholelithiasis are frequent complications. Some of the children show physical retardation, but all show marked improvement following splenectomy.

From time to time, the patients develop a sudden crisis. This is characterized by malaise, anorexia, and mild fever in association with bouts of jaundice. There is a sudden destruction of the circulating erythrocytes, and also a decrease of erythropoiesis with maturation arrest in the bone marrow. The cause for these crises is not well understood, but they are frequently associated with infections.

Laboratory studies show increased osmotic fragility of the red cells. The fragility is increased because the spherocytes can absorb less water from hypotonic media than do normal cells. Similarly, erythrocytes from patients with hereditary spherocytosis show a markedly increased mechanical fragility. In 1941, Dacie reported that in hereditary spherocytosis such cells underwent lysis 5-10 times as rapidly as normal cells when incubated at body temperature for 48 hours. These cells take in sodium at about the same rate as do normal cells, but they lose potassium slightly more rapidly than do normal cells. The rate of cell destruction is slowed down if glucose is added to the defibrinated blood so that its concentration is approximately 500 mg/100 ml. Since cells from patients break down more easily after incubation at body temperature, this approach is frequently used to demonstrate increased osmotic or mechanical fragility in patients who show no abnormalities when the tests are done on fresh blood.

HEREDITY.—Hereditary spherocytosis is transmitted as an autosomal dominant characteristic, with most of the affected individuals being heterozygotes. It is not clear at present whether the dominance is complete, since there are fewer affected siblings than one would expect on a purely mathematical basis. Also, Young has encountered five patients whose parents, on repeated testing, showed no demonstrable hematologic abnormalities. Although these patients could represent fresh mutations, it is possible that the condition did not manifest itself in these parents. The homozygous form of spherocytosis has not yet been demonstrated with certainty, although its occurrence has been suspected in two families.

Hereditary spherocytosis occurs once in about 20,000 live births.

PATHOGENESIS.—Prankerd and associates have demonstrated that in hereditary spherocytosis there is a defect in intracellular glycolysis involving a smaller flux of P^{32} into ATP and 2,3-diphosphoglycerate with a concurrent increase in the flux into orthophosphate. The turnover of P^{32} into ATP and 2,3-diphosphoglycerate in the stromal fraction tends to be lower than normal. These changes can largely be restored to normal upon incubation of the cells with adenosine. Although the actual enzyme defect has yet to be described, Altman and Young have presented some preliminary findings suggesting that it may involve a disturbance of enolase, the enzyme which converts 2-phosphoglycerate to phosphoenolpyruvate. They have suggested that the maintenance of the biconcave shape of the normal erythrocyte requires an adequate availability of energy-rich phosphate bonds. Such bonds are apparently lacking in the erythrocytes of patients with hereditary spherocytosis, because these erythrocytes show a greater susceptibility to destruction and lysis upon the depletion of glucose or any of the metabolites necessary for energy production in vitro. The addition of adenosine in some way replaces this deficit, at least in part. Splenectomy improves the clinical picture, and one can therefore assume that passage of the blood cells through the spleen is in many ways similar to incubating the blood in vitro. Presumably, in patients with hereditary spherocytosis, the stagnation and

CHART 32

HEREDITARY SPHEROCYTOSIS

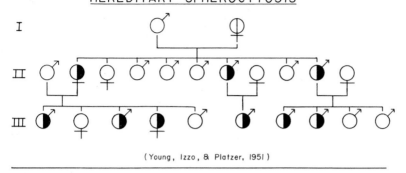

(Young, Izzo, & Platzer, 1951)

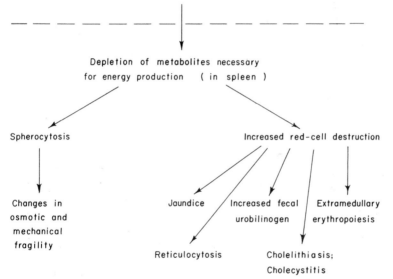

hemoconcentration in the spleen results in the erythrocytes being deprived of glucose and other energy-producing metabolites and the cells break down from "relative starvation." Splenectomy effectively removes this difficulty without fundamentally correcting the defect itself.

All of the signs and symptoms in hereditary spherocytosis can be attributed to the increased destruction of erythrocytes, as shown in Chart 32. The biochemical disturbances, such as the low potassium content found in these cells, the deficiency in phospholipids with an excess of cholesterol, and the increased transport of sodium across the cell membranes, must be regarded as secondary manifestations of the basic defect in glycolysis.

DIAGNOSIS.—The spherocytosis of the peripheral blood is characteristic. Also, the diagnosis is suggested by changes in the osmotic fragility (see Procedures 39 and 41) and the mechanical fragility (Procedures 40 and 41) of the erythrocytes.

TREATMENT.—Splenectomy after the age of 2 years effectively removes all of the complications of this defect and should be performed on every patient with hereditary spherocytosis. The operation should not be done in infancy because of the danger of recurrent infections, which have been reported.

*Dacie, J. V.: *The Haemolytic Anemias: Congenital and Acquired* (London: J. & A. Churchill, Ltd., 1954).

Motulsky, A. G.; Giblett, E.; Colman, D.; Gabrio, B. W.; and Finch, C. A.: Life span, glucose metabolism, and osmotic fragility of erythrocytes in hereditary spherocytosis, J. Clin. Invest. 34:911, 1955.

Prankerd, T. A. J.; Altman, K. I.; and Young, L. E.: Abnormalities of carbohydrate metabolism of red cells in hereditary spherocytosis, J. Clin. Invest. 34:1268, 1955.

Race, R. R.: On the inheritance and linkage relations of acholuric jaundice, Ann. Eugenics 11:365, 1942.

Selwyn, J. G., and Dacie, J. V.: Autohemolysis and other changes resulting from the incubation in vitro of red cells from patients with congenital hemolytic anemia, Blood 9:414, 1954.

Tabechian, H.; Altman, K. I.; and Young, L. E.: Inhibition of P^{32}-orthophosphate exchange by sodium fluoride in erythrocytes from patients with hereditary spherocytosis, Proc. Soc. Exper. Biol. & Med. 92:712, 1956.

*Young, L. E.: Hereditary spherocytosis, Am. J. Med. 18:486, 1955.

———; Izzo, M. J.; and Platzer, R. F.: Hereditary spherocytosis: I. Clinical, hematologic, and genetic features in 28 cases, with particular reference to the osmotic and mechanical fragility of incubated erythrocytes, Blood 6:1073, 1951.

9. HEREDITARY NONSPHEROCYTIC HEMOLYTIC ANEMIA

Hereditary nonspherocytic hemolytic anemia is characterized by macrocytosis, basophilic stippling, hepatosplenomegaly, and jaundice. In recent years, hematologists have been able to differentiate this disease from thalassemia, hereditary spherocytosis, hemolytic processes associated with the abnormal hemoglobins, and erythroblastosis fetalis by the distinctive laboratory findings.

CLINICAL FEATURES.—Patients with this disease usually come to the attention of physicians because of jaundice and anemia. In the very young age group, the condition is frequently mistaken for erythroblastosis fetalis, except that no blood-group incompatibility can be found and the reaction to the Coombs test is negative. In older people, there may be a history of intermittent jaundice, weakness, malaise, or right upper quadrant pain, sometimes accompanied by liver or splenic enlargement.

A study of the peripheral blood will reveal a moderate decrease of hemoglobin and red-cell count. Smears of the peripheral blood will show

CHART 33

HEREDITARY NONSPHEROCYTIC HEMOLYTIC ANEMIA

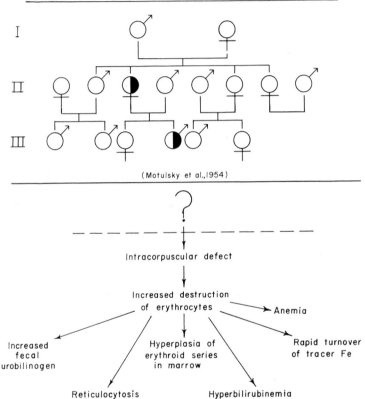

(Motulsky et al.,1954)

normal rouleaux formation; and there is no stippling, sickling, fragmentation, or other morphological changes. A mild anisocytosis and poikilocytosis is seen in all cases; however, careful studies will reveal all of the signs of a hemolytic process. There is a hyperplasia of the erythroid series in the bone marrow, reticulocytosis, hyperbilirubinemia, increased urobilinogen in the stools, and a rapid turnover of tracer iron in the plasma (Chart 33). There is no marked change in osmotic or mechanical fragility of the erythrocytes, although they tend to be more fragile after incubation for 24 hours. Electrophoretic studies show that the predominant hemoglobin is Type A, with a slight increase of Hgb F.

Patients with hereditary nonspherocytic hemolytic anemia are not greatly handicapped by the disease and lead relatively normal lives.

HEREDITY.—The condition has been reported in about a dozen families; it has been seen in both Europe and the United States. Undoubtedly, many more affected persons exist but have not been reported because clinically they appear to be so similar to persons with other hematological conditions.

Although genetic studies in the reported families are, as yet, incomplete, the condition appears to be transmitted as an autosomal dominant. However, there seems to be a variable degree of penetrance, and expressivity is usually incomplete.

Several workers have suggested that this group of patients is not homogeneous. For instance, in some families autohemolysis is not increased, but the addition of glucose does not reduce the amount of hemolysis to the degree that it does in a normal control. In other families there is an increased degree of autohemolysis which is not prevented by the addition of glucose.

PATHOGENESIS.—At the present time, at least two separate forms of hereditary nonspherocytic hemolytic anemia are known to exist: (1) in some patients there is a normal rate of glycolysis and P^{32}-orthophosphate exchange, but increased intracellular contents of 2,3-diphosphoglucose; and (2) in others there is a low content of ATP, deficient glucose consumption, and decreased P^{32}-orthophosphate exchange. Further studies are needed to decide whether we are dealing with a single disease or with two or more separate diseases.

DIAGNOSIS.—Hereditary nonspherocytic hemolytic anemia can be differentiated (1) from hereditary spherocytosis by the absence of spherocytes and essentially normal fragility tests; (2) from thalassemia by the clinical course, fetal hemoglobin content, and peripheral smear; (3) from the abnormal hemoglobins by electrophoretic and solubility studies; and (4) from erythroblastosis fetalis by blood-grouping studies.

TREATMENT.—None is required. Splenectomy is probably not helpful, and transfusions only serve to increase the degree of hemosiderosis.

Dacie, J. V.; Mollison, P. L.; Richardson, N.; Selwyn, J. G.; and Shapiro, L.: Atypical congenital haemolytic anemia, Quart. J. Med. 22:79, 1953.

Kaplan, E., and Zuelzer, W. W.: Familial nonspherocytic hemolytic anemia, Blood 5:811, 1950.

*Motulsky, A. G.; Crosby, W. H.; and Rappaport, H.: Hereditary nonspherocytic hemolytic disease, Blood 9:749, 1954.

———; Gabrio, B. W.; Burkhardt, J.; and Finch, C. A.: Erythrocyte carbohydrate metabolism in hereditary hemolytic anemias, Am. J. Med. 19:291, 1955.
Prankerd, T. A. J.: Inborn errors of metabolism in red cells of congenital
hemolytic anemias, Am. J. Med. 22:724, 1957.
Smiley, R. K.; Dempsey, H.; Villeneuve, P.; and Campbell, J. S.: Atypical
familial hemolytic anemia, Blood 11:324, 1956.

8

Disturbances in Endocrine Metabolism

DISTURBANCES IN ENDOCRINE METABOLISM may be divided into two groups: thyroid and adrenal.

FAMILIAL CRETINISM WITH GOITER

The biosynthesis of thyroid hormone takes place through a series of separate steps (Fig. 35): (1) Iodide and various forms of iodine enter the body through the intestinal tract and are distributed throughout the extracellular compartment of the body. (2) Some of the iodide is excreted through the kidneys, but most of it is trapped within the thyroid gland and oxidized to elemental, or free, iodine. The trapping process requires oxygen and is undoubtedly enzymatically controlled. A defect in this step results in *cretinism from a failure of organic iodine to form.* (3) The free iodine then reacts with tyrosyl residues to form monoiodotyrosine and diiodotyrosine. (4) Some of the iodinated tyrosyl residues condense to form iodinated thyronines—namely, thyroxine and triiodothyronine, which are the active hormonal products of the thyroid gland. This coupling process is probably also enzymatically controlled. A defect in this step results in *cretinism from a failure of iodotyrosines to couple.* (5) The remainder of the iodinated tyrosyl residues are dehalogenated by the enzyme "iodotyrosine deshalogenase" and returned to the thyroid iodide pool. This step is necessary for the proper conservation of iodine in the body. A defect in this system results in *cretinism from a failure of iodotyrosines to deiodinate.*

*Stanbury, J. B., and McGirr, E. M.: Sporadic or non-endemic familial cretinism with goiter, Am. J. Med. 22:712, 1957.

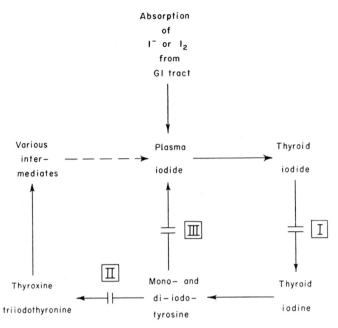

FIG. 35.—Biosynthetic pathway of thyroid hormone (postulated). A block at site I results in cretinism from failure of organic iodine to form; at site II in cretinism from failure of iodotyrosines to couple; and at site III in cretinism from failure of iodotyrosine to deiodinate.

I. CRETINISM FROM FAILURE OF ORGANIC IODINE TO FORM

CLINICAL FEATURES.—In 1950, Stanbury and Hedge reported on a 15-year-old girl who had both cretinism and goiter and who had lived on the seacoast of Massachusetts all of her life. In going over her history, they found that she had developed normally until about 6 months of age and thereafter had shown marked retardation. She had never walked, and she could not speak or feed herself at the time of the examination.

Signs of cretinism were noted at the age of 1 year. Skin was dry, cool, and coarse, with a spongy elasticity. The hair was slightly coarse. The bridge of the nose was depressed, and the lips were thick and protuberant.

At the age of 7 years she was noted to have a mass in the neck, which had slowly increased in size. Pathological examination of the gland showed intense compensatory hyperplasia, which was followed by degeneration and fibrous tissue replacement.

HEREDITY.—In this girl's family, the first three children were normal and the next four were all cretins. The parents were normal but were first cousins. In another family, 4 out of 13 children were found to be cretins. Since the condition affects individuals of both sexes, this would imply that the condition is transmitted as an autosomal recessive.

PATHOGENESIS.—Stanbury showed that, when labeled iodine (I^{131}) was given orally, a large fraction of it was accumulated rapidly in the thy-

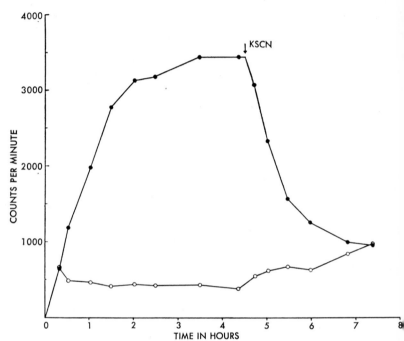

FIG. 36.—Radioactive iodine accumulation and discharge in a patient with cretinism from failure of organic iodine to form. At zero time, a tracer dose of 100 μc of I^{131} was given. The open circles are net counts per minute over the thigh; the closed circles, net counts per minute over the thyroid gland. When this had reached a plateau in 4 hours, an oral dose of 2 Gm. of potassium thiocyanate caused a striking and rapid disappearance of the labeled iodine from the gland (From Stanbury, J. B., and Hedge, A. N.: A study of a family of goitrous cretins, J. Clin. Endocrinol. 10:1471, 1950.)

roid gland. When this had reached a plateau in 4 hours, an oral dose of 2.0 Gm of KSCN caused a striking and rapid disappearance of the labeled iodine from the gland (Fig. 36). The same effect was not observed among controls.

The changes observed appeared to be identical with changes in patients who had received antithyroid drugs of the thiocarbamide group

Since it is known that the latter drugs inhibit the transfer of iodide to tyrosyl residues through an enzymatically controlled oxidative step, one may assume that this form of cretinism with goiter represents a metabolic block at this step. As a result, the thyroid gland contains iodide but is unable to convert it to iodine.

This defect causes a complete deficiency of thyroid hormone pro-

CHART 34

CRETINISM FROM FAILURE OF ORGANIC IODINE TO FORM

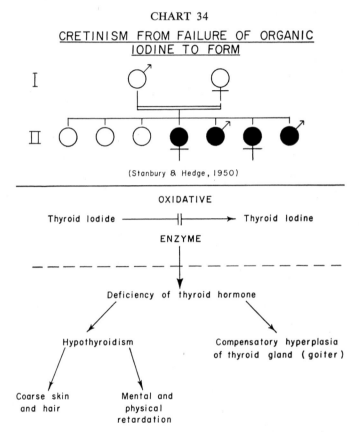

(Stanbury & Hedge, 1950)

duction. The gland tries to compensate for the deficiency by hypertrophy and hyperplasia, but this is largely unsuccessful and cretinism results (Chart 34).

DIAGNOSIS.—The diagnosis of cretinism from failure of organic iodine to form is established by the uptake and release of I^{131} in the thyroid gland and the typical response to KSCN (see Procedure 42).

TREATMENT.—Therapy with thyroid hormone early in life may help in preventing cretinism and mental retardation.

Schultz, A.; Flink, E. B.; Kennedy, B. J.; and Zieve, L.: Exchangeable character of accumulated I^{131} in the thyroid gland of a goitrous cretin, J. Clin. Endocrinol. 17:441, 1957.

Stanbury, J. B.: Cretinism with goiter: A case report, J. Clin. Endocrinol. 11:740, 1951.

———— and Hedge, A. N.: A study of a family of goitrous cretins, J. Clin. Endocrinol. 10:1471, 1950.

2. CRETINISM FROM FAILURE OF IODOTYROSINES TO COUPLE

CLINICAL FEATURES.—In 1955, Stanbury, Ohela, and Pitt-Rivers described a 25-year-old woman who showed retarded development and

CHART 35

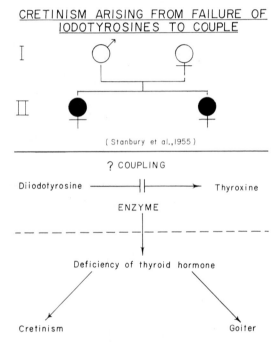

CRETINISM ARISING FROM FAILURE OF
IODOTYROSINES TO COUPLE

(Stanbury et al.,1955)

? COUPLING

Diiodotyrosine ————||————▶ Thyroxine

ENZYME

Deficiency of thyroid hormone

Cretinism   Goiter

goiter. Past history revealed that she had started talking at the age of 1 year and had started walking at 2½ years. Evidence of cretinism appeared at about the age of 4, with retarded growth and a thick and dry skin. She was sensitive to cold and was constipated. These symptoms seemed to improve upon the administration of thyroid.

At the time of her admission, the thyroid gland was enlarging rapidly. Pathological examination of the goiter showed marked hyperplasia with no colloid formation within the follicles.

HEREDITY.—A sister of the patient also showed evidence of cretinism with goiter. Both of the parents were normal and unrelated. Up until the present time, this is the only family with this type of cretinism which has been reported.

PATHOGENESIS.—Stanbury and his co-workers found that, although there was a rapid uptake of I^{131} by the thyroid, the administration of KSCN failed to discharge any of the retained labeled iodine. Direct analysis demonstrated labeled thyroxine and triiodothyronine in the blood but only a trace of thyroxine in the gland. On the other hand, labeled mono- and diiodotyrosine were found in the gland in abundance.

By measuring the rate of disappearance of labeled iodine from the gland and the urinary content of labeled and stable iodine before and during the administration of methimazole, a drug which blocks the incorporation of iodide with organic compounds, these investigators showed that more stable iodine was leaving the gland than could be accounted for by thyroxine and triiodothyronine production. They concluded that this represented a primary failure in the enzymatic coupling of iodotyrosines. This in turn caused a deficiency of thyroid hormone and a compensatory thyroid hyperplasia (Chart 35).

DIAGNOSIS.—The diagnosis is established by the kinetics of iodine metabolism with I^{131} administration before and during the administration of methimazole (see Procedure 43).

TREATMENT.—The administration of thyroid hormone may be of value in preventing the development of cretinism.

Stanbury, J. B.; Ohela, K.; and Pitt-Rivers, R.: The metabolism of iodine in 2 goitrous cretins compared with that in 2 patients receiving methimazole, J. Clin. Endocrinol. 15:54, 1955.

3. CRETINISM FROM FAILURE OF IODOTYROSINE TO DEIODINATE

CLINICAL FEATURES.—This condition was described first by Sir William Osler in 1897. Patients with this disease develop myxedema or goiter before the age of 3 years, and the physical changes are quite striking. In addition to a striking family likeness, most patients have the coarse, rather ugly facies of myxedema, as well as the supraclavicular pads, scanty eyebrows, and dry, lusterless hair. Most of the patients are markedly retarded in both physical and mental development, and usually they are unable to talk and are not toilet trained by adulthood. Their mental status is only slightly improved by thyroid therapy.

The pathological changes within the thyroid gland are highly variable. Some areas are characteristic of colloidal goiter, while other areas show little or no colloid formation; still other areas are filled with fibrous tissue. The changes suggest that, although there is an abundance of thyroid tissue and an adequate supply of iodine, there is an insufficient supply of thyroid hormone going to the tissues in the body.

HEREDITY.—Congenital hypothyroidism with goiter, resulting from failure of iodotyrosine to deiodinate, appears to be transmitted by an autosomal recessive gene. Consanguinity is a frequent occurrence, and the condition usually occurs among several of the siblings without the parents or other near relatives being involved.

Stanbury has recently shown that the near relatives of known patients show a decreased ability to deiodinate diiodotyrosine, and that a larger fraction of the I^{131} that is injected is excreted unchanged in the urine, as compared with normal individuals. It would appear, therefore, that the heterozygous carriers of the abnormal gene can be detected in this manner.

PATHOGENESIS.—The biosynthesis of thyroid hormone appears to take place by a series of separate steps: (1) the oxidation of iodide to iodine; (2) the iodination of tyrosine radicals within the thyroglobulin molecule to form mono- and diiodotyrosine; and (3) the coupling of two molecules of diiodotyrosine to give one molecule of thyroxine. Roche and his associates have shown that not all of the iodotyrosines formed in step 2 go to step 3. Instead, the unused portions are dehalogenated by a specific enzyme, iodotyrosine deshalogenase. This step is necessary for the proper conservation of iodine in the body and explains why mono- and diiodotyrosines are not found in the blood.

In 1955, Stanbury and his co-workers demonstrated the presence of both mono- and diiodotyrosine in the blood of a patient who had congenital hypothyroidism with goiter. They showed that intravenously administered mono- and diiodotyrosine were excreted in the urine either unchanged or as unidentified substances. There was no evidence of deiodination taking place. More recently they have shown that the enzyme "iodotyrosine deshalogenase" was actually absent in the thyroid tissue of a patient with familial goitrous cretinism.

The effects of the enzyme deficiency are shown in Chart 36. The deficiency of iodotyrosine deshalogenase results in the accumulation of mono- and diiodotyrosine within the blood and its loss through urinary excretion. The loss of iodine resulting from continuous excretion might be sufficient to prevent the formation of thyroid hormone in adequate amounts. This in turn is responsible for the signs of both cretinism and myxedema. The enlargement and hyperplasia of the thyroid gland is a compensatory mechanism for the thyroid hormone defect.

CHART 36

CRETINISM RESULTING FROM FAILURE OF IODOTYROSINE TO DEIODINATE

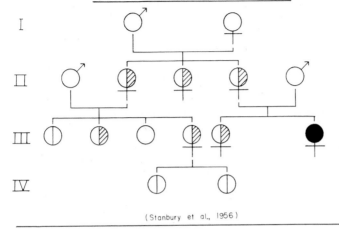

(Stanbury et al., 1956)

IODOTYROSINE DESHALOGENASE

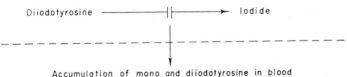

Diiodotyrosine ⟶ ⫴ ⟶ Iodide

Accumulation of mono and diiodotyrosine in blood

Excretion of mono and diiodotyrosine in urine

Inadequate formation of thyroid hormone

Compensatory hyperplasia of thyroid gland (goiter)

Hypothyroidism

Coarse skin and hair

Mental and physical retardation

DIAGNOSIS.—Congenital hypothyroidism with goiter is diagnosed by the presence of labeled mono- and diiodotyrosines in the blood following the administration of a tracer dose of I^{131} (see Procedure 44).

TREATMENT.—Early therapy with thyroid hormone may be helpful in preventing cretinism and mental retardation.

Hutchison, J. H., and McGirr, E. M.: Sporadic non-endemic goitrous cretinism: Hereditary transmission, Lancet 2:906, 1956.
Querido, A.; Stanbury, J. B.; Kassenaar, A. A. H.; and Meijer, J. W. A.: The

metabolism of iodotyrosines: III. Di-iodotyrosine deshalogenating activity of human thyroid tissue, J. Clin. Endocrinol. 16:1096, 1956.

Roche, J.; Michel, O.; Michel, R.; Gorbman, A.; and Lissitzyky, S.: Sur la déshalogénation enzymatique des iodotyrosines par le corps thyroide et sur son rôle physiologique: II. Biochim. et biophys. Acta 12:570, 1953.

Stanbury, J. B.; Meijer, J. W. A.; and Kassenaar, A. A. H.: The metabolism of iodo-tyrosines: II. The metabolism of mono and di-iodotyrosines in certain patients with familial goiter, J. Clin. Endocrinol. 16:848, 1956.

THE ADRENOGENITAL SYNDROME

The adrenogenital syndrome is an over-all term which can be applied to three separate conditions: (1) *adrenal hyperplasia with virilism only,* (2) *adrenal hyperplasia with hypertension,* and (3) *adrenal hyperplasia with electrolyte disturbances.* Although the three types appear to be clinically quite similar, genetic studies have shown that only one of the types is found among the affected members of a given family. Biochemical studies have shown that the first two types represent metabolic blocks at different sites in the normal pathway of compound F synthesis, as shown in Figure 37.

4. TYPE I, ADRENAL HYPERPLASIA WITH VIRILISM ONLY

Clinical features.—The picture differs depending on the sex of the patient.

In the female pseudohermaphrodite, the disorder begins in embryonic life and the sexual abnormalities are present at birth (Fig. 38). The characteristic findings are a hypertrophied phallus, which resembles a hypospadic penis, and a persistent urogenital sinus which communicates anteriorly with the urethra and posteriorly with the vagina, uterus, and tubes. The condition may occasionally be confused with true genetic intersexes, who may have testes, ovotestes, or ovaries. However, the latter do not show the marked increase of 17-ketosteroids in the urine.

In the male, there are no abnormalities of embryonic sex differentiation. However, macrogenitosomia praecox develops early in life. This is not true sexual precocity, since the testes remain small and immature. The Leydig cells do not appear, and the tubules do not show spermatogenesis. The elevation of urinary 17-ketosteroids differentiates the condition from sexual precocity.

In both sexes, there is a marked acceleration of both height and bone age during early childhood. However, because of the early closure of epiphyses, the final stature is usually less than average. There is also a premature appearance of pubic, axillary, and facial hair. Because of the

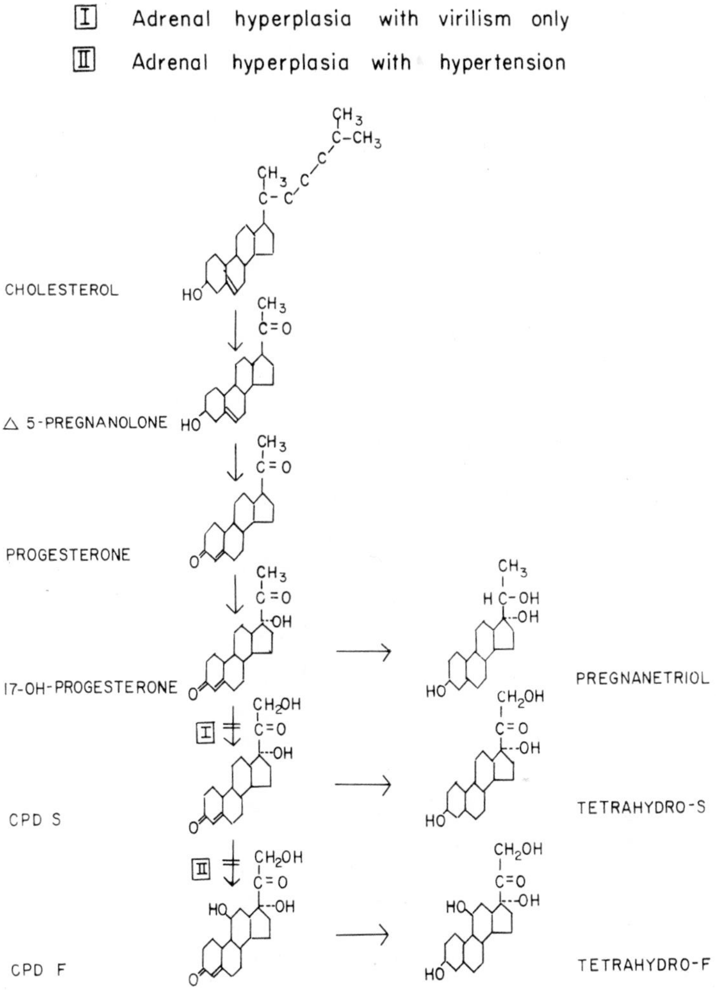

FIG. 37.—Biosynthetic pathway of compound F and sites of metabolic blocks in adrenogenital syndrome. (After Bongiovanni, A. M., and Eberlein, W. R.: Clinical and metabolic variations in the adrenogenital syndrome, Pediatrics 16:628, 1958.)

marked androgenic effects, female sexual development does not occur at the usual time in female pseudohermaphrodites.

The histological changes of the adrenal cortex consist of hyperplasia of the zona reticularis, the presumed site of androgen production.

Patients who have adrenal hyperplasia with virilism only do not develop hypertension or electrolyte disturbances, which is an important point in differential diagnosis in the adrenogenital syndrome.

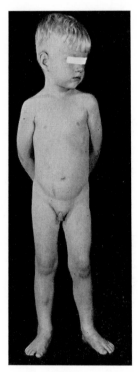

Fig. 38.—A female pseudohermaphrodite with marked increase in the size of the clitoris.

HEREDITY.—Adrenal hyperplasia with virilism only appears to be transmitted by a single autosomal recessive gene. Childs and his co-workers have found many more females were affected than males. They attribute this in part to the fact that genital abnormalities in the female are more striking, and the condition is, therefore, more likely to come to the attention of physicians. Childs has also estimated that the incidence of the disease in Maryland is about 1 in 67,000 births, which would make the incidence of heterozygotes as 1 out of 128 in the general population.

Attempts have been made to detect the effects of a possible gene in the parents, who are presumed to be heterozygotes. This was done by measuring pregnanetriol in the urine after the administration of 60-80 units of ACTH. The parents of known patients appear to excrete somewhat more of that compound than do the normal controls, the difference being significant at the 2-5% level.

PATHOGENESIS.—This has been clarified as a result of three fundamental discoveries: (1) in 1950, Wilkins and his associates showed that both the clinical manifestations and the excessive secretion of androgens can be effectively controlled by the administration of cortisone; (2) the following year, Bartter and his co-workers showed that adrenal hyperplasia probably represents a failure in the synthesis of compound F; and (3) in 1953, Bongiovanni and his fellow workers showed that patients with adrenal hyperplasia routinely excreted an excessive amount of pregnanetriol ($3\alpha,17\alpha,20\alpha$-pregnanetriol).

Bartter, in 1951, first postulated the normal pathway for the synthesis of compound F from cholesterol, as shown in Figure 37. The deficiency of compound F together with the excess of pregnanetriol indicates that the block must occur between 17-hydroxyprogesterone and compound S. It has been postulated that this block occurs as a result of a deficiency of an enzyme which hydroxylates carbon-21 to yield compound F, which might be referred to as "21-hydroxylase." The identity and characteristics of such an enzyme have just been demonstrated.

The effects of a deficiency of such an enzyme are shown in Chart 37. First, its absence would result in the accumulation of 17-hydroxyprogesterone, which in turn would be converted to pregnanetriol and excreted. This would also lead to a deficiency of compound F. The pituitary gland attempts to compensate for this deficiency by overproducing ACTH, and this results in the excessive production of androgens and the excessive excretion of 17-ketosteroids. The effects of the excessive androgens on the male are shown on the left side of the chart; precocious hair growth, accelerated stature, and macrogenitosomia praecox are prominent features. In the female, in addition to enlargement of the clitoris and early growth of hair and stature, there is a suppression of the female sex characteristics at puberty.

DIAGNOSIS.—The diagnosis of adrenal hyperplasia with virilism only is established by (1) the absence of hypertension and electrolyte disturbances; (2) the presence of pregnanetriol in the urine (see Procedure 45); and (3) increased 17-ketosteroids in the urine (see Procedure 46).

TREATMENT.—Wilkins and his co-workers have shown that small doses of cortisone (initial dosage of 50-100 mg daily, followed by 50 mg every 2 or 3 days) are effective in reducing the 17-ketosteroid excretion to normal levels. In female pseudohermaphrodites, this is effective in bringing about breast development and vaginal smears showing estrogen-

CHART 37

ADRENAL HYPERPLASIA WITH VIRILISM ONLY (TYPE I)

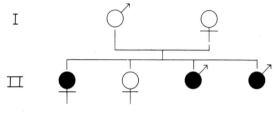

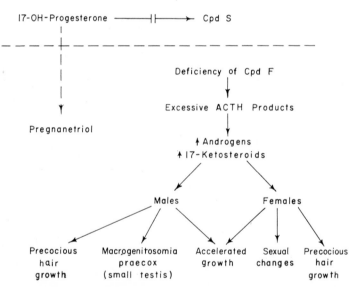

ic activity. In about half of the cases, normal menstruation will occur. In the older patients, there is no change in somatic growth because of early closure of the epiphyses. In some of the males there is an enlargement of the testes, suggesting that normal maturation is occurring.

Replacement therapy with cortisone should be started at an early age in order to insure proper somatic growth and development as well as normal sexual development.

Bartter, F. C.; Albright, F.; Forbes, A. P.; Leaf, A.; Dempsey, E.; and Carroll, E.: The effects of adrenocorticotrophic hormone and cortisone in the adrenogenital syndrome associated with congenital adrenal hyperplasia, J. Clin. Invest. 30:237, 1951.

Bongiovanni, A. M.: In vitro hydroxylation of steroids by whole adrenal homogenates of beef, normal man, and patients with the adrenogenital syndrome, J. Clin. Invest. 37:1342, 1958.

Childs, B.; Grumbach, M. M.; and Van Wyk, J. J.: Virilizing adrenal hyperplasia: A genetic and hormonal study, J. Clin. Invest. 35:213, 1956.

Eberlein, W. R., and Bongiovanni, A. M.: Partial characterization of urinary adrenocortical steroids in adrenal hyperplasia, J. Clin. Invest. 34:1337, 1955.

*Wilkins, L.: The diagnosis of the adrenogenital syndrome and its treatment with cortisone, J. Pediat. 41:860, 1952.

———; Crigler, J. F., Jr.; Silverman, S. H.; Gardner, L. I.; and Migeon, C. J.: Further studies on the treatment of congenital hyperplasia with cortisone: III. The control of hypertension with cortisone, with a discussion of variations in the type of congenital adrenal hyperplasia and report of a case with probable defect of carbohydrate-regulating hormones, J. Clin. Endocrinol. 12:1015, 1952.

5. TYPE II, ADRENAL HYPERPLASIA WITH HYPERTENSION

CLINICAL FEATURES.—In this type of adrenal hyperplasia, all patients show a persistent hypertension, which usually starts in the first few years of life and averages about 180 mm Hg systolic and 140 mm Hg diastolic without therapy. Occasionally the persistent hypertension will result in cardiac decompensation and cerebral vascular accident.

HEREDITY.—Childs has shown that two siblings of patients with this form of adrenal hyperplasia also showed the same condition. It is not clear whether this segregation in particular families is the result of different genes occurring as a system of alleles at one locus, or of different genes at different loci.

PATHOGENESIS.—Eberlein and Bongiovanni have shown that the principal metabolite excreted in the urine is a tetrahydro-S (pregnane-$3\alpha,17\alpha,20$-triol,20-one). There was a complete absence of the normal 11-oxygenated C-21 and 17-ketosteroids. Pregnanetriol was present, but in reduced quantities as compared with the first type. These investigators suggested that this hypertensive form of adrenal hyperplasia represented a metabolic block between compound S and compound F, resulting in the accumulation of both compound S and tetrahydro-S, as shown in Figure 37. These changes could be due to a deficiency of an adrenal enzyme concerned with the introduction of a hydroxyl group into the steroid molecule at C-11, and this could, therefore, be called the deficiency of "11-B-hydroxylase."

The results of this enzyme deficiency are shown in Chart 38, which essentially represents the same pedigree of causes as for adrenal hyper-

CHART 38

ADRENAL HYPERPLASIA WITH HYPERTENSION (TYPE II)

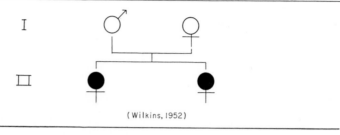

(Wilkins, 1952)

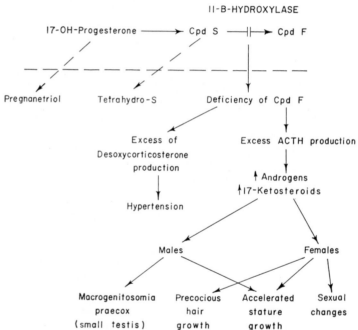

plasia with virilism only. The hypertension may be due to the secretion of desoxycorticosterone by the adrenal cortex, since metabolites of this substance have been partially identified in the urine of a patient with this condition.

DIAGNOSIS.—Adrenal hyperplasia with hypertension can be diagnosed by the presence of (1) persistent hypertension and (2) tetrahydro-S in the urine (see Procedure 47).

TREATMENT.—Cortisone in moderate doses will bring the blood

pressure down to normal levels and completely abolish the abnormal steroids in the urine.

Bongiovanni, A. M., and Eberlein, W. R.: Clinical and metabolic variations in the adrenogenital syndrome, Pediatrics 16:628, 1955.

Eberlein, W. R., and Bongiovanni, A. M.: Congenital adrenal hyperplasia with hypertension: Unusual steroid pattern in blood and urine, J. Clin. Endocrinol. 15:1531, 1955.

*Wilkins, L.: The diagnosis of the adrenogenital syndrome and its treatment with cortisone, J. Pediat. 41:860, 1952.

———; Crigler, J. F., Jr.; Silverman, S. H.; Gardner, L. I.; and Migeon, C. J.: Further studies on the treatment of congenital adrenal hyperplasia with cortisone: III. The control of hypertension with cortisone, with a discussion of variations in the type of congenital adrenal hyperplasia and report of a case with probable defect of carbohydrate-regulating hormones, J. Clin. Endocrinol. 12:1015, 1952.

6. TYPE III, ADRENAL HYPERPLASIA WITH ELECTROLYTE DISTURBANCES

CLINICAL FEATURES.—Certain infants with congenital adrenal hyperplasia develop serious disturbances in electrolyte metabolism. Characteristically, without treatment they become apprehensive and irritable and lose their appetite. Soon vomiting and weight loss occur. The serum electrolytes will show a sodium level of less than 120 mEq/L, a potassium level of more than 6 mEq/L, and a CO_2 level of less than 20 mEq/L. The changes in the serum chloride levels are more variable. If treatment is not promptly instituted, the infant will die from sodium loss and dehydration or from cardiac arrest due to hyperkalemia.

Pathological studies have shown that in some cases the zona glomerulosa of the adrenal is absent. This suggests that the Na-retaining hormone might be lacking, since it is believed to be secreted in that area.

HEREDITY.—The condition appears to be transmitted by a rare recessive gene. Childs has shown that all 11 siblings of 10 index patients with this form of adrenal hyperplasia were salt losers. Also, they found that, unlike Type I, there is less of a disproportion of females to males, possibly because the symptoms in these patients are much more striking and the infants are more likely to come to the attention of physicians.

PATHOGENESIS.—The metabolic block for adrenal hyperplasia with electrolyte disturbances has not been completely worked out. At the present time, there appear to be two types of deficiencies, which may be in some way related: (1) there is the usual deficiency of compound F, which is responsible for the virilization, the excess of 17-ketosteroids, and pregnanetriol; and (2) there is a deficiency of the Na-retaining hormone, which could be desoxycorticosterone. The latter deficiency is

CHART 39

ADRENAL HYPERPLASIA WITH ELECTROLYTE DISTURBANCES
(TYPE III)

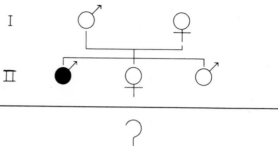

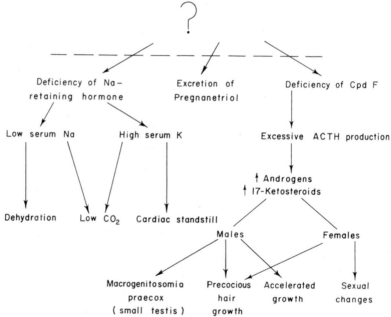

responsible for the loss of sodium and for hyperkalemia and acidosis, which are characteristic of this condition (Chart 39). Recently, Eberlein and Bongiovanni have shown that an essentially complete failure of hydrocortisone synthesis due to lack of 21-hydroxylase may be responsible for these marked changes.

DIAGNOSIS.—The diagnosis can be established by the disturbances of electrolyte metabolism in a patient with virilizing adrenal hyperplasia.

TREATMENT.—Prior to the advent of the corticotrophins, the administration of NaCl together with large doses of desoxycorticosterone

(DOCA) controlled the electrolyte disturbances but did not check the progressive virilization. Wilkins and his co-workers have found that, if cortisone is administered in sufficient amounts to suppress the excretion of 17-ketosteroids, less DOCA and NaCl are required. The exact amounts of steroids and salt to be given must be adjusted on an individual basis.

Butler, A. M.; Ross, R. A.; and Talbot, N. B.: Probable adrenal insufficiency in infant, J. Pediat. 15:831, 1939.

Crigler, J. F., Jr.; Silverman, S. H.; and Wilkins, L.: Further studies on the treatment of congenital adrenal hyperplasia with cortisone: IV. Effect of cortisone and compound B in infants with disturbed electrolyte metabolism, Pediatrics 10:397, 1952.

Eberlein, W. R., and Bongiovanni, A. M.: Steroid metabolism in the "salt-losing" form of congenital adrenal hyperplasia, J. Clin. Invest. 37:889, 1958.

Wilkins, L.: The diagnosis of the adrenogenital syndrome and its treatment with cortisone, J. Pediat. 41:860, 1952.

9

Disturbances in Pigment Metabolism

THE METHEMOGLOBINEMIAS

METHEMOGLOBINEMIA IS A condition in which a substantial proportion of the intracellular hemoglobin exists as methemoglobin, the ferric form of hemoglobin iron, which is incapable of transporting oxygen. When certain drugs, such as acetanilide, antipyrine, and phenacetin, are administered to normal people, a transient methemoglobinemia may result. The condition can also occur as a result of an inborn error of hemoglobin metabolism.

At least three types of congenital methemoglobinemia have been recognized, as described below:

I. CONGENITAL METHEMOGLOBINEMIA: TYPE I

CLINICAL FEATURES.—In Type I, the most common type, methemoglobinemia is present at birth and persists unchanged throughout life unless reversed by some special form of treatment. Most individuals with this condition appear to suffer no physical disability and lead normal active lives without specific treatment. A few show marked cyanosis and develop dyspnea on exertion, and sometimes a compensatory polycythemia. Occasionally, more serious disabilities, such as dwarfing and mental deficiency, are found in association with the defect.

One of the striking features is the fact that the abnormal pigment can be rapidly removed from the patient's blood after the administration of methylene blue, and somewhat more slowly by ascorbic acid and other oxidizing agents.

HEREDITY.—This type of congenital methemoglobinemia is transmitted as a rare recessive. In the pedigree described by Gibson and Harrison, 5 out of 9 brothers and sisters were definitely affected, although the parents and all near relatives did not appear to be. The family lived on a small farm in a remote and mountainous part of Ireland; and since the families of both parents had lived in the same village for generations, consanguinity was likely to have occurred to some degree. The heterozygous carriers of this gene have not been detected by chemical means.

The incidence of this type of congenital methemoglobinemia is not known. The condition is probably quite rare, since only about 50 families have been reported from all over the world.

PATHOGENESIS.—It is generally accepted that in normal blood there is a slow but continuous oxidation of hemoglobin to methemoglobin and that the reducing systems in the erythrocytes are sufficiently active so that

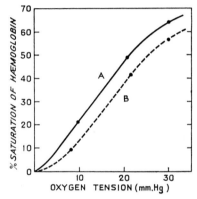

FIG. 39.—Oxygen dissociation curve of blood in Type I methemoglobinemia. *A*, with blood containing 4.2 Gm of methemoglobin per 100 ml of blood. *B*, with blood after removal of methemoglobin with methylene blue. (From Gibson, Q. H., and Harrison, D. C.: Familial idiopathic methaemoglobinaemia, Lancet 2:941, 1947.)

only about 0.4% of the erythrocytes consists of methemoglobin. In congenital methemoglobinemia, there is a defect in the reducing system within the erythrocytes, so that 20-50% of the red-cell pigment is present in the form of methemoglobin, as shown in Figure 39. The amount of methemoglobin does not continue to increase in the blood of affected persons to an unlimited extent because, as the concentration of methemoglobin rises, its rate of reduction with the nonspecific reducing agents in the blood also rises and an equilibrium becomes established. It is probable that, in this respect, ascorbic acid and glutathione are the most important reducing agents in the blood.

In the normal individual, methemoglobin is reduced as shown in Figure 40, pathway *A*. The conversion of glucose to lactate reduces coenzyme I (diphosphopyridine nucleotide); and the reduced coenzyme I together with a flavoprotein, diaphorase I, acts as a carrier in the conversion of methemoglobin to hemoglobin. Under normal circumstances, pathway *B* is of no importance because coenzyme II dehydrogenases do

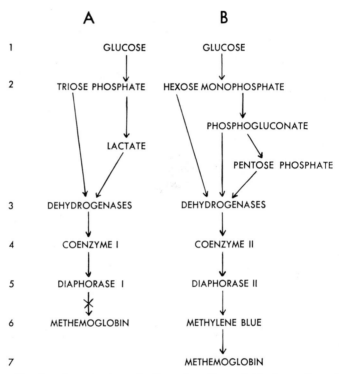

Fig. 40.—Reactions in the reduction of methemoglobin in erythrocytes. *A*, main normal pathway (blocked in idiopathic methemoglobinemia by deficiency of diaphorase I). *B*, effective alternative pathway in presence of catalyst methylene blue. (After Gibson.)

not play a significant part in the reduction of methemoglobin, probably because diaphorase II does not react with methemoglobin.

Gibson and his co-workers have demonstrated that in congenital methemoglobinemia there is a significant deficiency of diaphorase I, and that this results in the metabolic block of the conversion of methemoglobin to hemoglobin and in the accumulation of methemoglobin in the blood cells (Chart 40). When methylene blue is administered, this substance is capable of reacting rapidly with both diaphorase I and II and methemoglobin; and the reduction of the latter compound occurs as a result of both an

CHART 40

CONGENITAL METHEMOGLOBINEMIA: TYPE I

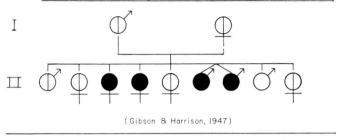

(Gibson & Harrison, 1947)

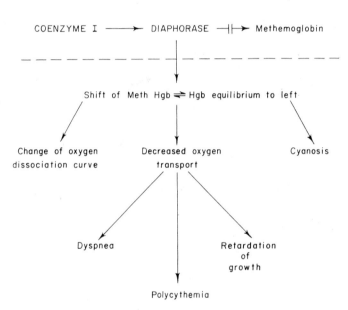

acceleration of pathway *A* and an opening-up of the new pathway *B,* using coenzyme II dehydrogenases.

DIAGNOSIS.—Congenital methemoglobinemia (Types I, II, and III) may be diagnosed by the presence of excessive amounts of methemoglobin in the erythrocytes (see Procedure 48). Type I may be differentiated by the absence or reduction of diaphorase I activity in the blood (see Procedure 49), and by an abnormal oxygen dissociation curve (Procedure 50).

TREATMENT.—Normally, no specific treatment is required. In a crisis, 50 mg of methylene blue will quickly convert the methemoglobin to normal hemoglobin. This form of therapy is of interest because it represents the first example of overcoming the defect by an alternative pathway of metabolism.

Darlington, R. C., and Roughton, F. J. W.: The effect of methemoglobin on the equilibrium between oxygen and hemoglobin, Am. J. Physiol. 137:56, 1942.

Gibson, Q. H.: The reduction of methemoglobin in red blood cells and studies on the cause of idiopathic methemoglobinemia, Biochem. J. 42:13, 1948.

———— and Harrison, D. C.: Familial idiopathic maethemoglobinaemia, Lancet 2:941, 1947.

Waisman, H. A.; Bain, J. A.; Richmond, J. B.; and Munsey, F. A.: Laboratory and clinical studies in congenital methemoglobinemia, Pediatrics 10:293, 1952.

2. CONGENITAL METHEMOGLOBINEMIA: TYPE II

In 1948, Hörlein and Weber reported a second type of congenital methemoglobinemia, which was distinct in a number of ways. Patients with this type of disease had some 15-20% of the red-cell pigment in the form of methemoglobinemia. This did not bother them, and they led normal lives. However, unlike the first type, the condition was transmitted

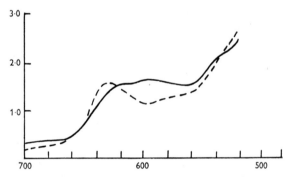

FIG. 41.—Absorption curve of abnormal Type II (*unbroken line*) and normal (*broken line*) methemoglobins. (From Hörlein, H., and Weber, G.: Über chronische familiäre Methämoglobinämie und eine neue Modifikation des Methämoglobins, Deutsche med. Wchnschr. 73:476, 1948.)

from parent to child for four generations, which suggested that the affected individuals were heterozygous for the condition and that it was transmitted as a dominant.

The methemoglobin in these patients had a different spectral absorption curve from that of Type I (Fig. 41). Hörlein and Weber split this protein into its heme and globulin components and recombined the components with fractions obtained from normal blood, and showed that the abnormality lay in the globulin component.

Finally, the administration of methylene blue or ascorbic acid failed to convert the pigment back to normal hemoglobin.

Gerald and his co-workers have reported on another family with the

CHART 41

CONGENITAL METHEMOGLOBINEMIA: TYPE II

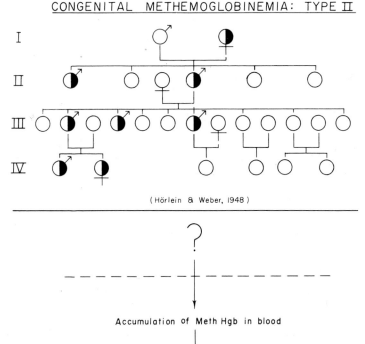

(Hörlein & Weber, 1948)

Accumulation of Meth Hgb in blood

Cyanosis

same spectral abnormality. They were able to separate the abnormal hemoglobin from normal adult hemoglobin electrophoretically, and they demonstrated that in the affected individuals both forms of hemoglobin were present. Because the defect lies in the globulin component, this abnormal hemoglobin has been included among the abnormal hemoglobins and designated "hemoglobin M." More recent work from Gerald's laboratory indicates that hemoglobin M should probably be subdivided into several varieties, depending on the absorption spectra.

These have been subclassified into the "Boston type" (Hgb M_B), "Saskatoon type" (Hgb M_S), and "Milwaukee type" (Hgb M_M).

Although the exact cause for this type of methemoglobinemia is not fully understood, the disturbance in the globulin structure may be similar to that of the abnormal hemoglobins (Chart 41).

Gerald, P. S.: The electrophoretic and spectroscopic characterization of Hgb *M*, Blood 13:936, 1958.

———; Cook, C. D.; and Diamond, L. K.: Hemoglobin *M*, Science 126:300, 1957.

Hörlein, H., and Weber, G.: Über chronische familiäre methämoglobinämie und eine neue Modifikation des Methämoglobins, Deutsche med. Wchnschr. 73:476, 1948.

Kiese, M.; Karz, H.; and Schneider, C.: Chronische Hämiglobinämie durch pathologischen Blutfarbstoff, Klin. Wchnschr. 34:957, 1956.

3. CONGENITAL METHEMOGLOBINEMIA: TYPE III

In 1949, Eder, Finch, and McKee reported a third type of congenital methemoglobinemia. The only known patient was a 23-year-old man who had been blue ever since early infancy. He had a methemoglobin level of 40% and a compensatory polycythemia but no evidence of excessive blood destruction. He was otherwise well and was able to lead a normal life. The family history revealed no similar cases among near relatives.

Unlike the other forms of methemoglobinemia, here the erythrocytes did not show the typical alteration by means of an oxygen dissociation curve. Also, the methemoglobin was quickly removed by both methylene blue and ascorbic acid. Preliminary studies suggest that the diaphorase I system in the erythrocytes of this patient was functioning satisfactorily. The pathogenesis is, therefore, not known.

Eder, H. A.; Finch, C.; and McKee, R. W.: Congenital methemoglobinemia: A clinical and biochemical study of a case, J. Clin. Invest. 28:265, 1949.

OTHER PIGMENT DISTURBANCES

4. HEPATIC PORPHYRIA

Hepatic porphyria may occur in three forms: intermittent acute porphyria; chronic cutaneous porphyria; and mixed porphyria, with both acute and chronic porphyria seen in the same family. The three conditions should probably be considered together.

INTERMITTENT ACUTE PORPHYRIA

As implied by the name, intermittent acute porphyria is characterized by individual attacks of longer or shorter duration, with periods of remission when the patient is completely free of symptoms. During attacks the symptoms vary a great deal. In some cases they are entirely abdominal; in others, nervous; but in most instances, both types of symptoms occur.

CLINICAL FEATURES.—Abdominal pain is often very severe; it takes the form of colic, and may involve all of the abdomen or may be highly localized. The condition has been mistaken for appendicitis, bowel obstruction, renal or biliary colic, perforated ulcer, and pancreatitis. Often there are no bowel movements for days on end.

The nervous manifestations may take four forms: (1) peripheral neuropathy, (2) bulbar symptoms, (3) psychic changes, and (4) autonomic involvement.

The peripheral neuropathy is characterized by pain in the limbs, especially in the legs; weakness; or marked flaccid paralysis. The latter comes on suddenly and may involve many parts of the body all at once, with an irregular distribution. For instance, some patients may show an ankle clonus without patellar reflexes in the same leg. Paralysis of the abdominal or other trunk muscles occurs less frequently, and the sensory system is never affected except for pain.

Bulbar signs are seen in the more severe cases. There is difficulty in swallowing, regurgitation, and aspiration. There may be vocal cord paresis, with a weak, hoarse, high-pitched voice. Tachycardia may be quite marked because of vagal nuclear involvement.

Among the psychic changes, a pseudohysteria is the most common finding. The patients are noted to be excessively "nervous" for years before the first attack. In some instances, acute porphyria has been wrongly diagnosed as schizophrenia or as a neurotic or depressed state.

It is difficult to determine exactly the autonomic nervous system involvement. A pigment is deposited in the autonomic ganglia; and the abdominal pain may be due to this rather than to a direct effect of porphyrin or porphobilinogen on the intestinal wall, as has been suggested. Hypertension is usually marked. In some cases, fatal relapses occur in association with pregnancy. In such instances the infant may show a "passive" porphyria, where the urine is port-wine colored and contains uroporphyrin and excessive coproporphyrin. This symptom persists for a few days and then disappears, suggesting that these substances were transferred across the placental barrier.

The characteristic biochemical finding in acute porphyria is the presence of abnormal quantities of porphobilinogen. There appears to be also an increased excretion of δ-aminolevulinic acid. However, most of the free porphyrins which at various times have been reported in the urine of such patients were probably mainly formed secondarily from excreted porphobilinogen.

HEREDITY.—The genetics of acute porphyria have been extensively studied by Waldenström in Sweden. The condition appears to be transmitted as an autosomal dominant. Penetrance is incomplete, partly because the age of onset is highly variable, onset seldom occurring before puberty. Acute porphyria has been seen in both members of a pair of concordant uniovular twins. The incidence of consanguinity is not increased. For some unexplained reason, the ratio of affected males to females is about 2 to 3.

Waldenström has shown that the incidence of acute porphyria is 1.4 per 100,000 in Sweden but increases to 1 in 100 in Lapland in the northern part of the country.

PATHOGENESIS.—Studies by Shemin, Rimington, Granick, and others indicate that the conversion of precursor pyrrole to porphyrins occurs as a result of the following steps (Fig. 42): (1) Two molecules of δ-aminolevulinic acid condense in the presence of a dehydrase to give the monopyrrole "porphobilinogen." (2) Porphobilinogen is then acted upon anaerobically by two enzymes. One enzyme is a deaminase, which condenses porphobilinogen to uroporphyrinogen I, which in turn is converted by auto-oxidation to uroporphyrin I. (3) A second enzyme is an isomerase, which, acting together with the deaminase, converts porphobilinogen to uroporphyrinogen III, which in turn is converted to uroporphyrin III. (4) Finally, a third enzyme fraction, a decarboxylase, converts uroporphyrinogen III to coproporphyrinogen III, which then is converted to coproporphyrin II.

Two pieces of evidence have been presented regarding the possible metabolic error in acute porphyria. Neuberger and his co-workers have shown that, when δ-aminolevulinic acid is administered orally to a normal

CHART 42

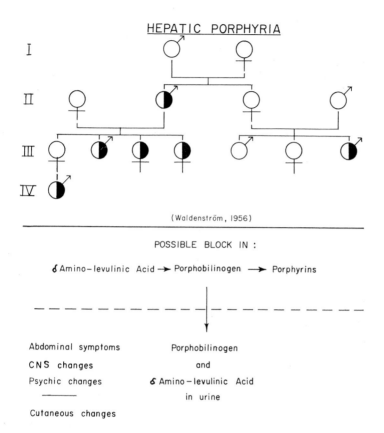

HEPATIC PORPHYRIA

(Waldenström, 1956)

POSSIBLE BLOCK IN :

δ Amino–levulinic Acid ⟶ Porphobilinogen ⟶ Porphyrins

Abdominal symptoms	Porphobilinogen
CNS changes	and
Psychic changes	δ Amino–levulinic Acid
———	in urine
Cutaneous changes	

adult, porphyria does not develop. However, when it is administered to patients with porphyria, it is converted to urinary porphobilinogen to a much greater degree. Also, Granick has reported the presence of rather large quantities of δ-aminolevulinic acid in the urine of a patient with acute porphyria during a clinical remission. This would suggest that a partial block above the porphobilinogen step might be responsible for porphyria (Chart 42). More recently, experimental porphyria has been produced in animals through the use of compounds with a chemical structure such as that shown on page 182.

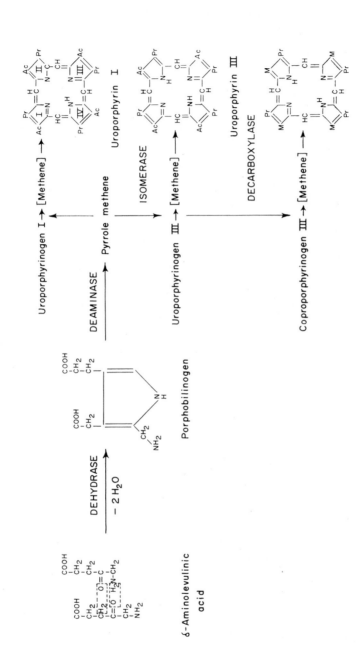

Fig. 42.—Conversion of pyrrole to porphyrins.

184

Although these chemical studies are very promising, they do not, unfortunately, help to explain the peculiar abdominal and central nervous system symptoms of porphyria. Explanations for these symptoms are yet to be determined.

DIAGNOSIS.—Acute porphyria can be diagnosed by the characteristic clinical picture and the presence in the urine (1) of porphobilinogen (see Procedure 51) and of δ-amino-levulinic acid and (2) lesser quantities of zinc complexes of uroporphyrin I and III (see Procedure 52) and coproporphyrin III (Procedure 53). The bone marrow in this form of porphyria is not affected.

TREATMENT.—Supportive and symptomatic treatment is all that can be given. Patients should also avoid alcohol, barbiturates, and hepatotoxins, which are likely to precipitate attacks. Death, when it occurs, is usually the result of a rapidly ascending paralysis which finally affects the medullary centers.

*Ciba Symposium on Porphyrin Biosynthesis and Metabolism (London: J. & A. Churchill, Ltd., 1955).

*Granick, S., et al.: Metabolism and Function of Iron, Report of the Nineteenth Ross Pediatric Research Conference (Columbus, Ohio: Ross Laboratories, 1955).

———— and Schrieck, H. G.: Porphobilinogen and delta amino-levulinic acid in acute porphyria, Proc. Soc. Exper. Biol. & Med. 88:270, 1955.

Neuberger, A.; Scott, J. J.; and Gray, C. H.: The metabolism of delta amino-levulinic acid in acute porphyria, Biochem. J. 58:xli, 1954.

Waldenström, J.: Studies on the incidence and heredity of acute porphyria in Sweden, Acta genet. et stat. med. 6:122, 1956.

————Studien über Porphyria, Acta med. scandinav., supp. 82, 1937.

CHRONIC CUTANEOUS PORPHYRIA

Chronic cutaneous porphyria usually appears in middle-aged adults. The patients often present a chronic eczematoid dermatitis and a lesser degree of the typical hydroa aestivale seen in porphyria erythropoietica (p. 67). The abdominal and nervous system symptoms are milder, although cirrhosis of the liver sometimes develops late in the course of the disease.

This type of porphyria is also familial and is transmitted as an autosomal dominant with incomplete penetrance.

The main chemical difference between this form of porphyria and the acute form is that porphobilinogen is absent from the urine in this form; whereas uroporphyrins I and III and coproporphyrin III are present and increased, just as in the acute form.

In clinical remission, there is a marked increase of protoporphyrin and coproporphyrin in the feces. This would suggest that this condition represents a disturbance in porphyrin metabolism which is quite unlike that found in congenital or acute porphyria. The nature of this disorder, however, is quite obscure.

Brunsting, L. A.; Mason, H. L.; and Aldrich, R. A.: Adult form of chronic porphyria with cutaneous manifestations, J.A.M.A. 146:1207, 1951.
Schmid, R.; Schwartz, S.; and Watson, C. J.: Porphyrin content of bone marrow and liver in the various forms of porphyria, Arch. Int. Med. 93:167, 1954.

MIXED PORPHYRIA

The term "mixed porphyria" applies to patients presenting both abdominal and nervous system symptoms in association with porphobilinogen in the urine during the course of chronic cutaneous porphyria. Several instances have been reported where both chronic cutaneous porphyria and intermittent acute porphyria are known to exist in the same family.

Brunsting, L. A.; Mason, H. L.; and Aldrich, R. A.: Adult form of chronic porphyria with cutaneous manifestations, J.A.M.A. 146:1207, 1951.
Dean, G., and Barnes, H. D.: Porphyria, Brit. M. J. 1:298, 1958.
Wells, Q. C., and Rimington, C.: Studies on a case of porphyria cutanea tarda, Brit. J. Dermat. 65:337, 1953.

5. CONGENITAL NONHEMOLYTIC JAUNDICE WITH KERNICTERUS

In 1952, Crigler and Najjar reported on a group of infants with a previously undescribed congenital abnormality characterized by the elevation of "indirect" bilirubin. All of these patients were from a large kindred in western Maryland, where there had been close inbreeding for several generations. Since extrapyramidal tract involvement is a prominent feature of the disease, the condition was named "congenital nonhemolytic jaundice with kernicterus."

CLINICAL FEATURES.—Infants with this condition develop jaundice early, frequently on the second day of life. The increase in bilirubin is limited to the "indirect" fraction, which gradually rises to levels of between 25 and 45 mg/100 ml. Opisthotonus, spasticity, and rigidity soon become apparent; and many of the infants with kernicterus die in the first year of life.

At postmortem, staining of the basal ganglia is a characteristic finding. Surprisingly, the liver shows no real abnormalities except for the presence of bile thrombi in the hepatic canaliculi.

Most of the laboratory tests are not remarkable. Blood-grouping studies reveal no incompatibilities. Fragility tests, bone marrow examinations, and reticulocyte counts are usually within normal limits. The liver funcion tests are negative; however, there is a marked inability of the patient to handle bilirubin, as shown by the bilirubin excretion test (see Procedure 54).

HEREDITY.—The condition has been seen in only two families: (1) in the large kindred in western Maryland and (2) in a single child of Italian ancestry. In both instances, consanguinity was noted. Congenital nonhemolytic jaundice with kernicterus is probably transmitted by a single autosomal recessive gene, which is expressed only in homozygous individuals.

Childs has recently demonstrated that the parents of such individuals show a decreased ability to form glucuronides following the administration of salicylates and other metabolites. This would suggest that they are heterozygous carriers of the abnormal gene.

PATHOGENESIS.—Schmid and his associates have shown that "indirect" bilirubin is converted to "direct" bilirubin by the following reaction:

Uridine diphosphate glucuronic acid (UDPGA) + Bilirubin ("indirect")

$$\xrightarrow[\text{Microsomes}]{\text{Liver}} \text{Bilirubin glucuronide ("direct")} + \text{Uridine diphosphate (UDP)}$$

This reaction is catalyzed by an enzyme system in the microsomes of mammalian liver which appears to be the same system that conjugates such substances as o-aminophenol or phenolphthalein with glucuronic acid.

The bilirubin from the serum of patients with congenital nonhemolytic jaundice with kernicterus has been crystallized by ammonium sulfate fractionation and found to be of the unconjugated type. Also, bilirubinuria is absent, and the bile in these patients is colorless and contains only traces of unconjugated bilirubin. Finally, the glucuronide formation of menthol, of salicylate, and of the metabolites of hydrocortisone is markedly depressed, which indicates that this condition represents a metabolic block at the stage of bilirubin conjugation and probably is due to a specific enzyme defect (Chart 43).

Extensive studies in vitro and in vivo have shown that a relationship exists between the elevation of "indirect" bilirubin in the serum and the kernicterus in erythroblastosis fetalis, premature infants, and those suffering from synkavit (menadiol) toxicity. The elevation of the bilirubin in this form is probably responsible for the brain damage in this disease. The reason for some infants getting kernicterus while others escape this complication is not known.

DIAGNOSIS.—Congenital familial nonhemolytic jaundice with kernicterus must be differentiated (1) from familial nonhemolytic jaundice

CHART 43

CONGENITAL NONHEMOLYTIC JAUNDICE
WITH KERNICTERUS

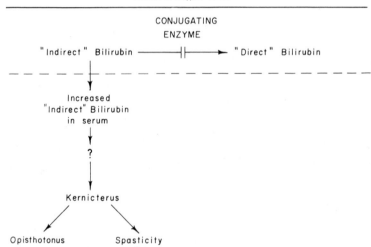

(Childs & Najjar, 1956)

CONJUGATING
ENZYME

"Indirect" Bilirubin ⟶ ‖→ "Direct" Bilirubin

Increased
"Indirect" Bilirubin
in serum

?

Kernicterus

Opisthotonus   Spasticity
&
Ataxia

Gilbert's disease) by the difference in age of onset and prognosis, (2) from chronic idiopathic jaundice with hepatic pigmentation (Dubin-Johnson syndrome) by the liver changes microscopically, and (3) from erythroblastosis fetalis by blood-grouping studies. The diagnosis is ultimately established by the ability of the liver to conjugate bilirubin (see Procedure 55).

TREATMENT.—Exchange transfusions temporarily lower the serum bilirubin levels and may be helpful during the first weeks of life, when the brain is presumably most susceptible to damage.

Billing, B. H., and Lathe, G. H.: The excretion of bilirubin as an ester glucuronide, giving the direct van den Bergh reaction, Biochem. J. 63:6P, 1956.
Childs, B.: The nature of direct bilirubin, Bull. Johns Hopkins Hosp. 97:333, 1955.
———— and Najjar, V. A.: Familial nonhemolytic jaundice with kernicterus, Pediatrics 18:369, 1956.
Crigler, J. F., Jr., and Najjar, V. A.: Congenital familial nonhemolytic jaundice with kernicterus, Pediatrics 10:169, 1952.
Rosenthal, I. M.; Zimmerman, H. J.; and Hardy, N.: Congenital nonhemolytic jaundice with disease of the central nervous system, Pediatrics 18:378, 1956.
Schmid, R.; Axelrod, J.; Hammaker, L.; and Rosenthal, I. M.: Congenital defects in bilirubin metabolism, J. Clin. Invest. 36:927, 1957.
————; Hammaker, L.; and Axelrod, J.: The enzymatic formation of bilirubin glucuronide, Arch. Biochem. 70:255, 1957.

6. FAMILIAL NONHEMOLYTIC JAUNDICE (Gilbert's disease)

Early in this century, Gilbert and his co-workers in France called attention to a nonhemolytic, acholuric icterus which was familial in nature. Subsequent workers felt that Gilbert and his associates were describing hereditary spherocytosis, a condition which was becoming known at that time, and little attention was paid to the condition "familial nonhemolytic jaundice" for many years. In the past decade, interest in this condition has been renewed, and some 350 cases are now recorded in the literature.

CLINICAL FEATURES.—The age of onset is not known. Most of the patients who come to the attention of physicians are between 15 and 25 years of age, but one might well assume that the symptoms have been present, although undetected, for some years previously.

Most patients with familial nonhemolytic jaundice are not aware that they are abnormal. They will frequently complain of weakness and lack of energy; but they attribute this state to overindulgence in alcohol, lack of sleep, overwork, excitement, or intercurrent infection. The jaundice appears only intermittently, and even then is usually mild in nature. The elevation of serum bilirubin is limited to the "indirect" fraction.

Other laboratory tests are within normal limits. There is no micro cytosis or spherocytosis; the osmotic and mechanical fragility of erythro cytes is not altered; and the bone marrow is normal. Quantitativ measurements of the urobilinogen in the stools have shown no evidenc of blood destruction. The reactions of the liver function tests are consis ently negative, and biopsies of the liver show only a slight fatty infiltratio of the liver cells. As in congenital familial nonhemolytic jaundice wit

CHART 44

FAMILIAL NONHEMOLYTIC JAUNDICE

(Dameshek & Singer, 1941)

CONJUGATING
ENZYME

"Indirect" Bilirubin ⟶ ⟶ "Direct" Bilirubin

Increased "indirect"
bilirubin

Fatigue
Weakness

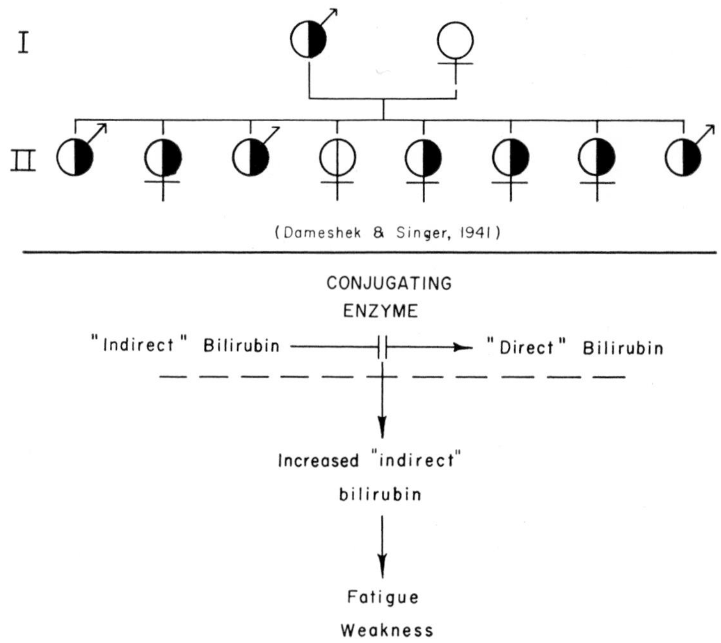

kernicterus, there is delayed excretion of bilirubin, as shown by the bil rubin excretion test.

HEREDITY.—Familial nonhemolytic jaundice is probably transmi ted as a dominant trait with incomplete penetrance. This is suggested i one study where half of the siblings and a quarter of the parents showe bilirubin levels in excess of 1.3 mg/100 ml. The exact hereditary pa tern is difficult to determine because some affected individuals do n show consistent hyperbilirubinemia and other, normal, persons sho slight icterus with fatigue or excessive intake of alcohol.

PATHOGENESIS.—The etiology of this disturbance is far less well understood than is that of congenital familial nonhemolytic jaundice with kernicterus. Dameshek and Singer have postulated that the disturbance may also represent a congenital inability to convert "indirect" bilirubin to "direct" bilirubin (Chart 44). Recently, Arias and London have shown that a deficiency of bilirubin glucuronyl transferase exists in a patient with Gilbert's disease. This raises the serious question of whether congenital familial nonhemolytic jaundice with kernicterus and Gilbert's disease are one and the same condition. If so, some explanation must be found for the marked differences in clinical symptoms and the mode of genetic transmission.

DIAGNOSIS.—For the present, familial nonhemolytic jaundice should be differentiated (1) from congenital familial nonhemolytic jaundice with kernicterus by the age of onset and severity of bilirubinemia; (2) from chronic idiopathic jaundice with hepatic pigmentation (Dubin-Johnson syndrome), where the diagnosis is made on the basis of liver biopsy and negative family history; (3) from hereditary spherocytosis by the absence of spherocytes and hemolysis; and (4) from jaundice due to liver disease by liver function tests.

TREATMENT.—None is required.

Alwall, N.; Laurell, C. B.; and Nilsby, I.: Studies on heredity in cases of nonhemolytic bilirubinemia without van den Bergh reaction (hereditary nonhemolytic bilirubinemia), Acta med. scandinav. 124:114, 1946.

Arias, I. M., and London, J. M.: Bilirubin glucuronide formation in vitro; demonstration of a defect in Gilbert's disease, Science 126:563, 1957.

Dameshek, W., and Singer, L.: Familial nonhemolytic jaundice: Constitutional hepatic dysfunction with indirect van den Bergh reaction, Arch. Int. Med. 67:259, 1941.

Gilbert, A.; Lereboullet, P.; and Herscher, M.: Les trois cholemies congenitales, Bull. et mém. Soc. méd. hôp. Paris 24:1203, 1907.

*Meulengracht, E.: A review of chronic intermittent juvenile jaundice, Quart. J. Med. 16:83, 1947.

10

Other Probable
Enzyme Disturbances

The present chapter covers four miscellaneous enzyme disturbances. Two of these are fully expressed and the other two become apparent only under unusual circumstances. Those in the former group are *hypophosphatasia,* which is caused by a deficiency of alkaline phosphatase, and *cystic fibrosis of the pancreas,* which is a generalized disease involving all of the exocrine glands. Those in the latter group are *deficiency of glucose-6-PO₄ dehydrogenase,* which appears only when the individual has been exposed to naphthalene, fava bean, or primaquine, and *deficiency of pseudocholinesterase,* which can be demonstrated only when the patient has been given suxamethonium or procaine.

I. HYPOPHOSPHATASIA

In 1948, Rathbun reported on a 3-week-old infant with rachitic bone lesions and a diminution of alkaline phosphatase activity despite adequate doses of vitamin D. He felt that this represented a new developmental anomaly, and suggested that the condition be called "hypophosphatasia."

CLINICAL FEATURES.—Patients with this condition show marked changes in the bones and teeth. The skeletal abnormalities include: marked knock knees, bowing of the femurs and tibias, enlarged wrists, Hansen's groove, and a protuberant abdomen. These changes are frequently present at birth; and sometimes, by x-ray studies, they can be shown to be present in utero. Spontaneous shedding of teeth prematurely is also a common feature of the disease.

Roentgenographic studies show poor mineralization of the long bones, ribs, jaws, and teeth. There are focal symmetrical defects in the metaphyses of the long bones. The spongiosa appears to be reduced, and the architecture of the cortex is coarse. There is a distinct brush border at the distal ends of the radius, tibia, and fibula.

At postmortem, many of the skeletal changes are found to be similar to those of rickets. The long bones are considerably shorter than the long bones of the normal infant of similar age. There is evidence of a deficiency of calcification, with the cartilaginous epiphyses separated from the diaphysis by a zone consisting mainly of osteoid tissue. Only vestiges of a zone of provisional calcification are present, and in most places the cartilage gives way to osteoid tissue without any calcification. There is also marked irregularity of the endochondral ossification, with islands and tongues of degenerate cartilage commonly present in the disorderly metaphyseal zones. Alkaline phosphatase is usually diminished or absent in the serum, tissues, and bone sections examined.

If the bone changes are marked, the affected infant may die in the neonatal period. If they are moderate, the infant will survive for a few years and die early in childhood, from either intercurrent infection or the complications of the bony deformities. A few individuals survive to adult life and are not greatly incapacitated by the defect.

HEREDITY.—Hypophosphatasia appears to be transmitted as an autosomal recessive. The condition is usually seen among siblings, and not in different generations. A history of consanguinity has been noted in some of the affected families.

The heterozygous carriers of the abnormal gene can be detected in two ways: (1) the known parents of affected children frequently, although not always, show a decrease of alkaline phosphatase in the serum; and (2) these same individuals usually show an increased excretion of phosphoethanolamine, an abnormal metabolite, in the urine.

The frequency of hypophosphatasia in the population is not known. The condition is probably not rare, however, since some 20 affected families have been described in England and at least an equal number in the United States.

PATHOGENESIS.—The primary metabolic defect in hypophosphatasia appears to be a deficiency or absence of alkaline phosphatase, a disturbance which is genetically determined. This defect appears to be responsible for the principal bone changes in this disease: (1) deficient calcification, (2) excess of osteoid tissue, and (3) irregularity of endochondral ossification (Fig. 43).

In 1955, McCance, Morrison, and Dent in England, and Fraser, Yendt, and Christie in Canada, simultaneously observed that phosphoethanolamine was present in the urine of all patients with hypophosphatasia. More recently Prankerd has shown, in a preliminary way, that adenosinemonophosphate may also be in the urine of these patients.

At the present time it is difficult to postulate how these three biochemical defects are interrelated. There appears to be no real disturbance in

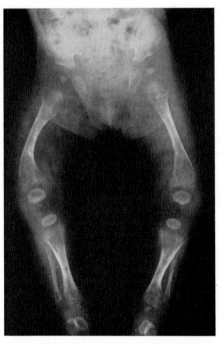

FIG. 43.—Pelvis and extremities in hypophosphatasia. There is poor ossification at the metaphysial ends of the bones with slight irregularity of the epiphysial-metaphysial junctions; also, spotty areas of incompletely ossified bone in the tibias.

the handling of phosphoethanolamine. One current view is that the deficiency of bone alkaline phosphatase results in the accumulation of the natural substrate for that enzyme, which may well be phosphoethanolamine (Chart 45).

DIAGNOSIS.—Hypophosphatasia may be diagnosed by a decrease of alkaline phosphatase in the serum (see Procedure 56) and the presence of phosphoethanolamine in increased amounts in the urine. (see Procedure 57).

TREATMENT.—The treatment is mainly supportive. There is no indication that vitamin D has any therapeutic value in this disease.

CHART 45

HYPOPHOSPHATASIA

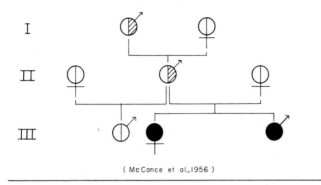

(McCance et al.,1956)

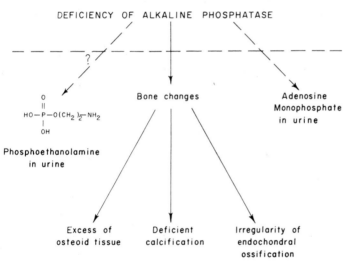

DEFICIENCY OF ALKALINE PHOSPHATASE

Bone changes

Adenosine
Monophosphate
in urine

$$HO-\overset{\overset{\text{O}}{\|}}{\underset{\underset{\text{OH}}{|}}{P}}-O(CH_2)_2-NH_2$$

Phosphoethanolamine
in urine

Excess of
osteoid tissue

Deficient
calcification

Irregularity of
endochondral
ossification

*Fraser, D.: Hypophosphatasia, Am. J. Med. 22:730, 1957.
———; Yendt, E. R.; and Christie, F. H. E.: Metabolic abnormalities in hypophosphatasia, Lancet 1:286, 1955.
McCance, R. A.; Fairweather, D. V. I.; Barrett, A. M.; and Morrison, A. B.: Genetic, clinical, biochemical and pathological features of hypophosphatasia, Quart. J. Med. 25:523, 1956.
———; Morrison, A. B.; and Dent, C. E.: The excretion of phosphoethanolamine and hypophosphatasia, Lancet 1:131, 1955.
Rathbun, J. C.: Hypophosphatasia, Am. J. Dis. Child. 75:822, 1948.
Sobel, E. H.; Clark, L. C., Jr.; Fox, R. P.; and Robinow, M.: Rickets, deficiency of "alkaline" phosphatase activity, and premature loss of teeth in childhood, Pediatrics 11:309, 1953.

2. CYSTIC FIBROSIS OF THE PANCREAS

Cystic fibrosis of the pancreas is a congenital defect in which the clinical evidences of the celiac syndrome, resulting from pancreatic exocrine insufficiency, are combined with severe pulmonary disease and disturbances in the secretion of the sweat and salivary glands.

CLINICAL FEATURES.—The earliest and most severe manifestation of fibrocystic disease is *meconium ileus* in the newborn infant. In this condition, the meconium fails to liquefy because of a marked deficiency or absence of pancreatic enzymes. The thick, tenacious meconium forms plugs, causing intestinal obstruction; and the terminal ileum becomes greatly distended and hypertrophied. Failure to correct this condition soon after birth results in intestinal perforation and meconium peritonitis. On the other hand, after surgical correction prognosis in such children is similar to that in other children with cystic fibrosis of the pancreas. About 15% of all affected children develop meconium ileus at birth.

If the deficiency of pancreatic enzyme is not complete, the infants do not develop meconium ileus, but the initial symptoms result from poor intestinal digestion or respiratory tract infections. These infants appear to be normal at birth but soon fail to gain weight despite adequate food intake. In fact, many show an increased appetite. Also, the parents notice that the infant passes foul-smelling, bulky stools, a symptom which becomes worse following the addition of cereal or starchy foods.

The respiratory symptoms start off first as a severe nonproductive cough, which later becomes spasmodic and productive and at times is followed by vomiting. Because of these symptoms, many of the infants are believed to be suffering from pertussis. The absence of the thin, watery secretions of mucus, which normally lubricate the cilia of the bronchial epithelium, causes the ciliary movement to be abolished. This results in the formation of thick, tenacious mucus within the trachea and bronchi, and the child coughs to try to expel the material. The lack of ciliary action also permits secondary bacterial invasion of the lungs by Staphylococcus aureus of comparatively low virulence. The pulmonary infiltration gives a characteristic x-ray picture which is diagnostic of the disease (Fig. 44).

In 1951, Kessler and Andersen reported that a number of infants with fibrocystic disease suffered from heat prostration during a heat wave in New York City. Two years later, Sant'Agnese and his co-workers showed that such prostration is caused by a depletion of salt. The concentration of sodium and chloride in the sweat of these infants was from 2 to 4

times that of normal controls. Similar changes were observed in the secretions of the salivary glands. In 1955, Sant'Agnese reported a fourth
defect, that of mucoproteins in the duodenal fluid. Precipitates of these
mucoproteins by an ethanol-benzene mixture are not readily soluble in

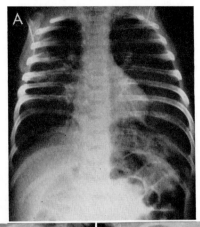

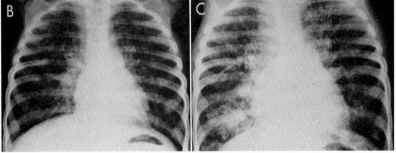

Fig. 44.—Anteroposterior views of patient with cystic fibrosis of pancreas.
A, some pneumatic infiltrate in right midlung field with bilateral emphysema and
a small amount of pulmonary fibrosis. *B,* 1½ years later, diffuse pulmonary fibrosis and emphysema progressing. *C,* 1½ years later, heart slightly enlarged; marked
progression of the pulmonary fibrosis; and pneumonic consolidation in the right
lower lobe.

water, whereas the precipitates from normal individuals are water soluble.
These observations have led to the conclusion that fibrocystic disease of
the pancreas represents a generalized disturbance of many—and perhaps all—of the exocrine glands.

Infants with this disease show marked retardation in physical
growth, signs of vitamin deficiencies due to poor absorption of fats,
bronchiectasis, and cor pulmonale. Cirrhosis of the liver is also a compli-

cation. Death usually occurs in the first year or two of life, but life expectancy has been greatly prolonged through the combined use of high-protein diets, pancreatin preparations, and wide-spectrum chemotherapeutic agents.

During the past few years a number of reports have appeared showing the existence of partial pancreatic insufficiency. The affected individuals frequently show only one of the several manifestations usually seen in fibrocystic disease of the pancreas. Some individuals develop a progressive decrease of pancreatic enzymes without pulmonary symptoms. Others show changes in sweat electrolytes. These cases appear to be examples of a partial manifestation of cystic fibrosis, and the affected individuals are not thought to represent heterozygous carriers of the abnormal gene.

HEREDITY.—Cystic fibrosis of the pancreas is transmitted as an autosomal recessive trait. Several large studies in both England and the United States suggest that the condition is fully penetrant. The disease affects siblings but not parents or collateral relatives. Since the gene is so common in the population, one does not find an increased incidence of consanguinity.

The heterozygous carriers of the abnormal trait are detectable in two ways: (1) many of the parents of affected children show an intermediate elevation of sweat electrolyte levels, and (2) some of them also demonstrate a decrease in duodenal enzymes. The former change appears with much greater regularity.

Population surveys have shown that the incidence of cystic fibrosis is between 0.7 and 1.0 cases per 1,000 live births. This means that 1 out of every 16-20 persons are carriers for the abnormal gene, a surprisingly common one. Since the homozygotes for cystic fibrosis always die before the age of reproductivity, geneticists have raised the question: How is this high gene frequency maintained? Two theories have been proposed: either (1) the heterozygotes have greater survival value or reproductive fitness, or both, compared with the general population; or (2) there is a high mutation rate for this gene. Since there is no specific evidence to support the former, we have to assume that the latter is the case.

PATHOGENESIS.—Gochberg and Cooke have postulated the mechanism responsible for fibrocystic disease. They feel that it may be caused by a genetically determined deficiency of an enzyme, coenzyme, or substrate, with a consequent alteration in the release of energy. As a result, the composition of secretion is abnormal. This may be reflected by the decrease of free-water clearance in this disease.

In any event, the generalized disturbance of exocrine gland function

CHART 46

CYSTIC FIBROSIS OF THE PANCREAS

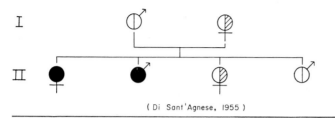

(Di Sant'Agnese, 1955)

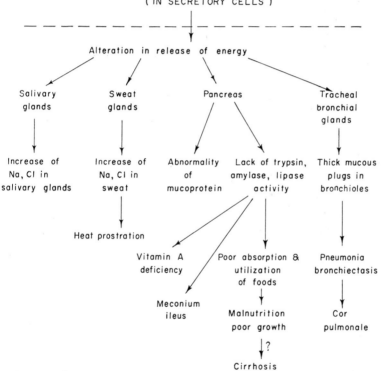

? DEFICIENCY OF ENZYME, COENZYME OR SUBSTRATE
(IN SECRETORY CELLS)

Alteration in release of energy

| Salivary glands | Sweat glands | Pancreas | Tracheal bronchial glands |

| Increase of Na, Cl in salivary glands | Increase of Na, Cl in sweat | Abnormality of mucoprotein | Lack of trypsin, amylase, lipase activity | Thick mucous plugs in bronchioles |

Heat prostration

Vitamin A deficiency

Poor absorption & utilization of foods

Pneumonia bronchiectasis

Meconium ileus

Malnutrition poor growth

Cor pulmonale

↓ ?

Cirrhosis

appears to be responsible for all of the signs and symptoms of the disease (Chart 46). The changes in the electrolyte content of the sweat cause heat prostration. The lack of pancreatic enzymes causes meconium ileus in the young infant and poor absorption and utilization of food in the older child. This exocrine disturbance is also probably responsible for the changes in mucoproteins. The lack of mucous gland secretions accounts for the pulmonary changes and, in turn, cor pulmonale.

From these facts one can conclude that deficiencies of trypsin and amylase are not the fundamental enzyme defects in this disease but that they merely reflect a more basic process.

DIAGNOSIS.—Although many tests are available for establishing the diagnosis of fibrocystic disease, probably the most valuable ones are those showing (1) abnormal composition of sweat electrolytes (see Procedure 58); (2) decrease of duodenal enzymes (this can be screened by the stool gelatin test [see Procedure 59], and more accurately ascertained by duodenal intubation [see Procedure 60]); and (3) changes in mucoprotein characteristics (Procedure 61).

TREATMENT.—Early diagnosis, together with proper therapy, can frequently prolong the life expectancy greatly. In meconium ileus, surgical intervention is indicated. When the condition appears in infancy, the following regimen is recommended: (1) normal diet with avoidance of excessive fat; (2) twice the recommended dose of water-miscible vitamins; (3) viokase powder, ¼-½ teaspoonful with each meal; (4) Aureomycin® or Achromycin® 5-15 mg per kilogram body weight daily; (5), in advanced cases, aerosol consisting of 100,000 units of aqueous penicillin and 250 mg streptomycin in 4 cc saline or detergent three times daily.

*Bodian, M.: Fibrocystic Disease of the Pancreas (New York: Grune & Stratton, Inc., 1953).

*Fibrocystic Disease of the Pancreas, Eighteenth Ross Pediatric Research Conference (Columbus, Ohio: Ross Laboratories, 1955).

Gochberg, S. H., and Cooke, R. E.: Physiology of the sweat gland in cystic fibrosis of the pancreas, Pediatrics 18:701, 1956.

Di Sant'Agnese, P. A.: Fibrocystic disease of the pancreas with normal or partial pancreatic function, Pediatrics 15:683, 1955.

————; Darling, R. C.; Perera, G. A.; and Shea, E.: Abnormal electrolyte composition of sweat in cystic fibrosis of pancreas, Pediatrics 12:549, 1953.

————; Dische, Z.; and Danilczenko, A.: Physicochemical differences of mucoproteins in duodenal fluid of patients with cystic fibrosis of the pancreas and controls, Pediatrics 19:252, 1957.

Kessler, W. R., and Andersen, D. H.: Heat prostration in fibrocystic disease of pancreas and other conditions, Pediatrics 8:648, 1951.

*Shwachman, H.; Leubner, H.; and Catzel, P.: Mucoviscidosis, Advances Pediat. 7:249, 1955.

PART IV

Disturbances in Renal
Transport Mechanisms

A NUMBER OF hereditary diseases arise because of defects in specific renal transport mechanisms. Before describing these disturbances in detail, it might be useful to review briefly how the mechanisms work in normal persons.

Urine is formed by two separate processes within the kidney: (1) A protein-like ultrafiltrate of plasma is prepared within the glomeruli; this appears to be a purely physical process and does not require any specialized transport mechanisms. (2) All but a minute fraction of this ultrafiltrate is reabsorbed in the proximal convoluted tubules; the remainder is excreted as urine. The process of reabsorption takes place because of specific renal transport mechanisms across the cell membranes. It has been shown that a number of distinct transport mechanisms are present in the tubular epithelium and that each of these operates more or less independently. For example, certain substances, such as water and electrolytes, are reabsorbed in sufficient proportions to maintain isotonicity with the extracellular fluid. Other substances, like glucose and the amino acids, must work against concentration gradients of a hundredfold or more.

At the present time, it is not entirely clear how these renal transport mechanisms function. Presumably, each one is governed by a separate gene which synthesizes either a special enzyme or an enzyme-like substance, which in turn controls the reabsorption of a particular substance. However, no such enzymes have yet been isolated, and this may prove to be too simple an explanation. On the other hand, we are aware of at least six inborn errors of metabolism which result from a defect in one or another of the renal transport mechanisms, as shown in Table 3. The first four represent defects of a single mechanism; the last two involve several such mechanisms. The latter suggest that the genes for these renal transport mech-

TABLE 3.—RENAL TRANSPORT DEFECTS

	RENAL TRANSPORT MECHANISMS					
			Amino Acids			
CLINICAL CONDITIONS	H₂O	Glucose	Dibasic	Others	P	K
1. Nephrogenic diabetes insipidus	+					
2. Renal glycosuria		+				
3. Resistant rickets					+	
4. Cystinuria			+			
5. Fanconi syndrome	(+)	+	+	+	+	(+)
6. Cystinosis	(+)	+	+	+	+	(+)

+ Mechanism involved. (+) Mechanism sometimes involved.

anisms may be located close to one another, or may even represent multiple alleles at the same locus. With the passage of time and the improvement of techniques for study, additional defects will undoubtedly be described.

These primary defects of renal transport mechanisms should not be confused with secondary renal disturbances. For example, the aminoaciduria in Wilson's disease and galactosemia are secondary manifestations of a more basic defect elsewhere. In these cases, the disturbances in renal transport are usually not present at birth and can frequently be abolished upon correcting the primary metabolic error.

11

Renal Transport Defects

SINGLE DEFECTS IN RENAL TRANSPORT MECHANISMS

I. NEPHROGENIC DIABETES INSIPIDUS

In nephrogenic diabetes insipidus there is a congenital failure of the renal tubules to reabsorb water, a condition which does not respond to antidiuretic hormone. The disease was first described by Waring, Kadji, and Tappan in 1945.

CLINICAL FEATURES.—The disease becomes apparent in early infancy, when it is characterized by a failure of the infant to thrive and develop normally and by attacks of unexplained fever, vomiting, and constipation. Polyuria may not be so noticeable as in an older child, although the mother may remember, in retrospect, that the baby's diaper always seemed to be wet. Thirst, too, is not an easily recognizable symptom in a young infant, although water, if offered between feedings, may be taken avidly.

There is a continual excretion of a large volume of dilute urine, as well as excessive thirst; and if sufficient water is not consumed, the patient will rapidly become dehydrated and feverish. During hot weather, infants may occasionally die from dehydration.

HEREDITY.—The condition is transmitted as a sex-linked recessive. All of the reported cases except one have been in males. The single affected girl was born out of wedlock, and the possibility that this child may be the offspring of a union that was consanguineous should be kept in mind.

It has always been noted that the mothers of known patients, who are presumed to be carriers, have suffered from excessive thirst and

polyuria. Recently, Carter and Simpkiss investigated four families having the disease, and they found that the administration of Pitressin® did
not reduce the polyuria or affect the specific gravity of the urine. However, simple measurements of urine concentration after withholding fluid
intake for 12 hours gave reasonably good discrimination between normal
individuals and presumed heterozygotes.

PATHOGENESIS.—All of the signs and symptoms can be attributed to

CHART 49

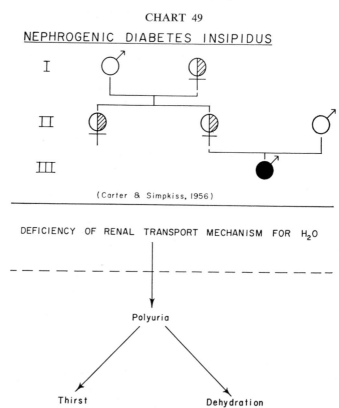

NEPHROGENIC DIABETES INSIPIDUS

(Carter & Simpkiss, 1956)

DEFICIENCY OF RENAL TRANSPORT MECHANISM FOR H₂O

Polyuria

Thirst   Dehydration

a specific defect of the renal tubules which renders them unable to reabsorb water (Chart 49). The patients also fail to respond to antidiuretic
hormone.

DIAGNOSIS.—The diagnosis is suggested by the large urine volume
and the failure to concentrate above pH 1.004. The patient should be
given the Pitressin® test (see Procedure 63). A failure to concentrate
after Pitressin® indicates nephrogenic diabetes insipidus.

TREATMENT.—Adequate fluid intake is necessary to maintain life.

Carter, O. C., and Simpkiss, M.: The "carrier" state in nephrogenic diabetes insipidus, Lancet 2:1069, 1956.

Waring, A. J.; Kadji, L.; and Tappan, V.: A congenital defect of water metabolism, Am. J. Dis. Child. 69:323, 1945.

Williams, R. H., and Henry, C.: Nephrogenic diabetes insipidus: Transmitted by females and appearing during infancy in males, Ann. Int. Med. 27:84, 1947.

2. RENAL GLYCOSURIA

Renal glycosuria is a benign condition characterized by the excretion of glucose in the urine when the blood sugar is normal.

CLINICAL FEATURES.—Patients with this condition are completely well and remain free of symptoms. Some of the individuals with renal glycosuria have been followed for many years, and none have developed diabetes mellitus or any of the other complications attributable to the sugar in the urine. The condition is important only as a point of differential diagnosis in diabetes mellitus.

HEREDITY.—The condition is transmitted as an autosomal dominant.

CHART 50

RENAL GLYCOSURIA

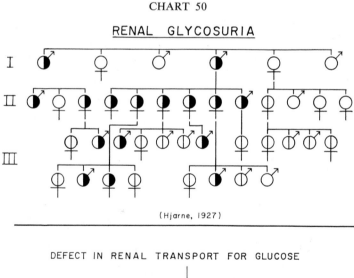

(Hjarne, 1927)

DEFECT IN RENAL TRANSPORT FOR GLUCOSE

GLYCOSURIA

In a survey based on one large family over several generations, Hjarne found that 34 out of 199 blood relatives were affected.

Renal glycosuria is a rare disorder. Only about 0.3% of all cases of melituria can be attributed to it.

PATHOGENESIS.—The condition is believed to represent a congenital defect of the renal transport mechanism for glucose (Chart 50). Normally, glucose passes freely into the glomerular filtrate and is almost completely reabsorbed by the proximal convoluted tubules. In renal glycosuria, however, this mechanism appears to be in some way inefficient, and the glucose passes into the urine. Some years ago, Friedman showed that, when the blood sugar was in the normal range of 100-200 mg/100 ml, these patients spilled glucose into the urine. More recently, Reubi has measured the ratio of Tm_G/C_T (maximal reabsorptive capacity for glucose divided by glomerular filtration rate). In the normal individual, this equals 2.41 ± 0.35. In patients with renal glycosuria on a hereditary basis, it is reduced to between 1.2 and 1.7 and remains low with increasing glucose loads of up to 600 mg/minute (Fig. 46). This finding is in distinct contrast to the findings in other nonfamilial types of renal glycosuria, in which the ratio rises with increased loads. The transport defect is limited to glucose alone; other clearance tests are perfectly normal in such individuals.

Recent evidence suggests that the transport mechanism for glucose involves the stepwise phosphorylation and dephosphorylation of glucose in the cells of the proximal convoluted tubule. This would involve: (1) the utilization of phosphate bond energy; (2) the interaction of the transport compound and the cellular element involving carboxyl mechanism; and (3) certain interdigitations with acetate metabolism, which should be apparent. If this is actually the case, a deficiency of one of the tissue phosphatases in the kidney could well account for the metabolic defect in renal glycosuria.

DIAGNOSIS.—The proper diagnosis of renal glycosuria requires: (1) that glucose be present in appreciable quantities in the urine on several occasions, both when fasting and postprandially; (2) that blood sugar levels and glucose tolerance curves be consistently normal; (3) that moderate doses of insulin exert little or no effect upon the glycosuria; and (4) that both carbohydrate and fat utilization be normal.

TREATMENT.—None is required.

Friedman, M.; Selzer, A.; Sugannan, J.; and Sokolov, M.: Renal blood flow, glomerular filtration rate, and degree of tubular reabsorption of glucose in renal glycosuria, Am. J. M. Sc. 204:22, 1942.

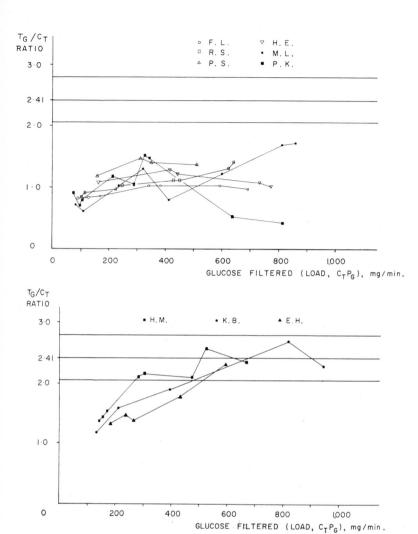

FIG. 46.—*Top*, ratio of T_G/C_T to glucose load $C_T P_G$ in six renal glycosuric patients. The ratio remains far below the normal range of 2.41 ± 0.35 even for high values of filtered glucose. *Bottom*, ratio of T_G/C_T to glucose load $C_T P_G$ in three other glycosuric patients. The ratio is below normal range for low values of filtered glucose $C_T P_G$ but increases rapidly and almost linearly when the amount of filtered glucose is raised, becoming normal at high levels of blood glucose.

Hjarne, V. A.: Study of orthoglycemic glycosuria with particular reference to its heredity, Acta med. scandinav. 67:422, 1927.

Houston, J. C., and Merivale, W. H. H.: Renal glycosuria in a family, Guy's Hosp. Rep. 98:233, 1949.

Marble, A.: Renal glycosuria, Am. J. M. Sc. 183:811, 1932.

Reubi, F. C.: Glucose titration in renal glycosuria, in *Ciba Foundation Symposium on the Kidney* (Boston: Little, Brown & Company, 1954), p. 96.

Taggart, J. V.: Some biochemical features of tubular transport mechanisms, in *Ciba Foundation Symposium on the Kidney* (Boston: Little, Brown & Company, 1954), p. 65.

3. RESISTANT RICKETS (refractory rickets; raised late rickets; resistance to vitamin D; essential hypophosphatasia rickets)

The term "resistant rickets" describes a clinical condition which is indistinguishable from ordinary rickets except that the signs occur despite an adequate intake of vitamin D in the diet. Resistant rickets is believed to occur because of a defect in the renal transport mechanism for phosphorus.

CLINICAL FEATURES.—While ordinary rickets is uncommon in patients beyond the eighteenth month, refractory rickets persists or may

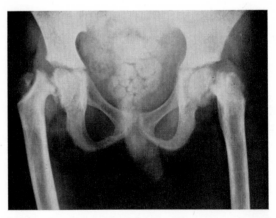

FIG. 47.—Pelvis of patient with resistant rickets. Note the bilateral slipped femoral heads. The width of the epiphysial-metaphysial junction is increased because the osteoid failed to convert to bone.

even manifest itself for the first time in childhood. The clinical findings are those of florid rickets, with bossing of the frontal bones, beading of the ribs, narrow flaring chest, prominent abdomen, swelling of the epiphyses of the wrists and ankles, and bowing of the legs and pronation of the feet. Progression of the defect in mineralization will lead to retarded growth and skeletal deformities (Fig. 47). Adults with this condition are usually in good general health but may suffer from bone pains, especially in the lower back region. There may be a severe muscular weakness, which sometimes causes confusion with muscular dystrophy. Tetany, however, never occurs.

The primary feature of the disease is its refractoriness to treatment with ordinary doses of vitamin D.

HEREDITY.—The condition is usually transmitted as a sex-linked dominant. In the past, geneticists thought that the dominance was incomplete in its manifestations, since quite a few cases seemed to occur in families in which both parents appeared to be perfectly healthy and normal. It was felt that these cases could not all be caused by fresh mutations. Recently, Graham has clarified the situation in some studies on a large kindred in North Carolina. He found that a low serum phosphorus level was transmitted as a dominant with complete manifestation but that not all of the affected individuals showed clinical signs of rickets.

No figures are available on the incidence of resistant rickets in the population. The disease is probably quite rare, since less than 100 cases have been reported from all over the world.

PATHOGENESIS.—Resistant rickets represents a congenital defect in the renal transport mechanism for phosphorus (Chart 51). The lack of reabsorption of phosphorus has the effect of keeping the plasma phosphate concentration at a permanently low level, usually in the order of 2 mg/100 ml. This in turn leads to a failure of normal bone development, manifested by most of the classical features of rickets.

The action of vitamin D on this condition is the subject of considerable dispute. Albright and his co-workers have expressed the view that in normal individuals the rising phosphorus level following the administration of vitamin D should be attributed to a decreased parathyroid activity resulting from the rise in serum calcium. They visualize the following sequence of events occurring after the administration of vitamin D: increased calcium absorption, rising calcium levels in the blood, decreased parathyroid activity, decreased urinary excretion of phosphorus, and, finally, a rise in serum phosphorus levels. Dent, on the other hand, feels that vitamin D in massive doses exerts its effects directly on the renal tubules. Simultaneous determinations of the rates of glomerular filtration and of phosphorus clearance before treatment and when healing was well advanced have shown that the rise of serum inorganic phosphorus coincides with an increased efficiency of the tubular epithelium in reabsorbing phosphorus from the glomerular filtrate.

DIAGNOSIS.—The diagnosis can be established by the finding of a persistently low serum phosphorus level (2 mg/100 ml) despite adequate vitamin D therapy.

TREATMENT.—Very large doses of vitamin D are required. As a rule, daily dosages of 200,000-400,000 units of oral calciferol are needed to cure the radiological signs and to prevent recurrence. It should be careful-

CHART 51

RESISTANT   RICKETS

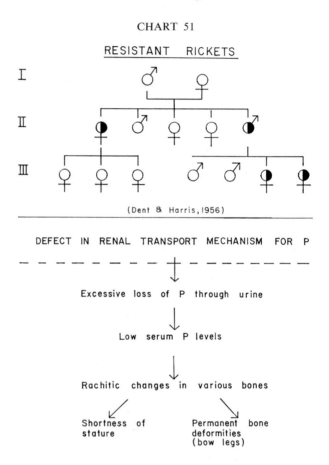

(Dent & Harris, 1956)

DEFECT IN RENAL TRANSPORT MECHANISM FOR P

Excessive loss of P through urine

Low serum P levels

Rachitic changes in various bones

Shortness of
stature

Permanent bone
deformities
(bow legs)

ly noted that the toxic dose of vitamin D may not be much greater than the therapeutic dose; this is because the resistance to vitamin D in this disease applies only to its antirachitic action, not to its toxic action. It is not uncommon to find persistent hypophosphatemia even in the face of active healing in the bones. Sufficient calciferol should be given to raise the serum phosphorus level to more than 2.5 mg/100 ml, but the serum calcium to no more than 11.5 mg/100 ml and the urine calcium to no more than 400 mg/24 hours.

Albright, F.; Burnett, C. H.; Parson, W.; Reifenstein, E. C., Jr.; and Roos, A.: Osteomalacia and late rickets, Medicine 25:399, 1946.

Dent, C. E.: Rickets and osteomalacia from renal tubular defects, J. Bone & Joint Surg. 34B:266, 1952.

*——— and Harris, H.: Hereditary forms of rickets and osteomalacia, J. Bone & Joint Surg. 38B:204, 1956.

*McCune, D. J.: Refractory rickets, Am. J. Dis. Child. 77:112, 1949.

Robertson, B. R.; Harris, R. C.; and McCune, D. J.: Refractory rickets: Mechanism of therapeutic action of calciferol, Am. J. Dis. Child. 64:948, 1942.

*Winters, R. W.; Graham, J. B.; Williams, T. F.; McFalls, V. W.; and Burnett, C. H.: A genetic study of familial hypophosphatemia and vitamin D resistant rickets, with a review of the literature, Medicine 37:97, 1958.

4. CYSTINURIA

A congenital defect in the reabsorption of the dibasic amino acids in the renal tubules appears to be responsible for the clinical condition known as "cystinuria." This disease is of historic interest because it is one of the original four inborn errors of metabolism described by Sir Archibald Garrod.

CLINICAL FEATURES.—The first case of cystinuria was probably described by Wollaston in the *Philosophic Transactions* of the Royal Society in 1810. However, it was not until over a century later that it became known that renal calculi are composed almost entirely of cystine. More recently, Dent and Rose have shown that the abnormality in the urine is not limited to cystine alone but that three other dibasic amino acids— lysine, arginine, and ornithine—are also involved. On the average, a patient with cystinuria will, in the course of a day, excrete 0.73 Gm of cystine, 1.8 Gm of lysine, 0.83 Gm of arginine, and 0.37 Gm of ornithine; and these amounts persist throughout his life relatively uninfluenced by dietary intake. Stone formation occurs in such patients because cystine is one of the least soluble of the amino acids. In urine of pH 5-7, cystine is soluble only to the extent of 300-400 mg/L. It can be seen that when the urine volume decreases, particularly at night, this amino acid is likely to come out of solution, and renal calculi may form. Since lysine, arginine, and ornithine are freely soluble, they do not become incorporated in stone.

Harris and his associates have recently suggested that patients with cystinuria may be divided into two phenotypes: (*a*) those who show a greatly increased excretion of cystine, lysine, arginine, and ornithine in their urine and who often develop cystine stones; and (*b*) those who show only a moderate increase of cystine and lysine but no increase of arginine in the urine and who never develop cystine stones.

HEREDITY.—Family studies indicate that cystinuria occurs as two separate genotypes: In Type I, which is transmitted by an autosomal recessive gene, the mode of inheritance is suggested (1) by the fact that abnormal individuals are found only in a single sibship in each family, with the parents, children, and other near relatives being normal, and (2) by the increased incidence of consanguinity among the parents. The individuals who are homozygous for the cystinuric gene belong to phenotype (a) and have large increases of all four amino acids in the urine and have cystine stones. No urinary abnormalities may be demonstrated among the heterozygous carriers of this abnormal gene. In Type II, which is also transmitted by an autosomal recessive gene, the individuals who are homozygous again belong to phenotype (a) and frequently have cystine stones. However, the heterozygotes of this type show changes in the urine which are characteristic of phenotype (b), and they can clearly be differentiated from individuals who are completely normal.

It would appear that these two types represent the effects of separate genes rather than those of a single gene affected by modifiers. The absence of any instances of a child with a group (a) pattern being derived from normal parents or from a parent with (b) pattern is rather in favor of the genes being located at two different loci.

In the past, it was felt that cystinuria was a comparatively rare metabolic disorder. Garrod stated that Simon encountered only one instance of cystine sediment in 15,000 urines examined. In 1932, Lewis threw a completely new light on the situation. By using reliable chemical tests for cystine, he was able to demonstrate that gross cystinuria could occur in individuals without either the appearance of cystine crystals or formation of cystine stones. In a systematic experiment involving over 10,000 students, he found that 18 gave positive reactions to chemical tests for cystine but that only 4 showed cystine crystals in the urine. He estimated that approximately 1 in 600 of the general population excreted abnormally large quantities of cystine, even though it is not clear at present how many of the affected individuals are homozygotes and how many are heterozygotes.

PATHOGENESIS.—Although early workers have suggested that cystinuria occurs as a result of some kind of block in the intermediary metabolism of cystine or methionine, Dent and his associates have clearly demonstrated that the primary defect is at the site of transport for cystine and the other dibasic amino acids in the renal tubules (Chart 52). They

CHART 52

CYSTINURIA

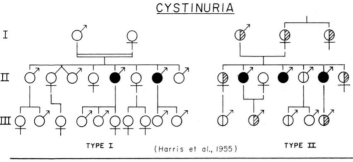

TYPE I   (Harris et al., 1955)   TYPE II

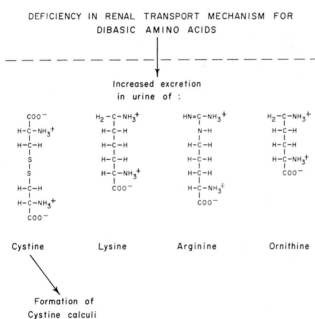

DEFICIENCY IN RENAL TRANSPORT MECHANISM FOR
DIBASIC AMINO ACIDS

Increased excretion
in urine of :

Cystine   Lysine   Arginine   Ornithine

Formation of
Cystine calculi

have shown that in cystinurics the cystine levels in plasma and other body
fluids are comparable to, or even lower than, the levels in normal controls. There is no excessive accumulation of cystine in the cystine-rich
tissues such as hair and nails. The feeding of large amounts of cystine,
methionine, and cysteine to these patients and to normal individuals produced no differences in the intermediary metabolism of these substances.
Finally, they have shown that the clearance of cystine in cystinurics is
often more than 30 times that found in normal individuals, and thus is

about the same as the expected rate of glomerular filtration. It seems probable that cystinuria can be explained on the basis that little or no renal tubular reabsorption of cystine takes place in these patients. Presumably, the same difficulties in reabsorption apply to lysine, arginine, and ornithine.

DIAGNOSIS.—Cystinuria can be diagnosed by the presence of excessive amounts of cystine in the urine (see Procedure 64). The condition can be differentiated from cystinosis in two ways: (1) by determining the type of aminoaciduria and (2) by the clinical pattern. By the use of paper-partition chromatography (see Procedure 65), it is possible to demonstrate that in cystinuria the aminoaciduria is limited to the four dibasic amino acids, with the other amino acids being excreted in normal quantities, while in cystinosis the aminoaciduria is a generalized one. Clinically, cystinosis is a systemic disease with deposits of cystine in the eyes, liver, kidneys, and long bones; and rickets is a common finding. None of these phenomena are present in cystinuria.

TREATMENT.—Therapy should be directed toward reducing the formation of cystine stones in the kidneys. This can be done by greatly increasing the fluid intake, especially at night, and by making the urine alkaline with sodium bicarbonate or lactate.

Dent, C. E.; Heathcott, J. G.; and Joron, G. E.: The pathogenesis of cystinuria: I. Chromatographic and microbiological studies of the metabolism of sulfur-containing amino acids, J. Clin. Invest. 33:1210, 1954.
———— and Rose, G. A.: Amino acid metabolism in cystinuria, Quart. J. Med. 20:205, 1951.
———— and Senior, B.: Studies in the treatment of cystinuria, Brit. J. Urol. 27: 317, 1955.
Harris, H.; Mittwoch, U.; Robson, E. B.; and Warren, F. L.: Phenotypes and genotypes in cystinuria, Ann. Eugenics 20:57, 1955.
*———— and Robson, E. B.: Cystinuria, Am. J. Med. 22:774, 1957.
Lewis, H. B.: The occurrence of cystinuria in healthy young men and women, Ann. Int. Med. 6:183, 1933.
Stein, W. H.: Excretion of amino acids in cystinuria, Proc. Soc. Exper. Biol. & Med. 78:705, 1951.

MULTIPLE DEFECTS IN RENAL TRANSPORT MECHANISMS

Although many variants of defects in the reabsorption of phosphates, glucose, amino acids, and sometimes potassium and water have appeared in the literature, the defects can usually be classified into two general groups: (1) those with renal tubular dysfunction but without cystine deposits, usually called "Fanconi syndrome"; and (2) those with both renal tubular dysfunction and cystine deposits, known as "Lignac's disease." At the present time, there is considerable controversy as to whether the Fanconi syndrome and Lignac's disease are one and the same condition. We feel that deposits of cystine in the body tissues are sufficiently unique to require that they be considered as a separate condition.

5. FANCONI SYNDROME

In 1931, Professor Fanconi in Zurich briefly described finding rickets and stunted growth in a child with albuminuria and glycosuria. Two years later, de Toni in Italy reported on a dwarfed child who had vitamin D resistant rickets and spontaneous fractures and who showed a low level of serum phosphorus, acidosis, pronounced glycosuria, and albuminuria. A little later, Debre reported a similar case from France. In 1936, Fanconi collected all these cases, added two more of his own, and established a new syndrome, which he called "nephrotic glycosuric dwarfism with hypophosphatemic rickets." The third feature of this condition, aminoaciduria, was described by Dent in England and the Fanconi syndrome became a definite clinical entity.

CLINICAL FEATURES.—The Fanconi syndrome can clinically be divided into two types: *infantile* and *adult*. Although physiologically and pathologically these types appear to be identical, they may represent different gene mutations.

In the *infantile* type, the infant grows and develops normally during the first 6-8 months of life. The parents then note his refusal of feedings other than liquids, the development of polyuria, and a cessation of growth. The infant may be brought into the hospital in a crisis, with fever, dehydration, and acidosis. In older children the bone deformities due to rickets are often striking and there is a marked shortening of stature. Physical examination may disclose florid rickets which develops despite adequate vitamin D prophylaxis; and there may be severe malnutrition, variable fever associated with dehydration, and occasional enlargement of the liver, as well as dwarfism. The skeletal musculature may be very flabby and hypotonic. The blood pressure is usually normal initially but may rise as the renal disease progresses.

In contrast, in the *adult* type the patients seldom show any manifestations until the second or third decade of life. The initial complaints are: severe pain in the back, shoulder, ribs, and thighs and spontaneous fractures. Laboratory studies usually show glycosuria and aminoaciduria. Whether or not the renal changes have been present since birth is not known, but the possibility that the disease develops in later life is very real. Death usually occurs after a crisis characterized by hypokalemia and uremia.

The only consistent changes noted at postmortem are in the kidneys.

The epithelial cells lining the tubules are, in many places, extremely large, practically blocking the lumen; but this is not a cloudy, swollen type of enlargement, and there is no evidence of degeneration.

HEREDITY.—The condition is probably transmitted by an autosomal recessive gene. The affected individuals are usually found in a single sibship, with parents, offspring, and near relatives being unaffected. There is sometimes a history of consanguinity; and at least one example of involvement in both members of a pair of identical twins has been reported to date.

It is not clear whether the adult type of the Fanconi syndrome and the *infantile* type are one and the same condition. Within individual families one sees only one or the other type, and this suggests that different abnormal genes may be involved. It is interesting to speculate whether these genes are at different loci or are alleles. If the latter is the case, then the underlying biochemical disturbances leading to the clinical syndrome would be qualitatively very similar, although different in degree.

PATHOGENESIS.—All of the clinical signs and symptoms can be explained on the basis of a defect in the proximal convoluted tubules. This is shown first by the fact that the functions classically relegated to the distal portions of the nephrons—namely, production of ammonia and acid—are relatively well preserved in the majority of cases. Secondly, Clay and his co-workers have shown that, if the nephron is dissected free throughout its entire length, the glomeruli appear to be uniform and normal throughout but that there is a "swan neck" appearance of the first portion of the tubule. There is also a shortening of the proximal convoluted tubules, including their narrow portion. It is not clear whether this is a developmental defect in the morphological sense or whether it represents secondary changes due to a chemical defect. However, there appears little doubt that the proximal portion of the convoluted tubule is disturbed. Finally, Stowers and Dent, and Cooke and his associates, have shown, by Gomori's stain, a complete absence of phosphatase in the proximal convoluted tubules, and this may represent the genetically determined enzyme defect responsible for this condition.

Regardless of the cause, the primary defects lie in the renal transport mechanisms for glucose, phosphates, amino acids and, to a less marked extent, for water and potassium. The pedigree of causes for the Fanconi syndrome is shown in Chart 53. The loss of phosphates is responsible for the rickets and bony changes; the loss of amino acids, probably for the cirrhosis and fatty infiltration of the liver; and the loss of water and potassium, in the terminal hypokalemia.

DIAGNOSIS.—The diagnosis of the Fanconi syndrome is difficult be-

CHART 53

FANCONI SYNDROME

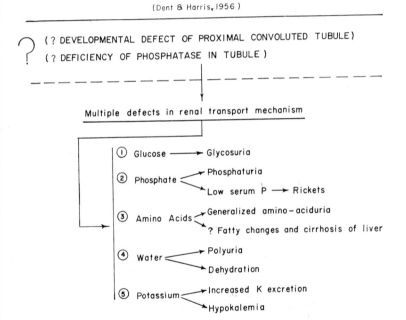

(Dent & Harris, 1956)

(? DEVELOPMENTAL DEFECT OF PROXIMAL CONVOLUTED TUBULE)
(? DEFICIENCY OF PHOSPHATASE IN TUBULE)

Multiple defects in renal transport mechanism

① Glucose ────► Glycosuria

② Phosphate
    ► Phosphaturia
    ► Low serum P ──► Rickets

③ Amino Acids
    ► Generalized amino-aciduria
    ► ? Fatty changes and cirrhosis of liver

④ Water
    ► Polyuria
    ► Dehydration

⑤ Potassium
    ► Increased K excretion
    ► Hypokalemia

cause no one change is specific for the condition. Some of the laboratory findings which suggest the diagnosis are: (1) polyuria with fixed specific gravity, (2) albuminuria, (3) glycosuria, (4) phosphaturia, (5) amino-aciduria, (6) low serum phosphorus, (7) low serum potassium, and (8) acidosis.

Renal function tests may not be remarkable during the early part of the disease.

TREATMENT.—The adult form of the disease responds quite well to doses of potassium or sodium bicarbonate and vitamin D. The infantile form shows some response to this treatment, but the ultimate outlook is poor because most of the patients succumb eventually to renal failure.

Clay, H. D.; Darmady, E. M.; and Hawkins, M.: The nature of the renal lesion in the Fanconi syndrome, J. Path. & Bact. 65:551, 1953.

Cooke, W. T.; Barclay, J. A.; Govan, A. D. T.; and Nagley, L.: Osteoporosis associated with lowered serum phosphorus and renal glycosuria, Arch. Int. Med. 80:147, 1947.

Dent, C. E.: The amino-aciduria in Fanconi syndrome, Biochem. J. 41:240, 1947.

——— and Harris, H.: Hereditary forms of rickets and osteomalacia, J. Bone & Joint Surg. 38B:204, 1956.

Fanconi, G.: Der frühinfantile nephrotisch-glykosuriche Zwergwuchs mit hypophosphatämischer Rachitis, Jahrb. f. Kinderh. 147:299, 1936.

*McCune, D. J.; Mason, H. H.; and Clark, H. T.: Intractable hypophosphatemia rickets with renal glycosuria and acidosis, Am. J. Dis. Child. 65:81, 1943.

*Sirota, J. H., and Hamerman, D.: Renal function studies in an adult subject with the Fanconi syndrome, Am. J. Med. 16:138, 1954.

Stowers, J. M., and Dent, C. E.: Studies on the mechanism of Fanconi syndrome, Quart. J. Med. 16:275, 1947.

6. CYSTINOSIS (Lignac's disease)

In 1903, Abderhalden reported on some chemical examinations carried out on tissues from a 21-month-old Swiss infant dying of "inanition." He found that the white flecks on the liver and spleen, which were hexagonal or round, were deposits of cystine. Since two other siblings had died of identical complaints, he tested the urine sediments of all members of the immediate family and found that all showed cystine. He therefore labeled the disorder as a "familial cystine diathesis." Twenty years later, Lignac, a Dutch pediatrician, reported three similar cases between the ages of 14 months and 3 years. All these patients showed stunted growth, severe rickets, "severe renal disease," and progressive inanition. At autopsy, widespread cystine deposits were found in all three cases. Subsequently, one of Fanconi's cases of "nephrotic glycosuric dwarfism with hypophosphatemic rickets" was also found to have cystine deposits, and so the clinical entity of cystinosis was established.

CLINICAL FEATURES.—Clinically the patients have all of the manifestations described in the de Toni-Fanconi-Debre syndrome. Dwarfism, wasting, rickets, osteoporosis, polydipsia, polyuria, dehydration, and acidosis are prominent findings. In addition, photophobia is usually noted. Cystine crystals may be interstitial; but usually they are accumulated in the large phagocytic reticuloendothelial cells, primarily in the liver, spleen, kidneys, lymph nodes, and bone marrow (Fig. 48).

HEREDITY.—Bickel and Harris have postulated that the condition is transmitted as an autosomal recessive. This is suggested by these facts:

it has never been known to occur in different generations; there is often a history of consanguinity; and only siblings are involved in any given family. The heterozygotes cannot be detected by chemical means, not even by the newly developed lysine tolerance test (see Procedure 66).

Cystinosis is not genetically related to either cystinuria or the de Toni-Fanconi-Debre syndrome. Considerable confusion has arisen

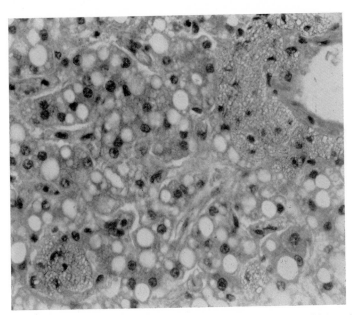

FIG. 48.—Photomicrograph of liver section from a patient with cystinosis. Deposits of cystine crystals occupy Kupffer's cells and hepatic cells, seen here as foamy groups of cells especially prominent adjacent to a venule. The hepatic cells also show coarse cytoplasmic vacuoles, indicative of fatty metamorphosis.

over the fact that Abderhalden described the heterozygotes of his original pedigree as being cystinurics. This does not seem to be likely, because (1) no cases of cystinosis have since been found among pedigrees of cystinuria and (2) no examples of cystinuria with characteristic urinary amino acid patterns have ever been found among families with cystinosis.

The frequency of cystinosis in the general population is estimated to be roughly 1 in 40,000, with a gene frequency of 1 in 200.

PATHOGENESIS.—The pathogenesis of the rickets, renal changes, and electrolyte disturbances is identical to that of the de Toni-Fanconi-Debre syndrome. The etiology for the cystine deposits is completely unknown

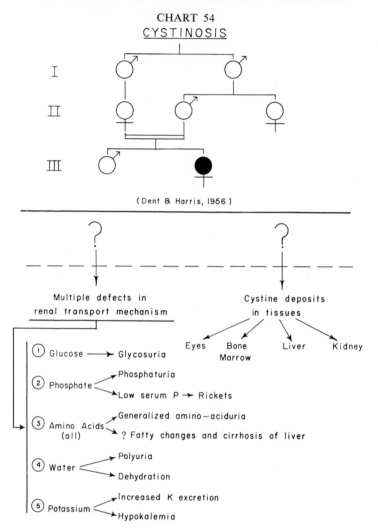

CHART 54
CYSTINOSIS

(Dent & Harris, 1956)

(Chart 54). At least three theories have been proposed: (1) that there is a failure of oxidative degradation of cysteine to sulfate along the metabolic pathway proposed by Brand and his associates (Fig. 49), which results in its increased oxidation to cystine; (2) that there is a defect in the utilization of amino acids in the kidneys which results in cystine storage; and (3) that there is a defect in the intracellular metabolism of amino acids within the reticuloendothelial system, resulting in cystine deposits. No proof has come forth for any of these theories, and we are

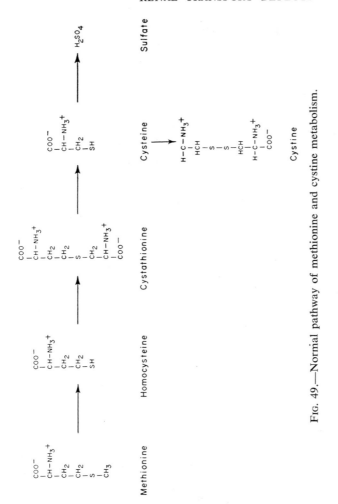

Fig. 49.—Normal pathway of methionine and cystine metabolism.

left only with the knowledge that cystine appears to be present in the serum in normal amounts, that cystine is excreted through the urine in slightly greater amounts, but no more so than any of the other amino acids, and that something has happened to the cystine in transit.

DIAGNOSIS.—The diagnosis can be established by identifying cystine (see Procedure 67) in the bone marrow, liver, or kidney. Clinically, cystine can easily be seen in the eyes with the aid of a slit lamp.

TREATMENT.—Patients are helped by treatment with citric acid, sodium citrate, and moderately high doses of vitamin D. Potassium chloride should be added also, to prevent hypokalemia. The prognosis is universally poor in children.

Abderhalden, E.: Familiäre Cystindiathesis, Ztschr. physiol. Chem. 38:557 1903.

*Bickel, H.: Cystine storage disease with amino-aciduria and dwarfism (Lignac-Fanconi disease), Acta paediat. (supp. 90), 42:1, 1952.

Brand, E.; Cahill, G. F.; and Harris, M.: Cystinuria: II. The metabolism of cystine, cysteine, methionine, and glutathione, J. Biol. Chem. 109:69, 1935.

Lignac, G. O. W.: Über den Cystinstoffwechsel, München. med. Wchnschr. 71:1016, 1924.

Robson, E. B., and Rose, G. A.: The effect of intravenous lysine on the renal clearances of cystine, arginine, and ornithine in normal subjects, in patients with cystinuria, in Fanconi syndrome, and in their relatives, Clin. Sc. 16:75, 1957.

*Worthen, H. G., and Good, R. A.: The de Toni-Fanconi syndrome with cystinosis, A.M.A. J. Dis. Child. 95:653, 1958.

PART V

Disturbances in Which the Etiology is Unknown

WE SHALL NOW CONSIDER some of the hereditary diseases about whose primary gene effect we know relatively little. These diseases will, therefore, be grouped according to the presenting symptoms, with the thought that their classification will be changed when more is known about the chemical defects responsible for each of these inborn errors of metabolism.

These disturbances will be arbitrarily divided into (1) disturbances in lipid metabolism, (2) the muscular dystrophies, and (3) miscellaneous metabolic disorders.

12

Disturbances in Lipid Metabolism

IN THIS CHAPTER, we shall take up the disturbances involving lipid metabolism. These include: (1) *idiopathic hyperlipemia*, (2) *primary hypercholesteremia*, (3) *Gaucher's disease*, (4) *Niemann-Pick disease*, (5) *amaurotic familial idiocy*, and (6) *lipochondrodystrophy*.

*Crocker, A. C.: Skin xanthomas in childhood, Pediatrics 8:573, 1951.
*Herndon, C. N.: Genetics of the lipidoses, Proc. A. Res. Nerv. & Ment. Dis 33:239, 1954.

I. IDIOPATHIC HYPERLIPEMIA (Buerger-Grütz disease)

In 1932, Buerger and Grütz described a new clinical syndrome in children which was characterized by the following triad: (1) sporadic attacks of acute abdominal pain, (2) a xanthomatous type of skin lesion, and (3) a fasting serum which is milky white. About 40 such cases have been reported from all over the world. Since the condition is frequently familial, it is customarily included among the inborn errors of metabolism.

CLINICAL FEATURES.—Affected children usually first come to the attention of the physician because of peculiar attacks of abdominal pain, characterized by extreme tenderness, boardlike rigidity, and sometimes collapse. Such an attack is accompanied by fever, polymorphonuclear leukocytosis, and anorexia; and it is sometimes mistaken for a surgical emergency. It lasts from 1 to 4 days and then terminates spontaneously, with a decrease of the serum lipid levels.

Another prominent feature is the presence of cutaneous xanthomas (Fig. 50). These consist of soft yellow papules and nodules, commonly located in the extensor aspects of the knees and elbows, on the buttocks and thighs, and also on the trunk, face, hands, and feet. Xanthelasmatosis (of the eyelids) does not seem to occur in such patients. When the blood

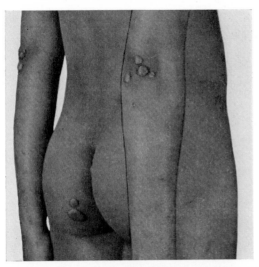

Fig. 50.—Cutaneous xanthomas in patient with idiopathic hyperlipemia. (From Boggs, J. D.; Hsia, D. Y. Y.; Mais, R.; and Bigler, J. A.: The genetic mechanism of idiopathic hyperlipemia, New England J. Med. 257:1101, 1957.)

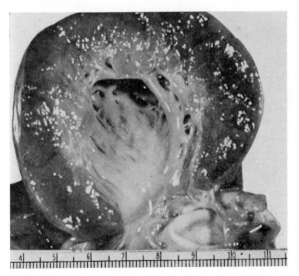

Fig. 51.—Heart in a patient with idiopathic hyperlipemia, opened to expose the left ventricular endocardium and base of aorta. Endocardial and myocardial fibrosis is apparent, and left ventricular myocardium shows hypertrophy.

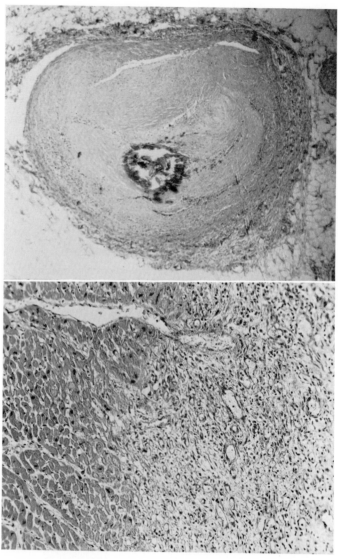

Fig. 52.—Photomicrographs of sections of heart shown in Figure 51. *Top,* left coronary artery. Advanced atherosclerosis has reduced the vascular lumen to a narrow slit. Focal calcification is seen in the atheroma. *Bottom,* margin of the myocardial infarct. Young, still moderately vascular scar tissue has replaced a portion of the myocardium.

lipid levels rise excessively, lipemia retinalis can be seen easily. Episodes of relapsing pancreatitis and atherosclerosis are the principal complications, and many affected individuals suffer from angina pectoris or myocardial infarction in the teens or twenties (Figs. 51 and 52).

HEREDITY.—Idiopathic hyperlipemia is transmitted by an autosomal recessive gene. The condition has been noted among siblings in at least eight different families, and consanguinity has been reported once. Some of the asymptomatic relatives, who are presumably heterozygous carriers

CHART 55

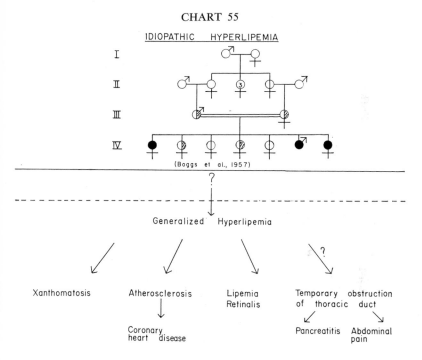

of the abnormal gene, have been found to have slight, but definite, increases in serum lipid levels.

The condition has been reported among both whites and Negroes and has been seen in different parts of the world. Although the exact incidence of this disease is not known, the condition probably occurs fairly rarely. In this era of frequent blood tests, it is unlikely that many cases are missed, because of the striking appearance of the serum.

PATHOGENESIS.—Some unknown defect in fat metabolism is responsible for idiopathic hyperlipemia (Chart 55). Thannhauser and Stanley have shown that when I[131]-labeled neutral fat is administered to affected individuals, the disappearance of iodine from the blood serum is considerably prolonged, as compared with normal subjects. In 1940, Goodman made the interesting observation that the blood from one such patient would not cause a splitting of olive oil, suggesting an absence of lipase in the blood.

The cause of the recurrent episodes of abdominal pain is also not known. Ahrens has postulated that they occur as a result of temporary obstructions of the thoracic duct with chylous fluid, and of exudation of chyle into retroperitoneal tissues and the mesenteric root. Distention of these tissues would probably produce pain and occasionally vascular collapse. Ahrens has shown that the attacks are not related to the blood lipid levels as such. Rather, the anorexia accompanying such an attack is frequently responsible for significant falls in the level of serum lipids.

DIAGNOSIS.—The diagnosis of idiopathic hyperlipemia is suggested by the milky white appearance of the serum (see Procedure 68) and the increase of total lipids (see Procedure 69). Laboratory tests reveal the following changes in the serum lipids:

	NORMAL RANGE* (mg/100 ml)	IDIOPATHIC HYPERLIPEMIA* (mg/100 ml)
Turbidity (units)	1.9-4.5	26
Total fatty acids	190-300	2,696
Neutral fat	0-400	2,116
Total cholesterol (see Procedure 70)	160-290	614
Free cholesterol	50-100	273
Esterified cholesterol	120-220	377
Phospholipids (see Procedure 71)	160-310	575

*Based on the figures of Lever, W. F.; Smith, P. A. J.; and Hurley, N. A.: Idiopathic hyperlipemic and primary hypercholesteremic xanthomatosis: I. Clinical data and analysis of the plasma lipids, J. Invest. Dermat. 22:33, 1954.

Electrophoretic analyses of the plasma show that either the alpha-2 peak alone or both the beta-1 and alpha-2 peaks are elevated. Highspeed centrifugation at 18,000 rpm at $-5°$ C induces partial or complete clearing of the plasma, with an accumulation of a creamy layer of lipid material on the top, a decrease in the size of previously elevated alpha-2 and beta-1 peaks, and a considerable decrease of neutral fat, cholesterol, and phospholipids.

The condition can easily be differentiated from primary hypercholesteremia by the milky appearance of the serum.

TREATMENT.—The reduction of fat in the diet causes some reduction in the plasma levels, but not sufficient to bring them down to normal. Lever has shown that the intravenous injection of 50-100 mg of heparin causes a change in the appearance of the electrophoretic pattern and will, if the injections are continued for long periods, result in considerable decrease of turbidity and of lipid values in the serum. In time the cutaneous xanthomas will also disappear. This form of therapy is indicated if the patient has a predisposition to atherosclerosis.

Boggs, J. D.; Hsia, D. Y. Y.; Mais, R.; and Bigler, J. A.: The genetic mechanism of idiopathic hyperlipemia, New England J. Med. 257:1101, 1957.

Buerger, M., and Grütz, O.: Über hepatosplenomegale Lipoidose mit xanthomatosum Veränderungen in Haut und Schleimhaut, Arch. Dermat. u. Syph. 166:542, 1932.

Holt, L. E., Jr.; Aylward, F. X.; and Timbres, H. G.: Idiopathic familial lipemia, Bull. Johns Hopkins Hosp. 64:279, 1939.

Lever, W. F.; Herbst, F. S. M.; and Hurley, N. A.: Idiopathic hyperlipemia and primary hypercholesteremic xanthomatosis: IV. Effects of prolonged administration of heparin on serum lipids in idiopathic hyperlipemia, A.M.A. Arch. Dermat. 71:150, 1955.

————; Smith, P. A. J.; and Hurley, N. A.: Idiopathic hyperlipemic and primary hypercholesteremic xanthomatosis: I. Clinical data and analysis of the plasma lipids, J. Invest. Dermat. 22:33, 1954.

Thannhauser, S. J., and Stanley, M. M.: Serum fat curves following oral administration of I131 labelled neutral fat to normal subjects and those with idiopathic hyperlipemia, Tr. A. Am. Physicians 62:245, 1949.

2. PRIMARY HYPERCHOLESTEREMIA (essential hypercholesteremic xanthomatosis)

Primary hypercholesteremia is characterized by an increase in the total cholesterol in the serum, frequently associated with the formation of xanthomas in various tissues.

CLINICAL FEATURES.—The condition can be differentiated from idiopathic hyperlipemia by the following characteristics: (1) the fasting serum is always clear; (2) the distribution of the xanthomas tends to be different (xanthelasmatosis is present in about a quarter of all affected individuals, while xanthoma tuberosum lesions are not quite so frequently seen on the extensor surfaces); (3) the tendons are frequently involved, with xanthomas being frequently seen in the Achilles tendon, the extensor tendons of the hand, and the patellar tendon; (4) the atheromatous changes take place early in life, and death from xanthomatous infiltrations of the aortic valve and coronary arteries frequently occur during childhood; and (5) the genetic factor seems to be much more prominent, with many of the close relatives of affected persons also showing the same elevations of serum cholesterol levels.

The pathology of the xanthoma tuberosum lesion has been described by Pollitzer and Wile, who sampled skin lesions at various stages of maturity in a single patient. The earliest changes appear in the adventitial connective-tissue cells of the smallest blood vessels. When lipid is present in excess in the blood, these cells pick it up, proliferate, and increase in size, forming xanthoma cells. This represents an "irritative connective-tissue hyperplasia." In the next stage, the lesion becomes surrounded by a fibroblastic reaction, which, combined with a saturation of the cells near the blood vessels with lipid, is believed to serve as a self-limiting check on the size of the xanthomatous lesion. At postmortem the patients frequently show: multiple xanthomas in subcutaneous tissues of the arms and elbows; cholesterol plaques in the aorta and coronary, innominate, and subclavian arteries; and, frequently, cholesterol plaques in the valves of the heart in young adults.

HEREDITY.—Primary hypercholesteremia appears to be transmitted as a dominant trait with incomplete penetrance. Some workers have suggested that xanthoma tuberosum multiplex represents the homozygous state for the inherited factor, which when heterozygous produces only hypercholesteremia. Others have suggested that atheromatous or coronary heart disease represents the homozygous state.

Proper genetic analysis has been handicapped because the upper limits of total serum cholesterol varies between males and females and tends to rise at an irregular rate until late middle age; however, despite these limitations, Adlersberg and his co-workers have found hypercholesteremia in about half of the siblings and a quarter of the offspring of individuals with elevations of serum cholesterol. This is a considerably higher value than that among the population as a whole, and indicates that the cholesterol levels are, to a great extent, genetically determined.

PATHOGENESIS.—Very little is known about the etiology of this disease (Chart 56). Chaikoff and his associates have shown that such patients show a normal blood lipid response after the ingestion of 100 ml of olive oil. This suggests that the defect is not exogenous but is related to the storage of fat. In view of the similarity of this disease to other inborn errors of metabolism, Adlersberg has suggested that it represents a disturbance in the genetically determined enzymatic chain reactions, which leads to abnormal metabolic pathways and results in the accumulation of lipid substances in the blood and in the tissues.

DIAGNOSIS.—The elevation of total cholesterol in the serum (see Procedure 70) is the most prominent chemical feature of the disease. The rise is usually moderate, averaging about 500 mg/100 ml (normal range, 160-290 mg/100 ml). Both the free and the esterified fractions of the cholesterol show this increase, and the ratio between the two remains unchanged. There is also a slight, but not striking, increase in phospholipids and total fatty acids, and no increase in neutral fat.

Electrophoretic analysis of plasma shows a constant increase of the beta-1 peak, and fractionation of the plasma proteins reveals a marked increase in the beta-1 lipoproteins. High-speed centrifugation, however, induces no changes in the electrophoretic patterns.

TREATMENT.—A reduction of fat or cholesterol in the diet does not significantly lower the serum cholesterol levels. Recently, some workers

CHART 56

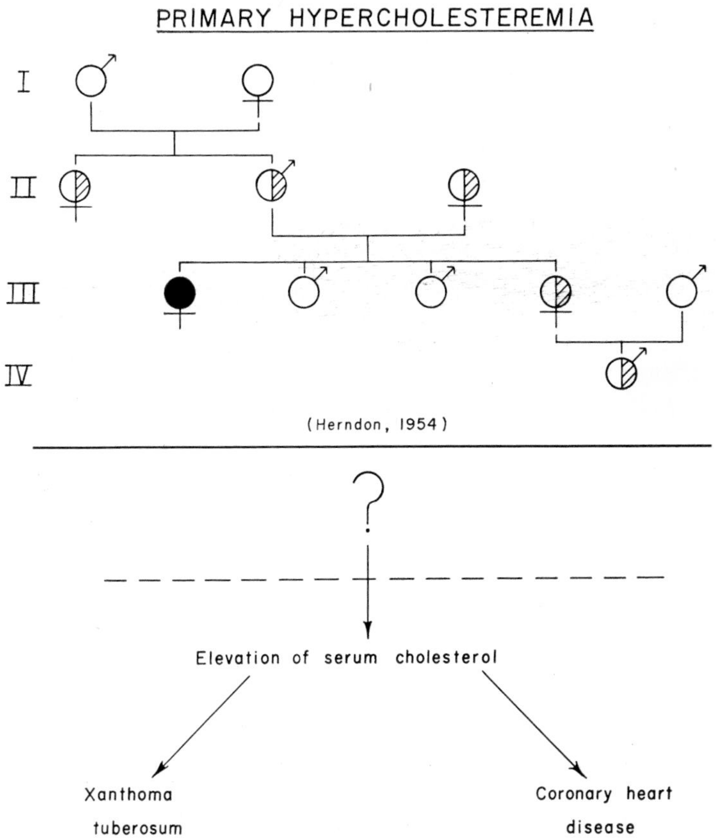

PRIMARY HYPERCHOLESTEREMIA

(Herndon, 1954)

have advocated the use of lipotropic substances such as sitosterol, high vegetable-oil diet, nicotinic acid, estrogens, and soybean phosphatides in the treatment of this condition. Although it is still too early to assess the long-term effects of such therapy, the results so far have not been dramatic.

Adlersberg, D.: Inborn errors of lipid metabolism: Clinical, genetic and chemical aspects, A.M.A. Arch. Path. 60:481, 1955.
Cook, C. D.; Smith, H. L.; Giesen, O. W.; and Beidez, G. L.; Xanthoma tu-

berosum, aortic stenosis, coronary sclerosis, and angina pectoris, Am. J. Dis. Child. 73:326, 1947.

Fliegelman, M. T.; Wilkinson, C. F.; and Hand, E. A.: Genetics of xanthoma tuberosum multiplex, Arch. Dermat. & Syph. 58:409, 1948.

*Herndon, C. N.: Genetics of the lipidoses, Proc. A. Res. Nerv. & Ment. Dis. 33:239, 1954.

Pollitzer, S., and Wile, U. J.: Xanthoma tuberosum multiplex, J. Cut. Dis. 30:235, 1912.

Schaefer, L. E.; Drachman, S. R.; Steinberg, A. G.; and Adlersberg, D.: Genetic studies on hypercholesteremia: Frequency in a hospital population and in families of hypercholesteremic index patients, Am. Heart J. 46:99, 1953.

3. GAUCHER'S DISEASE

This disease was first described in 1882 by Phillipe Charles Ernest Gaucher, a French dermatologist. In a thesis submitted to the Faculty of Medicine in Paris, entitled *De l'epithelioma primitif de la rate,* he reported on a patient in whom the splenic pulp had been entirely replaced by large, pale cells. At first he attributed this condition to a primary epithelioma of the spleen, but later he recognized it as a systematized storage disease of the reticuloendothelial system.

CLINICAL FEATURES.—Gaucher's disease tends to occur in two forms: (1) an acute, or *infantile,* type; and (2) a chronic, or *adult,* type.

The *adult* type, the more common form, becomes evident at any age. Classically, the patients have moderate to marked splenomegaly, anemia, and other evidences of hypersplenism, as well as patchy brown pigmentation of the skin, especially over the anterior surfaces of the legs and the malar region. Pingueculas of the conjunctivas are often seen in adults.

The bones show changes characteristic of failure of tubulation. There is a flaring of the ends of the femurs (so-called "Erlenmeyer-flask appearance") with thinning of the cortex. There is also a widening of the medullary cavities; and osteoporosis may occur in the vertebrae, pelvis, tibiae, and humeri, which may lead to pathological fractures and severe deformities. Many of the patients also suffer from epistaxis, anemia, and purpura, which are frequently relieved by splenectomy. The prognosis is variable; but many affected individuals lead long, nearly unhandicapped lives, especially after splenectomy.

In contrast, the *infantile* type pursues a rapid and malignant course. The infant, who is usually normal at birth, soon exhibits apathy together with progressive physical and developmental retardation. The abdomen becomes enlarged, with first the spleen and later the liver increasing in size. Subsequently, neurological symptoms begin to appear; and these become quite marked, with hypertonia and opisthotonus. Dysphagia, choking spells, severe cough, and intermittent cyanosis are frequently present and are aggravated by increasing pulmonary infiltrations with Gaucher cells. Cachexia becomes marked, and death usually occurs during the first year of life.

HEREDITY.—Gaucher's disease is usually transmitted by an autosomal recessive gene, with the homozygote being affected. The condition has been noted among siblings in a number of families, and at least one instance of consanguinity has been reported. We have recently found that when one affected individual has central nervous system involvement, all affected siblings in that family would be similarly involved.

In 1948, Groen demonstrated that the asymptomatic father of one of the patients showed Gaucher-like cells in the sternal marrow, and he suggested that this factor might represent a carrier state for the disease. This finding requires confirmation.

PATHOGENESIS.—Laboratory studies show that in Gaucher's disease the serum lipid and cholesterol levels are normal. Fat absorption studies show that there is no alteration by the usual laboratory tests. Furthermore, no measurable quantities of cerebrosides have been found in the serum of these patients.

On the other hand, at least three substances have been isolated in abnormal quantities within the tissues containing Gaucher cells (Chart 57): (1) a galactosiderocerebroside (kerasin), which is composed of lignoceric acid, sphingosine, and galactose; (2) a glucosiderocerebroside, in which the hexose is present in the form of glucose instead of galactose; and (3) a water-soluble glycolipid, which is made up of long-chain saturated fatty acids, sphingosine, or a sphingosine-like base, and one or more hexose residues. This last type of compound has been named a "polycerebroside."

Two explanations have been suggested for these changes. Pick has felt that this condition represents a primary disturbance of the intermediary lipid metabolism, which expresses itself in an accumulation of cerebrosides in the serum and leads secondarily to a storage of this abnormal substance in the reticulum cells of the affected organs. Thannhauser, on the other hand, feels that there is a dysfunction of the reticular cells themselves as a result of an enzymatic disturbance within the cell, which leads to an increased synthesis of cerebrosides and simultaneously to a storage of these substances within the cell.

Normally, ceramide (lignoceric sphingosine) combines with cholinphosphoric ester under the influence of phosphorylcholinesterase to form sphingomyelin. Also, ceramide combines with galactose or glucose to

CHART 57

GAUCHER'S DISEASE

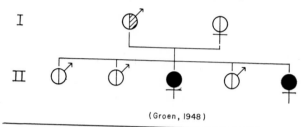

(Groen, 1948)

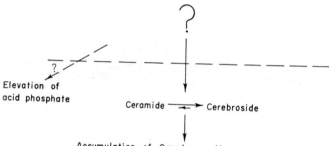

Elevation of acid phosphate

Ceramide ⇄ Cerebroside

Accumulation of Gaucher cells containing abnormal quantities of:

1) Galactosidero — cerebroside (Kerasin)
2) Glucosidero — cerebroside
3) Water-soluble glycolipid

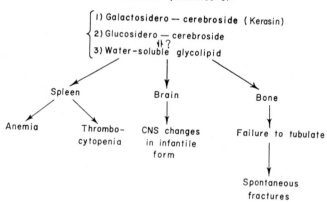

Spleen   Brain   Bone

Anemia   Thrombo-   CNS changes   Failure to tubulate
          cytopenia   in infantile
                          form

Spontaneous
fractures

240

form cerebrosides (Fig. 53). Thannhauser believes that in Gaucher's disease the balance of enzymes which leads to cerebroside formation or cerebroside disintegration is disturbed, with the result that cerebrosides accumulate in the organs involved. He has suggested that this may represent a perpetuation of a fetal mechanism after birth.

Uzman has shown that there is much less of the water-soluble glycolipid in the spleens of older patients with Gaucher's disease than in those

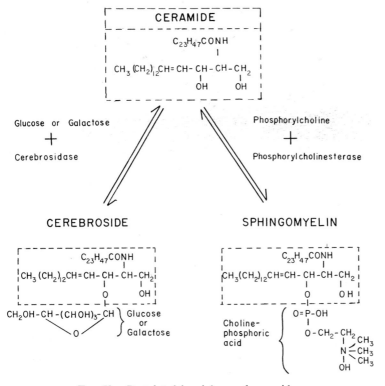

FIG. 53.—Postulated breakdown of ceramide.

of younger patients, although histologically both show heavy engorgement with Gaucher cells. He wonders if this compound represents a transitional stage which finally results in kerasin formation, since in Tay-Sachs disease there is great abundance of gangliosides in the central nervous system and since there is great similarity between gangliosides and polycerebrosides. This may help to explain the neurological changes in infantile Gaucher's disease.

Finally, Tuchman and his co-workers have shown an increase of acid phosphatase in the serum of patients with Gaucher's disease. The significance of this finding remains to be clarified.

DIAGNOSIS.—A positive diagnosis is established by demonstrating the characteristic accumulation of a pale, poorly staining material in large, often multinucleated cells with "wrinkled" cytoplasm (Fig. 54). Aspiration of the bone marrow is the safest and most frequently used method for finding the abnormal cells.

TREATMENT.—Splenectomy is sometimes helpful in relieving the ane-

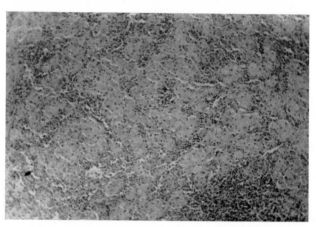

FIG. 54.—Photomicrograph of spleen in Gaucher's disease. Many large lipoid-filled cells occupy the pulp; a portion of a malpighian body occupies one margin.

mia and thrombocytopenia associated with hypersplenism. There is no treatment available for the basic defect.

Bigler, J. A.; Naylor, J. S.; and Hsia, D. Y. Y.: Gaucher's disease: report of a father-son transmission (to be published).

Gaucher, P. C. E.: De l'epithelioma primitif de la rate: Hypertrophie idiopathique de la rate sans leucemie (Paris, 1882).

Groen, J.: The hereditary mechanism of Gaucher's disease, Blood 3:1238, 1948.

Herndon, C. N., and Bender, J. R.: Gaucher's disease: Cases in five related Negro sibships, Am. J. Human Genet. 2:49, 1950.

Ottenstein, B.; Schmidt, G.; and Thannhauser, S. J.: Studies concerning the pathogenesis of Gaucher's disease, Blood 3:1250, 1948.

Tuchman, L. R.; Suna, H.; and Carr, J. J.: Elevation of serum acid phosphatase in Gaucher's disease, J. Mt. Sinai Hosp. New York 23:227, 1956.

Uzman, L. L.: Polycerebrosides in Gaucher's disease, A.M.A. Arch. Path. 55:181, 1953.

4. NIEMANN-PICK DISEASE (lipoid histiocytosis)

In 1914, Niemann described a new clinical syndrome which had many clinical features in common with Gaucher's disease but which appeared to spread more diffusely through all the organs. A few years later, Pick presented the characteristic pathological features, and hence it is now generally given the combined name "Niemann-Pick disease." About 80 such cases have been reported from all over the world.

CLINICAL FEATURES.—The clinical changes usually begin early in life. Although the infant may appear to be normal at birth, he soon begins to show both physical and mental retardation. Gradually, increasing debility and neurological deterioration, wasting of the extremities, and marked protuberance of the abdomen become noticeable. Spleen and liver are both markedly enlarged, with the hepatomegaly being more prominent than in Gaucher's disease. The skin is usually clear; but occasionally it has been observed to have extensive brownish, molelike pigmented areas, or vague, irregular, bluish or brownish discoloration, or, rarely, eruptive xanthomas. A cherry-red spot is present in the macula lutea in somewhat less than half of the patients. Anemia is often marked; and vacuolization in the agranulocytes in the peripheral blood smear can sometimes be found. Before long, the infant becomes apathetic and dull, and the clinical pattern can be defined as that of an anemic and emaciated idiot with an enlarged abdomen. Death occurs after the child is 6 months old; seldom do children with this condition live beyond 5 years.

During recent years a few cases of an adult, or chronic, type of Niemann-Pick disease have been described. The patients have the characteristic Niemann-Pick cells in the liver, lungs, and lymph nodes but show none of the clinical signs and symptoms described above.

Pathologically, there is an extremely generalized distribution of large pale cells (Fig. 55) with foamy-appearing vacuolated cytoplasm which stains in varying degree with the Smith-Dietrich myelin stain. The liver, spleen, lung, lymph nodes, and bone marrow are primarily involved, but almost no organ escapes infiltration. Degenerative changes in the ganglion cells with swelling are found in the central nervous system and elsewhere. The great similarity in the involvement of the central nervous system in both Niemann-Pick and Tay-Sachs disease has led to speculation on a possible common etiology of the two conditions.

HEREDITY.—Niemann-Pick disease has been described in Europe, the United States, Japan, and Australia. The condition is thought to appear with somewhat greater frequency among Jews.

The disease is probably transmitted by an autosomal recessive gene. There are many reports of the condition occurring among siblings, and it has appeared in a pair of identical twins. The heterozygous carrier is not detectable. Pfändler has suggested that the infant with the malignant form may represent the homozygote for the trait and that the adult, or chronic, form may represent the heterozygote. This has not been confirmed to date.

PATHOGENESIS.—A slight increase in some of the serum lipids has occasionally been seen in Niemann-Pick disease, but this is not a characteristic or consistent feature of the disease. On the other hand, there is an

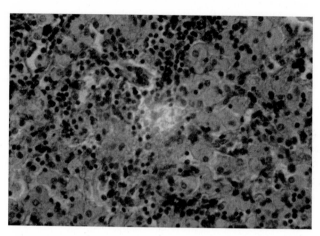

FIG. 55.—Photomicrograph of spleen in Niemann-Pick disease. The characteristic lipoid-filled cells occupy most of the pulp. The lipoid material and sphingomyelin distends the cytoplasm and displaces the nucleus peripherally.

immense intracellular accumulation of lipids, particularly sphingomyelin, in the tissues (Chart 58).

Thannhauser has postulated that in this disease the mechanism of conversion from ceramide to sphingomyelin is intact but the mechanism for reversing that step is defective (Fig. 53). As a result, sphingomyelin accumulates in the various tissues; and this results in hepatosplenomegaly, mental deterioration, and changes in the ganglion cells.

DIAGNOSIS.—The demonstration of the characteristic foam cells in the bone marrow or in a biopsy specimen of the spleen, liver, or lymph nodes is diagnostic of Niemann-Pick disease (Fig. 55).

TREATMENT.—None is of any avail.

*Crocker, A.: Niemann-Pick disease, Medicine 37:1, 1958.
Niemann, A.: Ein unbekanntes Krankheitsbild, Jahrb. f. Kinderh. 79:1, 1914.
Pick, L., and Bielschowsky, M.: Über lipoidzellige Splenomegalie (Typus Niemann-Pick) und amaurotische Idiotie, Klin. Wchnschr. 6:1631, 1927.
*Thannhauser, S. J.: Diseases of the nervous system associated with disturbances of lipid metabolism, Proc. A. Res. Nerv. & Ment. Dis. 32:238, 1953.
Videback, A.: Niemann-Pick disease: Acute or chronic type? Acta paediat. 37:95, 1949.

CHART 58

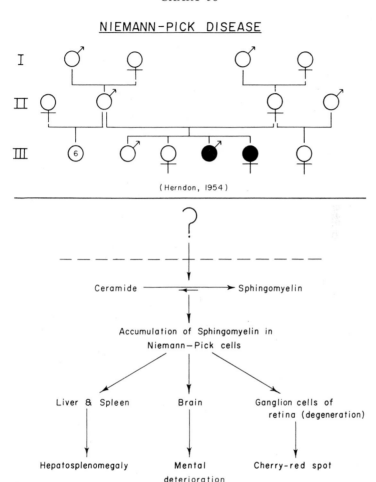

NIEMANN-PICK DISEASE

(Herndon, 1954)

5. AMAUROTIC FAMILIAL IDIOCY

"Amaurotic familial idiocy" is an over-all term applied to several distinct, but probably interrelated, disturbances in lipid metabolism. Generally, these are divided into the following types: (1) the infantile form (Tay-Sachs disease), (2) the late infantile form (Bielschowsky-Jansky disease), (3) the juvenile form (Spielmeyer-Vogt disease), and the late juvenile form (Kufs's disease).

INFANTILE AMAUROTIC FAMILIAL IDIOCY
(Tay-Sachs Disease)

In 1881, Tay described a familial disease of infants in which there appears in the maculae of both retinas during the first year of life a cherry-red spot which is surrounded by a fairly well-defined white area. A few years later, Sachs described autopsy findings and called the condition "amaurotic idiocy." It has subsequently been referred to as "Tay-Sachs disease," and over 100 cases of the condition have been reported in the world's literature.

CLINICAL FEATURES.—Affected children appear to be essentially normal up to the age of 4-6 months. The first noticeable changes are hyperacusis, irritability, and a plateauing of development. There is a progressive loss of muscle strength until the infant becomes completely helpless. Also, he no longer notices or recognizes the mother; the eyes cease to fix on objects; and gradually it becomes apparent that he sees badly, and he becomes blind later in the course of the disease. These symptoms are always accompanied by striking hyperacusis and sometimes by bursts of explosive laughter. Eventually the process advances to a state of complete idiocy. Early in the course of the disease, muscular spasticity and hyperflexion usually appear, with muscular twitchings and convulsions; this is followed by weight loss and emaciation; and, terminally, the infants have repeated respiratory infections with accumulation of secretions in the respiratory passages. There is also an increase of head size late in the disease which is not due to hydrocephalus. Most of the affected children die at about 2½-3½ years of age.

The ganglion cells of the retina are seriously affected by the degenerative process, which leads to an enlargement of the small red spot and allows more of the choroidal coat to show through; and the excess lipid in the ganglion cells produces the opaque whitish appearance of the zone surrounding the red spot, the color of the zone varying according to the intensity of the process. The brain is always firm and is frequently hard or leathery in consistency. The ganglion cells throughout the central nervous system are swollen, and the cytoplasm appears finely granular and sometimes vacuolated. Special stains demonstrate that the swelling and distortion of cells is due to the accumulation of lipid droplets. Defective primary myelination is noted together with cell destruction, and the microglia and astrocytes undergo proliferation and distention.

HEREDITY.—At one time, Tay-Sachs disease was believed to be limited to those of Hebrew ancestry. The occasional case that occurred in a non-Jewish child was thought to be either the result of racial mixing many generations ago or a matter of misdiagnosis. Experience with greater numbers of cases now indicates that about 10% of all Tay-Sachs patients are non-Jewish.

The disease appears to be transmitted by a rare recessive gene. Apart

CHART 59

TAY – SACHS DISEASE

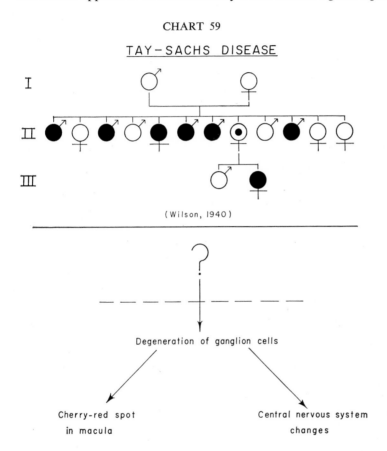

(Wilson, 1940)

Degeneration of ganglion cells

Cherry-red spot
in macula

Central nervous system
changes

from an increased incidence among siblings, the condition has been described in two sets of monozygotic twins, with both members of each pair being affected. Consanguinity is present in about 10% of the cases, the incidence being notably higher among non-Jews. This would seem to suggest that this rare recessive gene is present predominantly among Jewish people but that over the years it has spread slightly to the non-Jewish population through intermarriage. In agreement with this assumption, the homozygous form of the disease appears relatively frequently in random matings of Jewish parents but appears in non-Jews only when consanguinity occurs.

PATHOGENESIS.—The pathogenesis of this disease is completely unknown (Chart 59). The blood lipids do not appear to be disturbed. The only significant changes are in the nervous system, where there is a deposition of lipid material in the ganglion cells, eventually leading to their degeneration.

Many workers believe that Tay-Sachs disease and Niemann-Pick disease are interrelated, or may even be the same disease. Points in favor of this theory are: (1) both occur with increased frequency in the Jewish race; (2) the cherry-red spot and macular degeneration constitute a prominent feature in both conditions; (3) there are many points of similarity in the histological changes in the brain; and (4) cases of Tay-Sachs and Niemann-Pick disease have been described in siblings in the same families. However, sphingomyelin has not been a prominent component of the tissue in Tay-Sachs disease.

DIAGNOSIS.—Clinically, the condition is suggested by the presence of a cherry-red spot in the macula lutea without evidence of hepatosplenomegaly. The condition usually has to be confirmed by specific changes in the central nervous system at postmortem.

TREATMENT.—None is available.

*Rothstein, J. L., and Welt, S.: Infantile amaurotic idiocy, Am. J. Dis. Child. 62: 801, 1941.
Sachs, B.: On arrested cerebral development, with special reference to its cortical pathology, J. Nerv. & Ment. Dis. 14:541, 1887.
Slome, D.: The genetic basis of amaurotic familial idiocy, J. Genetics 27:363, 1933.
Tay, W.: Symmetrical changes in the region of the yellow spot in each eye of an infant, Tr. Ophth. Soc. U. Kingdom 1:55, 1881.
Wilson, S. A. K.: Neurology (Baltimore: Williams & Wilkins Company, 1940), vol. II, p. 877.
*Wynburn-Mason, R.: On some anomalous forms of amaurotic idiocy and their bearing on the relationship of the various types, Brit. J. Ophth. 27:145 and 193, 1943.

LATE INFANTILE AMAUROTIC FAMILIAL IDIOCY
(Bielschowsky-Jansky Disease)

The late infantile form of amaurotic idiocy was first described by Jansky and then by Bielschowsky. It is quite rare and seems to be intermediate between Tay-Sachs disease and Spielmeyer-Vogt disease.

CLINICAL FEATURES.—This form first appears at 3 or 4 years of age, and it runs a slower course than the infantile variety. In addition to the usual symptoms, children with this form of amaurotic idiocy develop ataxia and other cerebellar signs. The cherry-red spot in the macula is not found, but there is optic atrophy and pigmentation of the retina. There is some question whether the changes in the cases in this form are distinctive; this condition may merely be a variant of the infantile or the juvenile type.

HEREDITY.—The genetics of this form is not known. The type is not found predominantly in Jews.

PATHOGENESIS.—Unknown.

TREATMENT.—None is available.

Bielschowsky, M.: Über spät infantile familiäre amaurotische Idiotie mit Kleinhirn Symptomen, Deutsch. Ztschr. f. Nerv. 50:7, 1914.
Jansky, J.: Über einen bisher nicht publizierten Fall von familiärer amaurotische Idiotie, kompliziert mit Hypoplasie des Kleinhirns, Rev. de méd. Tchèque, Prague 1:58, 1908.

JUVENILE AMAUROTIC FAMILIAL IDIOCY
(Spielmeyer-Vogt Disease)

In 1903, Batten drew attention to the occurrence of "cerebral degeneration with symmetrical changes in the maculae in two members of a family." One patient developed symptoms at the age of 6 years, and his sister at the age of 5. The retinas showed generalized peppered pigmentary changes, and at each macula there was an irregular reddish black spot, with the region immediately surrounding the spot being paler. Shortly, Vogt and Spielmeyer reported further, with more detailed description of cases; and the condition has now become known as Spielmeyer-Vogt disease.

CLINICAL FEATURES.—The clinical course of Spielmeyer-Vogt disease is similar to that of Tay-Sachs disease but is distinguished by later onset and slower progression. The onset usually occurs between 3 and 10 years of age. Loss of vision is usually the first sign, and this is the only sign for about 2 years. It is followed by tonic and clonic convulsions and certain changes in mentality, including loss of emotional control, irritability, and alterations in personality. Definite mental deterioration follows, with progression to dementia. Muscle rigidity and signs of tremor start to appear, and paralysis follows. Sometimes athetosis is a prominent feature. Death occurs at about 15 years of age, following either convulsions or intercurrent infections.

The retinal lesions are often more diffuse than in Tay-Sachs disease, and there is often a dark brown pigmentation which can be mistaken for retinitis pigmentosa. There is also a secondary atrophy of the optic nerves with a rapid loss of vision.

HEREDITY.—Genetic studies have shown that Spielmeyer-Vogt disease is transmitted as an autosomal recessive; this is shown by a high incidence of the disease among siblings and in many cousin marriages in the reported cases. There is considerable evidence to suggest that the genes for Tay-Sachs disease and Spielmeyer-Vogt disease are not the same. For one thing, both conditions do not occur in the same family. Also, the latter does not occur predominantly among Jewish families.

PATHOGENESIS.—Klenk has shown that in this juvenile type of amaurotic idiocy there is present in the brain an unknown lipoid substance which has a melting point of 195° C and contains nitrogen and sugar. This lipoid material is regarded as composed of the same substances as those which enter into the formation of normal myelin and as being similar in many ways to the lipoidoses of Gaucher's and Niemann-Pick disease.

DIAGNOSIS.—This is usually made at postmortem because of the characteristic changes in the central nervous system.

TREATMENT.—None is available.

Klenk, E.: Beiträge zur der lipoidosen Niemann-Pickscher Krankheit und amaurotische Idiotie, Ztschr. physiol. Chem. 262:238, 1939.

Sjogren, T.: Die juvenile amaurotische Idiotie: Klinische und erblichkeitsmedizinische Untersuchungen, Hereditas (Lund) 14:197, 1931.

Spielmeyer, W.: Vom Wesen des anatomischen Prozesses bei der Familiären amaurotischen Idiotie, Jahrb. Psychiat. u. Neurol. 38:120, 1929.

Vogt, H.: Über familiäre amaurotische Idiotie und verwandte Krankheitsbilder, Monatsschr. Psychiat. u. Neurol. 18:161 and 310, 1905.

LATE JUVENILE AMAUROTIC FAMILIAL IDIOCY
(Kufs's Disease)

Also rare is the late juvenile form of amaurotic idiocy. It usually begins between the ages of 15 and 25 years and progresses very slowly. Convulsions and mental deterioration are the first-appearing symptoms. This state is followed by tremors, cerebellar ataxia, and muscular rigidity. As a rule, the patients do not suffer from loss of vision, but retinitis pigmentosa has been described in relatives.

The mode of transmission of this type of disease is unknown.

Kufs, H.: Über eine Spätform der amaurotischen Idiotie, Ztschr. d. ges. Neurol. u. Psychiat. 95:169, 1925.

It should be emphasized that one should take a flexible approach to this classification of types and that exceptions are not unusual. For instance, Wynburn-Mason has pointed out that the cherry-red spot may be seen in other than infantile cases, or that there may be an absence of the cherry-red spot in the infantile form, or that the infantile form may run a protracted clinical course. However, by such an arbitrary grouping one can differentiate the types with greater ease.

6. GARGOYLISM (Hurler's syndrome; lipochondrodystrophy)

This is a generalized disease process characterized by defects in the construction of the collagenous tissues within the body. The skeletal defects were first described by Hunter, an Englishman, in 1917; and the

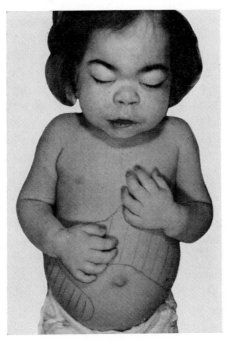

Fig. 56.—A typical gargoyle. Note the facies, the appearance of the hands, and the markings denoting the enlargement of the liver and spleen.

mental retardation and clouding of the cornea were noted by Hurler in Germany 2 years later. Over 250 cases of gargoylism have been described from all over the world.

CLINICAL FEATURES.—Patients with Hurler's syndrome can best be described by the term "grotesque" (Fig. 56). Changes are present in almost every part of the body.

The head is always enlarged and can be described as scaphocephalic. The lips are thick, and the teeth appear to be poorly formed and wide apart. The distance between the orbits is great. Many of the patients show a diffuse and spotty clouding of the cornea, which is thought to be due either to a corneal dystrophy or to a lipoid infiltration.

The skin is dry and coarse. The neck is short and the shoulders tend to be hunched, and so the head appears to be sitting directly on the chest. There is a dorsolumbar kyphosis, and the abdomen is large and protuberant. Hepatosplenomegaly is a frequent finding, and umbilical and inguinal hernias are sometimes present. Frequently a flexion deformity of the extremities is present, with limitation of extension; but this does not interfere with further flexion of the involved joints. Many gargoyles are mentally retarded, and deafness is a frequent complication.

Roentgenographic examination shows a widening of the suture lines, enlargement of the anterior fontanelle, and occasional bony ridges. In some cases the sella turcica is enlarged. In addition, the long bones, phalanges, and rib cage appear to be shorter and broader than usual; and sometimes there is a delay in the development of centers of epiphysial ossification (Fig. 57).

The principal pathological change consists of a widespread presence of vacuolated cells and an increase of collagen fibers and ground substance in various parts of the body, primarily in tissues of presumed fibroblastic origin. This causes an enlargement of the organs. In the brain there is a "ballooning" of the large ganglion cells of the cerebral cortex, basal ganglia, and the olivary bodies. In the heart there is a chronic endocarditis with fibrous thickening of the valves. Many of the patients die from cardiac failure.

HEREDITY.—Recent studies have shown that lipochondrodystrophy should probably be divided into two genetically distinct groups. Type 1 is transmitted by an autosomal recessive gene; both males and females are affected in equal numbers, and the incidence of consanguinity is comparatively high. The affected individuals show corneal clouding and dwarfism but seldom develop deafness. It is believed that about two thirds of all cases of Hurler's syndrome belong to this type. Type 2 is transmitted as a sex-linked recessive; only males are affected, and no consanguineous matings have been recorded. In Type 2, in contrast to the first type, corneal clouding is never seen, and only one third of the patients are dwarfed. On the other hand, about 43% of the patients are deaf.

The heterozygous carriers for gargoylism have not been detected by chemical tests.

PATHOGENESIS.—The storage substance in lipochondrodystrophy ap-

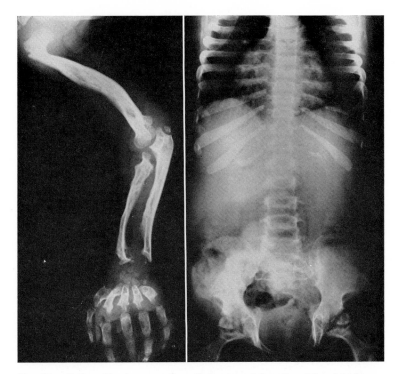

FIG. 57.—Deformities in gargoylism. *Left,* gross deformity of the right humerus, radius, and ulna, with gross irregular development of the epiphyses. The metacarpals and phalanges are bizarre in shape and show loss of modeling. The hands are broad, and the bones shortened and thickened. *Right,* lower thoracic ribs— narrow at the vertebral border and broader toward the periphery. Marked chondrodysplastic changes around the hip joints consist of incompletely developed acetabula and femoral heads and irregularity of the epiphysial-metaphysial junction. Bilateral coxa valga and enlarged liver and spleen are present.

pears to be made up of two distinct chemical entities (Chart 60). Brante has identified one of them as a mucopolysaccharide which is similar to or identical with chondroitin (or Mucotin®) sulfuric acid. This component appears to be made up of 3.9% sulfur, 27% hexosamine, and 26% glucuronic acid. It was found to be soluble in water but insoluble in ethanol and other organic solvents. It shows metachromasia with toluidine blue, which is characteristic of the storage substance in this condition. Recently, Dorfman and his associates have identified a similar mucopolysaccharide in the urine of patients with lipochondrodystrophy.

In 1955, Uzman identified a second storage substance in these tissues, a water-soluble glycolipid. This compound is soluble in ethanol but insol-

CHART 60

GARGOYLISM (HURLER'S SYNDROME)

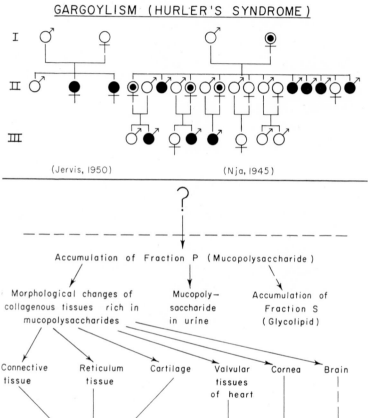

uble in other organic solvents. It is electrophoretically homogeneous at pH 8.6 and 7.0 but unhomogeneous at lower levels of pH. The chief constituents of this fraction appear to be fatty acids, sphingosine, neuraminic acid, hexuronic acid, hexosamines, glucose, and galactose.

Uzman has defined the mucopolysaccharide substance as fraction P and the glycolipid as fraction S. It is generally felt that the accumulation of fraction P is the primary metabolic defect and that fraction S is present as a consequence of the interference of normal function in involved cells resulting from the deposition of the first. This defect in the metabolism of a structural polysaccharide in proportion to protein growth and differentiation leads to morphological anomalies in tissues normally rich in polysaccharides, resulting in the formation of abnormal connective tissue, reticular tissue, cartilage, valvular tissues of the heart, and Bowman's layer of the cornea, which are the principal manifestations of gargoylism.

DIAGNOSIS.—The condition can usually be diagnosed by the typical grotesque facies and appearance. The diagnosis can be confirmed by the characteristic history and changes in the connective tissues.

TREATMENT.—None is of any avail.

Brante, G.: Gargoylism: A mucopolysaccharidosis, Scandinav. J. Clin. & Lab. Invest. 4:43, 1952.

Dorfman, A., and Lorincz, A. E.: Occurrence of urinary acid mucopolysaccharides in the Hurler's syndrome, Proc. Nat. Acad. Sc. 43:443, 1957.

Hunter, C.: A rare disease in two brothers, Proc. Roy. Soc. Med. 10:104, 1917.

Hurler, G.: Über einen Typ multipler Arbartungen vorwiegend am Skelet-system, Ztschr. Kinderh. 24:220, 1919.

Jervis, G. A.: Gargoylism (lipochondrodystrophy): A study of 10 cases with emphasis on the formes frustes of the disease, Arch. Neurol. & Psychiat. 63:681, 1950.

Nja, A.: A sex-linked type of gargoylism, Acta paediat. 33:267, 1945.

Uzman, L. L.: Chemical nature of the storage substance in gargoylism, A.M.A. Arch. Path. 60:308, 1955.

13

The Muscular Dystrophies

THE MUSCULAR DYSTROPHIES consist of a group of hereditary conditions characterized by a primary degenerative process within the skeletal muscles themselves. Unlike many of the neural and spinal muscular atrophies, there is no defect in the innervation of the affected muscles. In fact, one is frequently surprised to find pathologically that the muscular nerves and nerve endings are intact despite severe degeneration of the muscle fibers all around them. Clinically, the muscular atrophy is symmetrical in distribution, and the ability to respond to faradic excitability is retained in proportion to the remaining power of contraction. There are no sensory changes, and the cutaneous reflexes are preserved in this disease.

Although workers have described many separate and distinct types of muscular dystrophy, we shall limit the discussion to the following main groups: (1) *severe generalized familial muscular dystrophy*, (2) *mild restricted muscular dystrophy*, (3) *progressive dystrophia ophthalmoplegia*, and (4) *myotonia dystrophia*.

*Adams, R. C.; Denny-Brown, D.; and Pearson, C. M.: *Diseases of Muscle* (New York: Paul B. Hoeber, Inc., 1953), pp. 239-254.

I. SEVERE GENERALIZED FAMILIAL MUSCULAR DYSTROPHY
(Duchenne's pseudohypertrophic muscular dystrophy)

The severe generalized familial muscular dystrophy is the most common form of muscular dystrophy. The condition usually begins early in childhood and follows a rapidly progressive course. The patients may or may not show pseudohypertrophy, but the outcome and prognosis are about the same.

CLINICAL FEATURES.—The two outstanding clinical findings in pseudohypertrophic muscular dystrophy are a progressive alteration in the size of the muscles and weakness. Attention is called to the former because of an unusual enlargement of the calf muscles, which is followed by enlargement of the infraspinatus and deltoid muscles. Eventually, most of the muscles in the body become affected. As the disease progresses, the hypertrophy tends to turn to atrophy; and terminally, the patients may give the appearance of wasting away.

Evidence of weakness is usually apparent for several years before the disease is recognized. The weakness may be suggested by an inability to walk or run at the usual age, or a tendency to fall easily. As the condition progresses, there is a bilateral weakness of the extensors of the hip and knee joints which interferes with such activities as arising from the floor or from a chair and climbing stairs. Ultimately, marked deformities and scoliosis may develop from the weakness.

Death usually occurs either because of persistent pulmonary infections or from cardiac hypertrophy and failure. Patients with this disease seldom survive past 20 years of age.

HEREDITY.—Pseudohypertrophic muscular dystrophy occurs 6 times as frequently in males as in females. The disease can also be transmitted by unaffected females. Because of this, it is generally agreed that the condition is transmitted as a sex-linked recessive.

The most extensive genetic studies on the disease were made by Julia Bell, who analyzed 1,228 cases from the literature and the files of the National Hospital in Queen's Square, London. The reader is referred to her excellent monographs on how a disease should properly be studied from the genetic standpoint.

PATHOGENESIS.—Numerous attempts have been made to discover a fundamental biochemical abnormality in progressive muscular dystrophy. So far, this research has led to several pieces of isolated information which may or may not prove to be important in the etiology of this disease (Chart 61).

First, most patients with progressive muscular dystrophy show an increase in the excretion of creatine and a decrease in the excretion of creatinine in the urine during the acute phase of the disease. In advanced dystrophy, the content of both the creatine and the creatinine in the urine decreases to below that of normal. Some investigators have also found an increase of creatine in the plasma while the creatinine remains within normal limits. It is believed that these abnormalities reflect changes in muscle mass and have little to do with the energy mechanisms in muscle contraction.

Second, Milhorat and others have shown that a deficiency of *l*-tocopherol (vitamin E) in rabbits causes a pathological condition not un-

CHART 61

SEVERE GENERALIZED FAMILIAL MUSCULAR DYSTROPHY

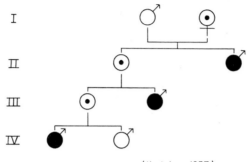

(Kostakow, 1937)

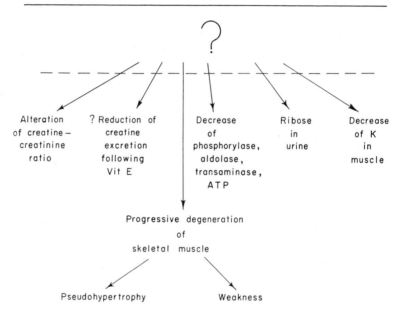

Alteration of creatine— creatinine ratio	? Reduction of creatine excretion following Vit E	Decrease of phosphorylase, aldolase, transaminase, ATP	Ribose in urine	Decrease of K in muscle

Progressive degeneration of skeletal muscle

Pseudohypertrophy   Weakness

like that of muscular dystrophy. However, the administration of vitamin E to patients with the disease does not in any way alter the muscular weakness or atrophy.

Third, chemical analyses of dystrophic muscles have shown that there is less creatine, phosphocreatine, and adenosinetriphosphate present than in normal muscle. More recently, Dreyfus and his associates have shown that in such muscle there is also a decrease in the activity of phosphorylase and aldolase. On the other hand, aldolase and glutamic oxalacetic transaminase are greatly increased in the serum of dystrophic patients.

Fourth, Minot and his co-workers have demonstrated the presence of a pentose in the urine (see Procedure 72) of the majority of patients with progressive muscular dystrophy.

Finally, Horvath and his associates have shown that there is an actual decrease of potassium in the muscles of such patients as compared with normal controls.

While it is still too early to speculate on the possible mechanisms responsible for this disease of skeletal muscle, these preliminary findings suggest that it represents a defect in either glycolysis or energy transfer, possibly at the membrane level.

DIAGNOSIS.—The diagnosis can be established on clinical grounds and confirmed by muscle biopsy.

TREATMENT.—Symptomatic therapy to prevent pulmonary and cardiac complications is needed late in the course of the disease.

*Bell, J.: On pseudohypertrophic and allied types of progressive muscular dystrophy, in *The Treasury of Human Inheritance* (London: Cambridge University Press, 1943), vol. 4, pp. 283-342.

Dreyfus, J. C.; Schapira, G.; and Schapira, F.: Biochemical study of muscle in progressive muscular dystrophy, J. Clin. Invest. 33:794, 1954.

Duchenne, G. B.: *De l'electrisatron localisee et son application a la pathologie et a la thérapeutique* (Paris: J. B. Baillière et fils, 1855).

Gowers, W. R.: *Pseudo-Hypertrophic Muscular Paralysis: A Clinical Lecture* (London: J. & A. Churchill, Ltd., 1879).

Horvath, B.; Berg, L.; Cummings, D. J.; and Shy, G. M.: Muscular dystrophy: Blood content of dystrophic muscles, J. Appl. Physiol. 8:22, 1955.

Kostakow, S., and Derix, F.: Familien forschung in einer muskeldystrophischen Sippe und die Erbprognose ihrer Mitglieder, Deutsches Arch. klin. Med. 180: 585, 1937.

Minot, A. S.; Frank, H.; and Dziewiatkowski, D.: Occurrence of pentose and phosphorus-containing complexes in the urine of patients with progressive muscular dystrophy, Arch. Biochem. 20:394, 1949.

Nevin, S.: A study of muscle chemistry in myasthenia gravis, pseudohypertrophic muscular dystrophy, and myotonia, Brain 57:239, 1934.

Pearson, C. M.: Serum enzymes in muscular dystrophy and certain other muscular and neuromuscular diseases: I. Serum glutamic oxalacetic transaminase, New England J. Med. 256:1069, 1957.

Proceedings of the 1st and 2nd Medical Conferences of the Muscular Dystrophy

Association, Inc., Held in New York April 14-15, 1951, and May 17-18, 1952 (ed. by A. T. Milhorat) (New York: Muscular Dystrophy Association of America, Inc., 1953).

*Shank, R. E.; Giler, H.; and Hoagland, L.: Studies on diseases of muscle: I. Progressive muscular dystrophy; a clinical review of 40 cases, Arch. Neurol. & Psychiat. 52:431, 1944.

2. MILD RESTRICTED MUSCULAR DYSTROPHY (facioscapulohumeral dystrophy of Landouzy and Déjerine)

Unlike the severe generalized familial muscular dystrophy, mild restricted muscular dystrophy is slow in progression, with long remissions and often complete arrest. It involves primarily the musculature of the shoulder and often of the face.

CLINICAL FEATURES.—The first symptoms of this condition are usually noted between the ages of 7 and 20 years. The most common initial complaint is the loss of ability to raise the arms above the head or to hold them in that position. Some patients note abnormal posture without noting this symptom.

As the disease progresses, there is atrophy and weakness of the facial muscles, resulting in an inability to pucker the lips and whistle and an in-co-ordination of the remainder of the facial muscles. The shoulder muscles also become involved, with the pectoralis major, rhomboids, and deltoids being most seriously affected. However, the weakness progresses very slowly, and most of the patients have a normal life span with only minor disability.

HEREDITY.—Mild restricted muscular dystrophy has been extensively studied by Tyler and Stephens in a Mormon family in which 159 out of 1,249 members are affected with the facioscapulohumeral type of dystrophy. They have concluded that the condition is transmitted as a simple autosomal dominant with complete penetrance but variable expression.

This form of muscular dystrophy, however, can also sometimes be transmitted as a recessive trait, as reported in a small restricted community in Switzerland by Minkowski and Sidler. Probably the term "mild restricted muscular dystrophy" should be applied to a variety of nearly similar muscular dystrophies, each caused by a separate gene abnormality; and thus, each would be expected to show a different mode of inheritance.

PATHOGENESIS.—It is not clear at present whether this type of muscular dystrophy has a common etiology with the type described in the preceding section. If so, much of the discussion above would be applicable here (Chart 62).

CHART 62

MILD RESTRICTED MUSCULAR DYSTROPHY

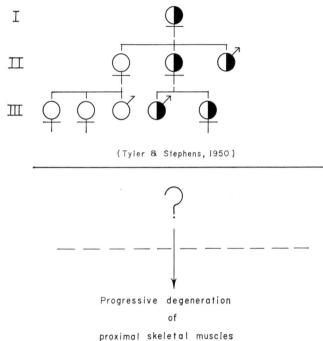

(Tyler & Stephens, 1950)

Progressive degeneration

of

proximal skeletal muscles

DIAGNOSIS.—The clinical signs and course are characteristic, and the diagnosis can be confirmed by muscle biopsy.

TREATMENT.—Usually, none is required.

andouzy, L., and Déjerine, J.: De la myopathie atrophique progressive (myopathie héréditaire) débutant dans l'enfance, par la face, sans altération du système nerveux, Compt. rend. Acad. sc. 98:53, 1884.

inkowski, M., and Sidler, A.: Zur Kenntnis der dystrophia musculorum progressiva und ihrer Vererbung, Schweiz. med. Wchnschr. 9:1005, 1928.

yler, F. H., and Stephens, F. E.: Studies in disorders of muscle: II. Clinical manifestations and inheritance of facioscapulohumeral dystrophy in a large family, Ann. Int. Med. 32:640, 1950.

3. PROGRESSIVE DYSTROPHIA OPHTHALMOPLEGIA

Progressive dystrophia ophthalmoplegia can develop at any age. The onset is usually insidious and the course progresses slowly.

CLINICAL FEATURES.—As a rule, ptosis of the eyelids is noted first.

This is followed by a progressive weakness of the lateral and vertic
movements of the eyes. In the advanced stage of the disease, all mov
ments are paralyzed and the eyes remain slightly divergent. Myotoni
cataracts, and other endocrine disturbances have not been observe
(Chart 63).

HEREDITY.—The condition occurs with about equal frequency i

CHART 63

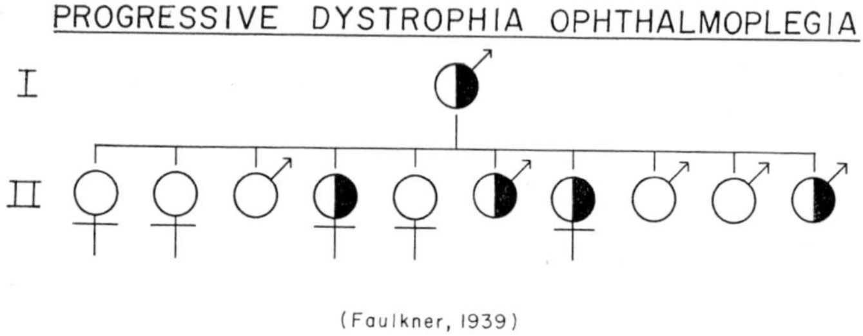

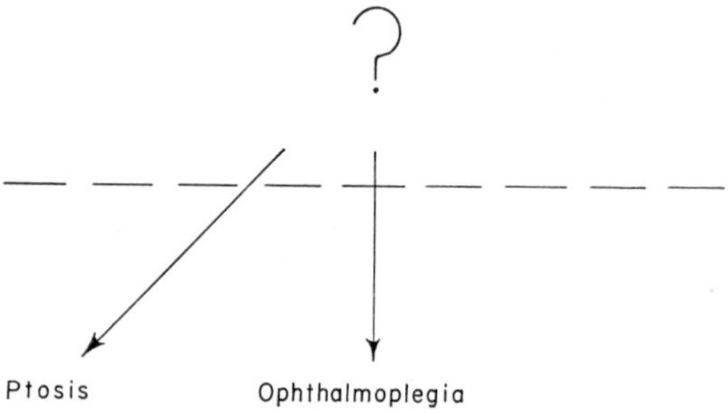

PROGRESSIVE DYSTROPHIA OPHTHALMOPLEGIA

(Faulkner, 1939)

Ptosis   Ophthalmoplegia

males and females. In about half of the families a history of ptosis o
ophthalmoplegia can be elicited.

The disease is usually transmitted as an autosomal dominant trai
but instances of recessive inheritance have also been described.

PATHOGENESIS.—Nothing is known.

DIAGNOSIS.—The clinical course is usually quite typical.

TREATMENT.—As a rule, none is required.

Bradburne, A. A.: Hereditary ophthalmoplegia in five generations, Tr. Ophth. Soc
U. Kingdom 32:142, 1912.
Faulkner, S. H.: Familial ptosis with ophthalmoplegia externa starting in adult life
Brit. M. J. 2:854, 1939.
Gates, R. R.: Human Genetics (New York: The MacMillan Company, 1936), vol
II, pp. 955-1009.

4. MYOTONIA DYSTROPHIA

Myotonia dystrophia is a familial disorder characterized by myotonia, trophy of the distal muscle compartments, cataracts, frontal baldness, nd various endocrinopathies.

CLINICAL FEATURES.—In most patients the myotonia precedes the uscular atrophy by 2 or 3 years. The prolonged contraction of skeletal muscles can be caused by external factors such as electrical or mechanal stimulation, or it can represent a delay in relaxation after a strong oluntary contraction. The latter state tends to be aggravated by cold and is more marked after the muscles have been at rest for some time.

The muscle atrophy follows a characteristic pattern and eventually involves the abduction of the thumb, the muscles of the forearm, the ternocleidomastoids, the facial muscles, the quadriceps, and the dorsiexors of the feet. One is frequently impressed by the thinness and lack f expression in the face, and there is a wasting-away of the masseters and ternocleidomastoids.

Myotonia dystrophia differs from the other forms of muscular dystrohy with regard to the endocrine glands. The most common disturbance testicular insufficiency, characterized by atrophy of the seminiferous bules, an absence of spermatogenic and Sertoli's cells, and normalppearing Leydig cells. This results in either reduced libido or impotnce in a considerable proportion of the reported cases, and most patients ith myotonia dystrophia fail to reproduce. Other endocrine disturbances clude deficiencies of the thyroid, adrenal, and pituitary glands. Frontal aldness and cataracts are also frequently seen.

HEREDITY.—The condition seems to be transmitted as an autosomal ominant. However, in some instances, both parents appear to be normal.

Fleischer and others believe that the disease may frequently occur an earlier age, and in a more severe form, in each succeeding generaon. They point out that in a given family the dominant inheritance may manifest itself in the first generation by a very slight sign, such as senile ataracts; in the next generation, by earlier onset of cataracts; in the next eneration, by the full syndrome of myotonia dystrophia; and that sterlity excludes the continued propagation of that trait. On the other hand, enrose feels that the degree of manifestation of the main gene for myonia dystrophia does not depend on this, but on the allelic gene which companies it.

PATHOGENESIS.—This is completely unknown at the present time. me preliminary studies suggest that the endocrinopathy does not in any

CHART 64

MYOTONIA DYSTROPHIA

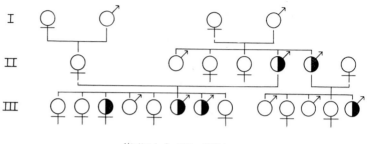

(Holland & Hill, 1956)

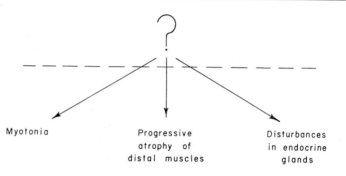

Myotonia   Progressive   Disturbances
atrophy of   in endocrine
distal muscles   glands

way appear to be related to the muscular defect in the patients (Chart 64).

DIAGNOSIS.—The clinical course usually suggests the diagnosis. Muscle and testicular biopsies may be helpful.

TREATMENT.—None is of any avail.

Fleischer, B.: Über myotonische Dystrophie mit Katarakt: Eine hereditäre familiäre Degeneration, Arch. Ophth. 96:91, 1918.

Holland, C. M., and Hill, S. R.: Myotonia dystrophica: Report of six cases in one family, with an analysis of the metabolic defects, Ann. Int. Med. 44:738, 1956.

Penrose, L. S.: The problem of anticipation in pedigrees of dystrophia myotonica, Ann. Eugenics 14:125, 1948.

*Ravin, A.: Myotonia, Medicine 18:443, 1939.

14

Miscellaneous Metabolic Disorders

WE SHALL NOW take up the disturbances which have not so far been classified into specific groups. The first three (*idiopathic spontaneous hypoglycemia, pituitary diabetes insipidus,* and *diabetes mellitus*) represent endocrine disorders; the last three (*gout, hereditary periodic paralysis, and congenital pancytopenia with multiple congenital anomalies*), disturbances in purine, electrolyte, and possibly peroxidase metabolism.

1. IDIOPATHIC SPONTANEOUS HYPOGLYCEMIA

In the 1954 presidential address before the American Pediatric Society, Dr. Irvine McQuarrie reported on 25 children with signs and symptoms which might best be described as those of "idiopathic spontaneous hypoglycemia." In many instances the condition appears to be familial in nature, and it should probably be included among the inborn errors of metabolism.

CLINICAL FEATURES.—Children with this condition suffer from fatigue, weakness, flushing, sweating, speech disturbances, and visual disturbances. There are also neurological manifestations, such as in-cordination, tremor, syncope, convulsions, and coma. In milder cases the changes may be confined to irritability, negativism, and behavior changes. There may also be hypothermia.

Idiopathic spontaneous hypoglycemia usually appears before the age of 2 years, and the symptoms tend to become milder as the child grows older. If the condition goes unrecognized—and this can easily be the case—permanent brain damage may be the result, characterized by epileptic seizures and mental retardation, complications which are irreversible.

HEREDITY.—Idiopathic spontaneous hypoglycemia appears to be

familial, since 11 of the 25 children studied by McQuarrie had brother or sisters with the same complaint. The condition is probably transmitte as an autosomal recessive with incomplete manifestation. Some of th milder cases probably go unrecognized because of the difficulties of bein absolutely certain of the diagnosis. Anderson has reported that some c the parents of affected children show an abnormal response to insulir

PATHOGENESIS.—The exact mechanism responsible for idiopathi

CHART 65

IDIOPATHIC SPONTANEOUS HYPOGLYCEMIA

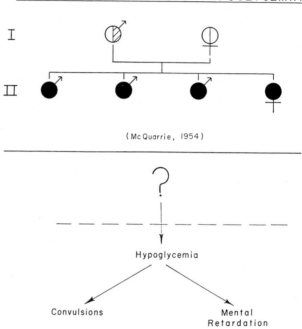

(McQuarrie, 1954)

spontaneous hypoglycemia is not well understood (Chart 65). When co ticotropin (plain ACTH) is given intramuscularly, the fasting bloc glucose level rises, the patient no longer suffers from hypoglycemia c convulsions, and normal mental development becomes possible. Th would suggest that the hypoglycemia is in some way related to an adren deficiency, which can be corrected by stimulation with pituitary hormon

DIAGNOSIS.—The oral glucose tolerance test (using 1.75 Gm of gl cose per kilogram of body weight, given by mouth in a fasting state shows either a flat response or a diabetic type of curve, which eventual drops to hypoglycemic levels with a true glucose value of less than 5

1g/100 ml. There is also unusual sensitivity to small doses of insulin. On the other hand, the blood sugar will show a characteristic response to drenalin, since there are adequate stores of glycogen.

Idiopathic spontaneous hypoglycemia should be differentiated from 1) true hyperinsulinism, which is caused by an adenoma, malignant tumor, or hyperplasia of the beta cells of the islets of Langerhans; (2) other specific causes, such as adrenal insufficiency, panhypopituitarism, hypothyroidism, and von Gierke's disease; and (3) functional disturbances of carbohydrate metabolism, such as the "dumping" syndrome.

TREATMENT.—ACTH, 5-10 mg every 2 or 3 days, appears to be the treatment of choice. Partial pancreatectomy or the production of diabetes mellitus by alloxan used to be tried as a means of controlling hypoglycemia; but since the introduction of the corticotropins, such therapy is no longer necessary.

Anderson, R. C.; Wright, W. S.; Bauer, E. G.; and McQuarrie, I.: Familial hypo-glycemosis of probable genetic origin, Am. J. Human Genet. 2:264, 1950.
McQuarrie, I.: Idiopathic spontaneously occurring hypoglycemia in infants, A.M.A. Am. J. Dis. Child. 87:399, 1954.
———; Bauer, E. G.; Ziegler, M. R.; and Wright, W. S.: Effect of pituitary adreno-corticotropic hormone in children with non-Addisonian hypoglycemia, Proc. Soc. Exper. Biol. & Med. 71:555, 1949.

2. PITUITARY DIABETES INSIPIDUS

Pituitary diabetes insipidus is a rare genetic condition characterized by an increase of thirst and the passage of large quantities of urine low in specific gravity. The symptoms can be relieved quickly by the adminis-tation of antidiuretic hormone preparations.

CLINICAL FEATURES.—Polydipsia and polyuria are the principal symptoms. During early infancy the child cries excessively and can only be quieted by being given large amounts of fluids to drink. If unrelieved, the infant quickly becomes dehydrated, and fever usually develops. In older children, nocturnal and diurnal polyuria is the rule, and enuresis is not an uncommon complaint. Thirst is accompanied by epigastric pain, hunger, and a sensation of a rise in temperature developing in the after-noon, with the lips developing the "sensation of fever blisters."

HEREDITY.—Several large pedigrees of families afflicted with this disease have been reported. In most instances, pituitary diabetes insipidus is transmitted as an autosomal dominant. However, Forssman has re-ported on two pedigrees in which this form of diabetes insipidus has been inherited as a sex-linked recessive. The heterozygous carriers of this ab-normality have not been detected by laboratory tests.

Pituitary diabetes insipidus is a rare disease. In 1914, Fitz collecte
the material from four hospitals and found 79 cases out of 553,007 pa
tients, or 14.5 per 100,000. From the Mayo Clinic, Rowntree has note
56 cases out of 428,000 patients.

PATHOGENESIS.—In 1913, von der Velden and Farini, working sep
arately, showed that the extracts of the posterior lobe of the pituitary hav

CHART 66

DIABETES INSIPIDUS

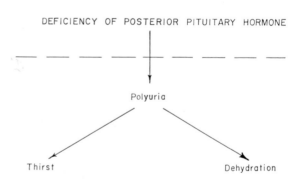

(Levinger & Escamilla, 1955)

DEFICIENCY OF POSTERIOR PITUITARY HORMONE

Polyuria

Thirst   Dehydration

an antidiuretic effect on patients with pituitary diabetes insipidus (Cha
66). This active substance was later identified as vasopressin.

The production of vasopressin depends on a complex functional un
which consists of the posterior lobe of the pituitary gland, part of the in

fundibular stalk, the nucleus paraventricularis, the nucleus supraopticus of the hypothalamus, and the nerve tracts connecting them. Damage to any part of this functional unit may cause a deficiency in the excretion of vasopressin, and diabetes insipidus may be expected to develop. Presumably, some disturbance in this basic mechanism is responsible for the hereditary form of pituitary diabetes insipidus.

The antidiuretic principle of the posterior lobe of the pituitary acts on the kidney tubules. A deficiency of this causes either a failure to reabsorb water preferentially or to avoid reabsorption of salt, or both (Chart 66).

DIAGNOSIS.—The diagnosis of pituitary diabetes insipidus is suggested by a failure to concentrate urine above a specific gravity of 1.008 despite withholding fluids to the point of discomfort in the patient. The condition must be differentiated from the following: psychogenic polydipsia, nephrogenic diabetes insipidus, and secondary pituitary diabetes insipidus. (1) Psychogenic polydipsia can be determined by observing the effect of an intravenous infusion of hypertonic saline solution on urine flow. The patient with true diabetes insipidus will not show the characteristic increased urinary output of the normal individual (see Procedure 63). (2) A patient with pituitary diabetes insipidus will show a cessation of diuresis and an increase of urine specific gravity after the administration of a 30 mg lozenge of posterior pituitary extract, while the patient with nephrogenic diabetes insipidus will show no such response (see Procedure 63). (3) Secondary pituitary diabetes insipidus is usually due to a specific cause, such as a pituitary tumor, encephalitis, Hand-Schüller-Christian disease, trauma, etc., and has no familial basis.

TREATMENT.—For the sake of convenience, lozenges of posterior pituitary, 30 mg each, are effective when taken every 4 hours. Patients will also respond to vasopressin tannate in oil or to posterior pituitary powder used as snuff.

Cannon, J. F.: Diabetes insipidus, A.M.A. Arch. Int. Med. 96:215, 1955.
Farini, A.: Diabete insipido ed optoterpia ipifisaria, Gas. d. opp. 34:1135, 1913.
Forssman, H.: On hereditary diabetes insipidus, Acta med. scandinav., suppl. 159, 1945.
Levinger, E. L., and Escamilla, R. F.: Hereditary diabetes insipidus, J. Clin. Endocrinol. 15:547, 1955.
von der Velden, R.: Die Nierenwirkung von Hypophysenextrakten beim Menschen, Berlin klin. Wchnschr. 50:2083, 1913.

3. DIABETES MELLITUS

In a book of this size, it is obviously impossible to give an adequate discussion on the diagnosis, pathogenesis, and treatment of diabetes mellitus. Instead, we shall take up only the genetic aspects of this inborn error of metabolism.

HEREDITY.—It is universally agreed that there is a large hereditary component in the causation of diabetes mellitus. In fact, in the preamble to Chapter 3 of *The Treatment of Diabetes Mellitus,* Joslin states that "heredity is the basis of diabetes." Disagreement arises, however, when an attempt is made to describe the exact nature of this component.

The first extensive studies on the hereditary nature of diabetes mellitus were done by Pincus and White in 1934. They presented the following evidence to support the hypothesis that the disease has a genetic origin: (1) the almost simultaneous occurrence of diabetes mellitus in both members of pairs of similar twins, (2) the greater incidence of diabetes mellitus in blood relatives of diabetics than in a controlled population, (3) the demonstration that Mendelian ratios of the recessive type are found in a large series of cases selected at random, (4) the demonstration of expected ratios in presumably latent cases, and (5) the observation, from genealogies, that diabetics behave as a recessive trait.

In the years that followed, there was considerable controversy over the mode of inheritance of diabetes mellitus. Opinions varied all the way from regarding the condition as a dominant with a penetrance of about 10%, to regarding it as an autosomal recessive, to considering it a sex-linked tendency in familial diabetes in a significant proportion of the families. In 1950, Harris suggested that many of the late-onset cases may be heterozygous for a gene which, in homozygous form, may give rise to the severe, early-onset type of case.

The recent studies of Steinberg and Wilder suggest that diabetes mellitus is transmitted by a single autosomal recessive gene, d. Individuals who are genetically liable to develop the disease are dd, and those who are not genetically liable to develop it are Dd or DD. These investigators have estimated that about 5% of the population of the United States belongs to dd. However, because of the variable age of onset and the difficulty of making the diagnosis clinically, only about 1% of the population is recognized as being diabetic.

Using this type of nomenclature, it is possible to calculate the probability of genetic susceptibility to diabetes mellitus in any given family. When Dd mates Dd, it is expected that 25% of the offspring will be dd. When Dd mates dd, where one parent is genetically liable to develop diabetes mellitus, 50% of the offspring will be dd. Finally, when dd mates dd, 100% of the offspring will be dd also. On this same assumption, it is possible to calculate the probability of any one individual in a given family being dd if one knows that certain other relatives in the same family have diabetes mellitus or may be dd.

We are still left with the problems of how to determine (1) which asymptomatic individuals are dd and (2) when they are likely to show symptoms of diabetes mellitus. Fajans and Conn have made progress toward answering the first question by devising a combined cortisone-glucose tolerance test. They found that 19% of 152 relatives of known diabetics showed an abnormality of the usual glucose tolerance test. However, if 50 mg of cortisone was administered 8 hours before, the incidence was increased to 24%. In contrast, only 1 of 50 control subjects with no history of diabetes mellitus in the family demonstrated an abnormality with the usual glucose tolerance test, and 1 of 37 control subjects demonstrated blood sugar changes by the cortisone-glucose tolerance test.

Woodyatt and Spetz have suggested that the onset of diabetes mellitus becomes earlier with each affected generation. Thus, if the grandfather developed diabetes mellitus at the age of 50, the father may develop symptoms at 30, and the offspring at 10. More recent studies suggest that, although such a trend may sometimes be present, there is no evidence of such a consistent relationship between parent and child, and the term "anticipation" should not be used.

In summary, present thinking indicates that diabetes mellitus is probably transmitted by a simple autosomal recessive gene. Individuals who are homozygous for this gene (dd) are liable to develop diabetes, but the age of onset is highly variable.

Fajans, S. S., and Conn, J. W.: An approach to the prediction of diabetes by modification of the glucose tolerance test with cortisone, Diabetes 3:296, 1954.

Harris, H.: The familial distribution of diabetes mellitus: A study of the relatives of 1241 diabetic propositi, Ann. Eugenics 15:95, 1950.

Pincus, G., and White, P.: On the inheritance of diabetes: II. Further analysis of family histories, Am. J. M. Sc. 188:159, 1934.

Steinberg, A. G., and Wilder, R. M.: An analysis of the phenomenon of "anticipation" in diabetes mellitus, Ann. Int. Med. 36:1285, 1952.

Woodyatt, R. T., and Spetz, M.: Anticipation in the inheritance of diabetes, J.A.M.A. 120:602, 1942.

4. GOUT

Gout is a hereditary constitutional disorder of purine metabolism characterized by increased amounts of uric acid in the blood and recurrent attacks of acute arthritis. If the articular inflammation becomes chronic, tophaceous deposits of sodium urate take place in many of the tissues.

The history of gout is a long and distinguished one. The early writings of Aretaeus of Cappadocia and Caelius Aurelianus indicate that the physicians of Greece and Rome had an intimate knowledge of its varied features. For instance, Aretaeus mentions that during the asymptomatic periods, a gouty subject was capable of winning in the Olympic games. Throughout the ages, members of the nobility seem to have been especially prone to develop the disease, and few royal lines appear to have escaped. Writers of fiction and biography have made classical descriptions of its dramatic appearance, the ensuing pathos, and the rapid recovery with or without treatment. Victims of gout were also the favored subjects of many caricatures during the nineteenth century.

CLINICAL FEATURES.—The best clinical description of an acute attack of gout was given in 1696 by Dr. Thomas Sydenham, himself a victim of the disease for 34 years. Since this account has not been improved upon, we shall quote from him directly:

He goes to bed and sleeps well, but about two a Clock in the Morning is waked by the Pain, seizing either his great Toe, the Heel, the Calf of the Leg or the Ancle; this Pain is like that of dislocated Bones, with the Sense as it were of Water, almost cold, poured upon the membranes of the Parts affected, presently shivering and shaking follow, with a feverish Disposition; the Pain is first gentle but increases by degrees . . . sometimes resembling a violent stretching or tearing those Ligaments, sometimes the gnawing of a Dog, and sometimes a weight; moreover the part affected has such a quick and exquisite Pain, that it is not able to bear the weight of the Cloths upon it, nor hard walking in the chamber; and the Night is not passed over in Pain upon this account only, but also by reason of the restless turning of the Part hither and thither, and the continual Change of its place . . . yet there is no ease to be had till two or three a Clock in the Morning . . . . And now being in a breathing Sweat, he falls asleep, when he wakes he finds the Pain much abated, and the Part affected swelled afresh; for before that there was only (which is usual in the Fits of those that have the Gout) visible, a swelling of the Veins intermixed with the affected Members. The next Day, and perhaps two or three after . . . the part affected will be in Pain, which will be violent towards Evening, but it will be eased about the time of the Cock's crowing; within a few Days the other Foot will be in Pain as the former was; and if the former have left off aking, the Weakness which rendered it infirm will presently vanish, Strength and perfect Health being so presently restored, as if it never had been out of order.

Recurrent attacks of acute arthritis are followed by remissions during which the patient experiences no arthritic symptoms. These periods become progressively shorter until acute episodes occur regularly once or twice a year. As the disease continues, more of the joints become affected. In addition to the first metatarsophalangeal joint, which is usually the first to become affected, other joints in the feet, hands, ankles, and wrists become involved. The infiltration of urates into periarticular and bursal tissues produces subcutaneous tophi, which are the cause of the knobby deformities of the knuckles and interphalangeal joints. Tophaceous deposits can also occur in nonarticular cartilages, such as the helix of the ear.

Attacks of acute gouty arthritis can sometimes be precipitated by trauma, food, and excessive alcoholic intake.

HEREDITY.—The exact incidence of gout is not known because statistics reported for various sections of the United States and other countries require interpretation. For instance, only a small fraction of 1% of the meat-eating people of the British Isles are afflicted; while 7% of the natives in India, who are largely vegetarians and teetotalers, have gout. These astonishing variations are due partly to the differences in the populations studied and in the diagnostic standards applied. It should be remembered that the diagnosis is frequently missed because the patients do not exhibit all of the classical features of chronic gout.

From the beginning, medical writers have believed that gout is a hereditary disease, but the mode of transmission was not well understood. In 1948, Smyth and his co-workers showed that asymptomatic hyperuricemia is caused by a single autosomal dominant gene but that only a fraction of those with hyperuricemia ever develop clinically recognizable gout. They explained the lower incidence of the disease in women in the following way. They estimated that the statistical upper limit of normal serum uric acid level in women is about 1 mg/100 ml lower than in men. As a result, levels of 5-6 mg/100 ml represent hyperuricemia among female relatives of gouty patients. These slight increases are sufficient to equalize the distribution of hyperuricemia between the sexes but are usually not sufficient to cause precipitation of urates in tissues and the symptoms of gout clinically.

At present, there is no way of determining which of the individuals with hyperuricemia will develop gout.

PATHOGENESIS.—Various theories have been advanced to explain the complex features of gout; but, unfortunately, none are compatible with all of the known facts about the disease (Chart 67). It should be mentioned that in most mammals uric acid is converted by means of an enzyme, uricase, to the more readily soluble allantoin. However, New World monkeys, the anthropoid apes, and men lack this uricolytic enzyme. As a result, uric acid either has to be disposed of through the gastric juice, bile, saliva, or sweat or has to be excreted via the kidneys. In healthy individuals these routes are sufficient; but in gout the body cannot excrete sufficient uric acid via these channels, and the uric acid begins to accumulate in the blood stream and becomes deposited in the various tissues.

Gutman and Yu have suggested that four mechanisms may be responsible for the deposition of urates in gout: (1) uricolysis may occur in lesser degree in the gouty than in the normal subject, thus permitting retention of urate; (2) urate production may be within the normal range or even low, but the capacity for disposal may be so reduced that urate is nevertheless retained; (3) the overproduction of urate may be so great

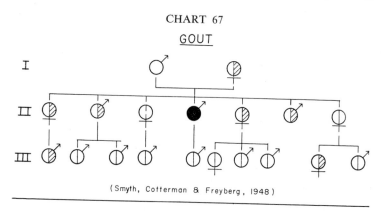

CHART 67

GOUT

(Smyth, Cotterman & Freyberg, 1948)

DISTURBANCE IN PURINE METABOLISM

(Overproduction or underexcretion

or both)

Increase of   Renal disturbances
uric acid
in blood

Deposit of urates
(tophi)

that, even if the disposal routes are of normal capacity, or indeed respond to the need by increasing their capacity, they are inadequate to the load, and excess urate therefore persists in the body; and (4) there may be both overproduction and reduced excretion of urate.

Considering these mechanisms in the order cited, we find, first, little to suggest that the oxidation of urate occurs at a rate less than normal in gout. At the most, such oxidation could represent only a minor accessory factor in the causation of chronic tophaceous gout.

Second, the evidence for a primary renal defect is also not very satisfactory. Some gouty individuals have been found to show albuminuria and impairment of renal function, especially of the glomerular filtration rate. However, this is by no means a consistent finding. Furthermore, studies on the clearance of uric acid itself reveal little or no significant difference between gouty and nongouty subjects. The renal changes could simply be due to secondary changes following urate retention and perhaps the disabilities of the tophaceous form of the disease.

Third, there is also controversy over the theory that hyperuricemia is the result of an overproduction of uric acid in the body. Some workers have pointed out that frequently the urinary urate excretion in gouty individuals is within, or even below, the normal range, and also that the inorganic phosphates in the urine show no evidence of being increased, a finding one would expect with an accelerated nucleoprotein breakdown. Benedict and his associates have argued that there is actually an overproduction of uric acid in these patients. In one experiment they injected N^{15}-labeled glycine, a precursor of uric acid. There was initially a greater rise and subsequently a more rapid fall in isotope concentration of uric acid than normal. They interpreted this as indicating that a portion of the uric acid excreted by this subject was formed from dietary glycine by a more rapid, and possibly more direct, process. This means that some of the glycine nitrogen was diverted from metabolic pathways ordinarily culminating in urea formation to other pathways leading to urate formation, and this action might represent the primary metabolic defect in gout.

Finally, it is possible that both the overproduction of urate and its reduced excretion may play a role in the pathogenesis of gout.

DIAGNOSIS.—Gout can be diagnosed by a constant elevation of serum uric acid levels (see Procedure 74) to 6 mg/100 ml or higher.

TREATMENT.—Attacks of acute gouty arthritis can be prevented by a diet low in purines and by restraint of alcohol consumption. Drugs that have been found helpful in reducing discomfort during acute attacks are: colchicine, salicylates, and, more recently, the corticotropins.

Benedict, J. D.; Roche, M.; Yu, T. F.; Bien, E. J.; Gutman, A. B.; and Stetten, D.: Incorporation of glycine nitrogen into uric acid in normal and gouty man, Metabolism 1:3, 1952.

*Gutman, A. B., and Yu, T. F.: Gout, a derangement of purine metabolism, Advances Int. Med. 5:227, 1952.

———— and ————: Current principles of management in gout, Am. J. Med. 13:744, 1952.

Smyth, C. J.; Cotterman, C. W.; and Freyberg, R. H.: The genetics of gou and hyperuricemia—an analysis of 19 families, J. Clin. Invest. 27:749, 1948.

Sydenham, T.: Tractatus de podagra et hydrope, in *The Whole Works of That Ex cellent Physician, Dr. Thomas Sydenham* (tr. by John Pechy) (London: R Wellington, 1696).

Talbott, J. H., and Coombs, F. S.: Metabolic studies on patients with gout J.A.M.A. 110:1977, 1938.

5. HEREDITARY PERIODIC PARALYSIS

Hereditary periodic paralysis is a rare clinical entity characterized by intermittent attacks of flaccid paralysis of the muscles of the extremities and loss of the deep tendon reflexes. These changes usually occur in association with a decrease in the concentration of potassium in the se-

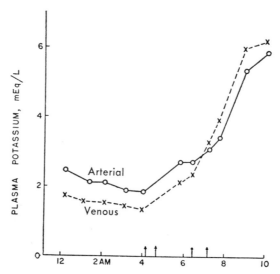

FIG. 58.—Arterial and venous plasma potassium concentrations during attack and recovery in a patient with hereditary periodic paralysis. (From Zierler, K. L. and Andres, R.: Movement of potassium into skeletal muscle during spontaneous attack in family periodic paralysis, J. Clin. Invest. 36:731, 1957.)

rum. The condition was probably first described by Musgrave in 1727, although contemporary literature usually attributes its first description to Cavere, a French clinician of the nineteenth century.

CLINICAL FEATURES.—Patients with hereditary periodic paralysis suffer from acute attacks of paralysis (Fig. 58). The attacks are frequently preceded by a prodromal period when the patients feel tired or irritable, or sometimes have a sense of apprehension for several hours before the actual attack. In the typical case, paralysis begins peripherally in the legs and progresses centrally until the patient becomes completely helpless and unable to move. The deep reflexes of the involved parts are greatly diminished or absent during these episodes, but there are no accompanying sensory or psychic disturbances beyond mild apprehension. At its height, electrical or mechanical excitability of the involved muscles is either absent or markedly impaired. In some instances, paralysis of the respiratory muscles leads to suffocation and death.

After a few hours the muscles begin to recover gradually, starting with the central muscles, which were the last to become affected, and followed by the more peripheral ones. Some residual stiffness or soreness may persist for a few days after an attack.

Episodes of paralysis may occur as often as several times weekly, or even daily in some affected individuals, while occurring infrequently or not at all in others. In some well-documented familial cases there have been only one or two spontaneous attacks during a long lifetime. Most commonly, the attacks occur during the early morning hours or in the forenoon, and then disappear later in the day. An attack can sometimes be induced following strenuous exercise, the ingestion of a high carbohydrate meal, or by the injection of epinephrine.

HEREDITY.—The condition appears to be transmitted as an autosomal dominant, and it sometimes skips a generation. Also, it tends to affect males more frequently than females. This suggests that the penetrance is not complete.

More than 400 cases of hereditary periodic paralysis have been reported from various parts of the world. In most instances, symptoms appear about the time of puberty. Very few examples are reported as beginning during early infancy or childhood.

PATHOGENESIS.—According to Talbott and to Gass and his co-workers, hereditary periodic paralysis is caused by an unknown defect in the metabolism of potassium which causes its mobilization beyond normal limits. This defect could be due to (a) a natural deficiency of potassium in the liver or other tissues, (b) an unexplained increased requirement for potassium in certain aspects of metabolism, or (c) a change in cellular permeability to potassium or other cations. In any event, when glucose is increased in the liver from the ingestion of carbohydrates or from the injection of epinephrine, three types of changes occur: (1) a decrease of potassium in the serum and urine; (2) a decrease of phosphorus in the serum and urine, which may be related to the disturbance of potassium metabolism; and (3) a decrease of potassium in the muscle, which is accompanied by paralysis of the peripheral muscles, cardiac arrhythmia,

CHART 68

HEREDITARY PERIODIC PARALYSIS

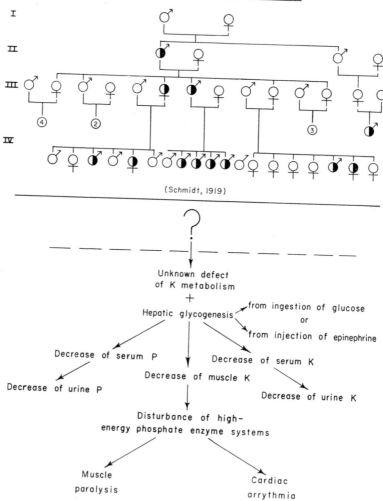

(Schmidt, 1919)

Unknown defect
of K metabolism
+
Hepatic glycogenesis → from ingestion of glucose
or
from injection of epinephrine

Decrease of serum P   Decrease of serum K

Decrease of urine P   Decrease of muscle K

Decrease of urine K

Disturbance of high-
energy phosphate enzyme systems

Muscle
paralysis

Cardiac
arrythmia

278

and electrocardiographic changes (Chart 68). All of these symptoms can be reversed upon the administration of potassium.

DIAGNOSIS.—Clinically, the condition can be diagnosed by flaccid paralysis, loss of reflexes, and loss of electrical excitability. Laboratory studies show a low serum potassium level during an attack.

TREATMENT.—The oral administration of 2-10 Gm of potassium chloride is effective in stopping an acute attack. The episodes can also be prevented by taking frequent low carbohydrate meals and prophylactically administering KCl at regular intervals.

Biemond, A., and Daniels, A. P.: Familial periodic paralysis and its transition into spinal muscular atrophy, Brain 57:91, 1934.

Gass, H.; Cherkasky, M.; and Savitsky, N.: Potassium and periodic paralysis: A metabolic study and physiological considerations, Medicine 27:105, 1948.

McQuarrie, I., and Ziegler, M. R.: Hereditary periodic paralysis: II. Effects of fasting and of various types of diet on occurrence of paralytic attacks, Metabolism 1:129, 1952.

Schmidt, A. K. E.: Die paroxysmale Lähmung. Monograph der Ges. Neurol. u. Psychiat., p. 18, 1919.

*Talbott, J. H.: Periodic paralysis, Medicine 20:85, 1941.

6. CONGENITAL PANCYTOPENIA WITH MULTIPLE CONGENITAL ANOMALIES (Fanconi type)

In 1926, Fanconi described three siblings who presented a syndrome consisting of multiple congenital anomalies, pancytopenia, and hypoplasia of the bone marrow. Nearly 30 examples of this condition have now been reported from all over the world.

CLINICAL FEATURES.—Patients with Fanconi's syndrome have a wide range of congenital anomalies. The most common finding is a patchy brown pigmentation of the skin, which has been shown to be due to a deposit of melanin. Other morphological changes include dwarfism, microcephaly, hypogenitalism, strabismus, anomalies of thumbs, absence of the radius and renal malformations. Mental retardation is also a common manifestation.

Laboratory studies show a pancytopenia characterized by marked anemia, leukopenia with the white cell count of less than 4,000/mm^3, and a decrease of platelets to below 100,000/mm^3. The bone marrow is hypoplastic, and there is no evidence of reticulocytes or regeneration. The erythrocytes show a normal life span by the Ashby technique.

The disease is fatal in about two thirds of the cases. Death usually occurs as a result of hemorrhage into either the brain or the gastrointestinal tract.

HEREDITY.—Fanconi's syndrome appears to be transmitted by an autosomal recessive gene with variable penetrance. The condition usually occurs in siblings and does not affect parents or other relatives. Consanguinity has been reported in at least two instances. No attempt has been made to detect the condition among heterozygotes.

PATHOGENESIS.—In 1953, Higashi and his associates made observations on the peroxidase activity of the erythrocytes in a patient with this condition and found a decrease of nuclear peroxidase in the normoblasts,

CHART 69

FANCONI'S ANEMIA

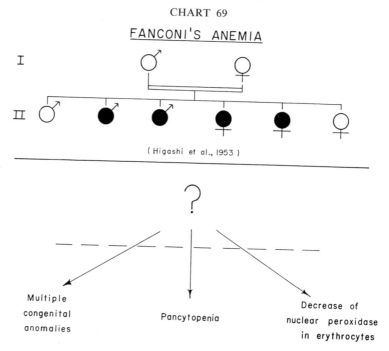

(Higashi et al., 1953)

Multiple congenital anomalies

Pancytopenia

Decrease of nuclear peroxidase in erythrocytes

which they interpreted as reflecting some constitutional defect in the red-cell precursors (Chart 69).

Fanconi's syndrome is of particular interest because it is one of the few inborn errors of metabolism in which a defect in metabolism is presumably present early in utero and is responsible for the morphological malformations. This same metabolic error appears to persist after birth and is reflected by changes in erythrocyte peroxidase activity.

DIAGNOSIS.—The diagnosis is suggested by a combination of pancytopenia and multiple congenital anomalies.

TREATMENT.—Multiple transfusions are useful in the control of anemia, and antibiotic therapy is indicated during periods of infection.

Some patients show a nonspecific improvement following splenectomy.

*Dawson, J. P.: Congenital pancytopenia associated with multiple congenital anomalies, Pediatrics 15:325, 1955.

Fanconi, H.: Familiäre infantile perniziösartige Anämie (perniziöses Blutbild und Konstitution), Jahrb. f. Kinderh. 117:257, 1927.

Higashi, O.; Koseki, E.; and Higuchi, M.: A case of Fanconi's syndrome with study of peroxidase activity of the erythron, Arch. Dis. Childhood 28:359, 1953.

Reinhold, J. D. L.; Neumark, E.; Lightwood, R.; and Carter, C. O.: Familial hypoplastic anemia with congenital abnormalities (Fanconi's syndrome), Blood 7:915, 1952.

PART VI

Extension of the Concept of "Inborn Errors of Metabolism" to Clinical Medicine

IN THIS BOOK, only those conditions which may clearly be regarded as inborn errors of metabolism have been discussed. However, as one thinks about disease processes in the broader sense, it becomes apparent that this concept may eventually be extended to cover much of clinical medicine.

15

The Future of Biochemical Genetics

It would be interesting to speculate on the future of hereditary diseases as they relate to clinical medicine. First, one might consider the group of hereditary conditions which are primarily morphological in nature (Table 4). It appears probable that the structural abnormalities in these diseases are the sequelae of a genetically induced chemical abnor-

TABLE 4.—Partial List of Genetic Conditions for Which There Has So Far Been Found Little Evidence of a Basic Chemical Cause

1. Acephaly
2. Aniridia
3. Arachnodactyly (Marfan's syndrome)
4. Arcus juvenalis
5. Arthro-onychodysplasia
6. Brachydactyly
7. Calvé-Legg-Perthes disease
8. Cataracts
9. Chondrodystrophy
10. Chondroectodermal dystrophy (Ellis-van Creveld syndrome)
11. Choroideremia
12. Cleft lip
13. Cleft palate
14. Clubfeet
15. Coloboma iridis
16. Congenital dislocation of hip
17. Craniofacial dysostosis (Crouzon's disease)
18. Disseminated sclerosis
19. Endocardial sclerosis
20. Epidermolysis bullosa
21. Epiloia (tuberous sclerosis)
22. Friedreich's ataxia
23. Hemiatrophy
24. Hemorrhagic telangiectasia (Osler's disease)
25. Hereditary spastic paraplegia

6. Huntington's chorea
7. Hydrocephalus
8. Hyperelastosis cutis (Ehlers-Danlos syndrome)
9. Hypertelorism
0. Hypertrophic neuritis
1. Ichthyosis
2. Intestinal polyposis (Jegher-Peutz syndrome)
3. Lindau's disease
4. Lobster-claw defect of hands and feet
5. Marie's (cerebellar) ataxia
6. Mandibulofacial dysostosis (Treacher-Collins syndrome)
7. Merzbacher-Pelizaeus cerebral sclerosis
8. Microcephaly
9. Microphthalmia
0. Multiple exostoses
1. Nadelung's deformity
2. Neurofibromatosis (Recklinghausen's disease)
3. Optic atrophy
4. Osteochondrodystrophy (Morquio's disease)
5. Osteogenesis imperfecta (Lobstein's disease)
6. Osteopetrosis (marble bones; Albers-Schönberg disease)
7. Otosclerosis
8. Pectus excavatum
9. Peroneal muscular atrophy (Charcot-Marie-Tooth disease)
0. Pleonosteosis
1. Polycystic kidneys
2. Polydactyly
3. Polyostotic fibrous dysplasia
4. Progressive lipodystrophy
5. Pseudohemophilia (von Willebrand's disease)
6. Psoriasis
7. Pterygium syndrome (Bonnevie-Ullrich syndrome)
8. Retinitis pigmentosa
9. Retinoblastoma (glioma retinae)
0. Schilder's disease
1. Situs inversus viscerum (Kartagener's syndrome)
2. Spina bifida aperte
3. Sprengel's deformity
4. Sturge-Weber-Dimitri disease
5. Syndactyly
6. Torticollis
7. Xeroderma pigmentosum

nality during the early stages of embryonic development. As a result of his insult, the individual is left with a deformity of bone, eye, or muscle. The chemical abnormality is no longer detectable after birth, and we cannot classify such conditions as inborn errors of metabolism in the strict sense. Yet, in their way, these conditions represent a hereditary condition resulting from a chemical abnormality.

At the present stage of our thinking, we cannot be too rigid in defining the lines that separate the morphological disturbances from the functional. For instance, there is increasing evidence that there may be a chemical basis for some of the muscular atrophies. As we learn more about the fundamental processes of transport across cell membranes and the energy mechanisms responsible for the processes, this group of conditions may turn out to be similar to some definitely known chemical disturbances, such as cystic fibrosis of the pancreas. Likewise, in conditions like Fanconi's anemia, the primary disturbance may be morphological, and the present evidence indicating a biochemical lesion may turn out to be incorrect.

Next, we might consider the group of biochemical disturbances in which genetics may play an etiological role (Table 5). On the basis of the presently available information, these disturbances cannot be classi-

TABLE 5.—PARTIAL LIST OF CONDITIONS WHICH MAY BE
GENETICALLY DETERMINED

1. Acatalasia	19. Laurence-Moon-Biedl syndrome
2. l-Amino-adipic-aciduria	20. Milroy's disease
3. Angioneurotic edema	21. Mongolism
4. Celiac disease	22. Myasthenia gravis
5. Cretinism	23. Oxalosis
6. Epilepsy	24. Oxaluria
7. Ethanolaminuria	25. Primary amyloidosis
8. Familial cirrhosis	26. Psychosis
9. Familial eosinophilia	27. Rickets
10. Familial hemophagocytic reticulo-cytosis	28. Secretors and nonsecretors of blood group substances
11. Familial hypoplastic anemia	29. Sexual precocity
12. Familial nephrosis	30. Succosuria
13. Familial neutropenia	31. Taste sensitivity to thiourea
14. Histidinuria in pregnancy	32. Thrombocytopenic purpura
15. Hydroxyphenuria	33. Urobilinuria
16. Hypochromic microcytic anemia	34. Xanthinuria
17. Idiopathic hypoparathyroidism	35. Xanthurenic aciduria
18. Idiopathic hypoproteinemia	

fied among the hereditary diseases in the classical sense. For instance, only about 5% of the brothers and sisters of children who have vitamin D-deficient rickets develop this complication. Yet, it does occur in such families with greater regularity than in other families where the diet is equally deficient in that vitamin. In such instances, it is difficult to decide to what extent the rickets occurs because of inadequate vitamin intake and to what degree it is due to familial tendencies. Similar examples may be found in such conditions as cretinism, familial nephrosis, and idiopathic hypoproteinemia. It appears probable that genetic factors play a role in such diseases; and they can, therefore, be regarded as inborn errors of metabolism in the broader sense.

One can carry this reasoning one stage farther. The ability of the individual to respond to certain situations may be genetically determined. In an earlier section (p. 201), we have discussed the disturbance in hemolysis which follows the ingestion of primaquine or fava beans and which is due to a hereditary deficiency of glucose-6-PO_4 dehydrogenase. Many other similar deficiencies must occur in the human race, and such individuals can only be detected when placed in certain environments or stresses. Eventually it may be possible to show that the individual response to such things as the common cold or an overdose of alcohol may in part be genetically determined.

Finally, we should bear in mind the large amount of work being done by Williams and others in "biochemical individuality." They have found that any given person tends to remain the same, from a biochemical point of view, throughout his life. He will tend to put out the same amount of lysine in his urine, show the same glucose tolerance curve, and have the same uric acid level from day to day regardless of the diet he is on or the type of work he is doing. These characteristics distinguish him from another person who may be of the same age, eating the same food, and working in the same office as the first man. Preliminary studies suggest that the biochemical individuality of a person may in part also be genetically determined. If so, this represents another approach to our thinking concerning the inborn errors of metabolism in man.

It is apparent that all of the problems regarding the inborn errors of metabolism are far from solved. In fact, we are just beginning to make an intelligent study of this vast and virgin field of medicine. We hope that this book has served its purpose in arousing interest in this area and that all physicians will henceforth think, not only about the specific patient he is treating, but also about the family background which produced the disease process.

Appendix

(The symbol ► indicates that the procedure has been checked and found to be satisfactory in our own laboratory)

Chapter 2

SICKLE CELL ANEMIA
AND THE OTHER ABNORMAL HEMOGLOBINS

► 1. TEST FOR SICKLING

REFERENCE: Hanno, H. A., and Margolies, M. P.: Science 112:109, 1950.

PROCEDURE: From 5 to 10 ml of venous blood is collected in an oxalated tube. The blood is transferred to an Erlenmeyer flask, and a stream of pure CO_2 is directed into the neck of the flask for 10-15 seconds. The flask is then immediately stoppered and the blood gently swirled for a few seconds. After the flask has remained stoppered for 5 minutes, the cork is removed and a drop of blood is quickly transferred, by means of a pipette, to a clean cover glass. A petrolatum-sealed preparation is immediately made on a slide, and the cells are examined under a microscope.

2. SOLUBILITY OF HEMOGLOBIN SOLUTIONS

REFERENCE: Itano, H.: Arch. Biochem. 47:148, 1953.

REAGENTS:

1. Blood specimens are obtained in citrate or oxalate. The erythrocytes are separated from the plasma and washed with 0.15 M NaCl. Following lysis of the erythrocytes with water, a one-third volume of toluene is added and shaken. The toluene and stromal layer are then removed by centrifugation.

2. The precipitating solution is prepared by dissolving anhydrous KH_2PO_4 crystals and K_2HPO_4 powder of reagent grade in water; it contains 1.62 M K_2HPO_4 and 1.18 M KH_2PO_4 per liter. Insoluble material is removed by filtering this solution through a sintered glass funnel. Anhydrous $Na_2S_2O_4$ powder is used to maintain the reduced state of the ferrohemoglobin during the solubility determinations.

PROCEDURE: The concentration of the original hemoglobin solution is determined at 540 mμ. in the Beckman Model B spectrophotometer. A slit width of 0.15 mμ. is used.

The solubility is then tested in 2.24 M phosphate. Into a 10 ml volumetric flask, 100 mg of $Na_2S_2O_4$ is weighed. Eight ml of the phosphate solution is delivered to the flask from a burette, and the contents are agitated until the $Na_2S_2O_4$ goes into solution. One ml of water is layered over this solution. A volume of hemoglobin solution containing 50 mg of hemoglobin is then added, with a measuring pipette, into the superficial water layer. Care is taken at this stage to avoid the precipitation of hemoglobin. The flask is immersed in a water bath at 25° C. Finally, water is added to the 10 ml mark, and the contents are completely mixed by inversion several times.

If a solid phase appears, the mixture is transferred and centrifuged at 17,000 × g for 20 minutes at 25° C. Following centrifugation, a long hypodermic needle is inserted through the superficial layer and 3-4 ml of the solution phase is removed and the hemoglobin determined spectrophotometrically.

If precipitation does not occur in the flask following 8 ml of phosphate solution, the procedure is repeated with 9.2 ml of solution.

INTERPRETATION: The solubility of the hemoglobin present can be calculated from the difference between the original hemoglobin solution and the amount of hemoglobin left in solution after precipitation.

► 3. PAPER ELECTROPHORESIS

REFERENCE: Chernoff, A.: New England J. Med. 253:322, 1955.

REAGENTS:

1. From 2 to 3 ml of unclotted venous blood is prepared and diluted to 5 Gm/100 ml of hemoglobin.

2. Barbital buffer, pH 8.8, ionic strength 0.06. A stock solution, ionic strength 0.24, is prepared by dissolving 98.9 Gm of Na barbital and 11.1 Gm of barbituric acid in distilled water and diluting to 2,000 ml. To prepare a 0.06 ionic strength solution, this is diluted with 1 part buffer and 3 parts water.

ELECTROPHORESIS APPARATUS: A sheet of filter paper is inserted between two glass plates. Siliconized glass plates, 9-15/16 × 14 × ½ inch, are suspended between two buffer chambers made of Plexiglas. Each buffer chamber is divided by a partition into two sections, which are connected by a series of glass bridges. Carbon or platinum electrodes are placed in the outer receptacles, and the paper dips into the inner containers. Direct current of 300-400 volts is used to supply the necessary power.

PROCEDURE: Veronal® buffer is placed in each of the four compartments and equalized. The smooth side of a sheet of Whatman No. 3 MM paper is soaked in the buffer solution and blotted almost dry. From 0.002 to 0.005 ml of the hemoglobin solution is applied at the cross-mark, and approximately 350 volts of direct current is applied. With a paper width of 9½ inches, 14-16 milliamperes of current will be drawn. The electrophoretic run is permitted to proceed for 6-8 hours. The paper is then dried rapidly. For a permanent record, the paper may be stained with bromphenol blue.

Chapter 3

OTHER "STRUCTURAL" DISTURBANCES

THALASSEMIA

4. DETERMINATION OF BLOOD PLASMA IRON

REFERENCE: Kitzes, G.; Elvehjem, C. A.; and Schuette, H. A.: J. Biol. Chem. 155:653, 1944.

REAGENTS:

Trichloroacetic acid, 25% solution in water. Redistill if not free from iron.

Hydrochloric acid, 6 N, redistilled.

Ammonium hydroxide, approx. 6 N.

Buffer solution, pH 4.58, 27.2 ml of C.P. glacial acetic acid, and 33.4 Gm of C.P. sodium acetate (anhydrous) dissolved in water and made to a volume of 250 ml.

Thioglycolic acid, Eastman's practical grade.

p-Nitrophenol, 0.1% solution in water.

a,a'-Bipyridine, 0.2% solution in 5% acetic acid. Dissolve 0.2 Gm of the reagent in 5 ml of C.P. glacial acetic acid and dilute to 100 ml with water.

Standard iron solution. Dissolve iron wire (99.8%) in a mixture of nitric acid and hydrochloric acid and dilute with water to give a concentration of 1 mg per ml. From this stock solution, standard solutions are made of 100 and 1γ per ml.

Iron-free water. Distilled water should be redistilled from glass. All equipment should be thoroughly cleaned and rinsed with iron-free water.

Plasma iron may be determined with a maximum error of $\pm 10\%$ for blood plasma containing 30-90% iron, with a maximum error of $\pm 5\%$ for blood plasma containing $100\text{-}200\gamma$ per 100 ml of iron.

PROCEDURE: From 3 to 5 ml of blood plasma containing about $3\text{-}9\gamma$ of inorganic iron is pipetted into an ungraduated Pyrex 15 ml conical centrifuge tube. Three ml of redistilled water is added and mixed with the plasma.

A blank consisting of all the reagents used is also prepared.

Place the tubes in boiling water for 2-3 minutes or until the solution becomes opaque. Cool the tubes in cold water.

Add 2 ml of 25% trichloroacetic acid solution and stir thoroughly so that the acid is intimately mixed with the plasma. Use a small blunt-end stirring rod in order not to break through the bottom of the tubes.

Place the tubes in a water bath at $90°\text{-}95°$ C for 3 minutes, stirring the solution once or twice.

Remove from the bath and cool in cold water. Centrifuge at 2,000-3,000 rpm and decant the supernatant liquid into a 15 ml graduated centrifuge tube.

Add 4 ml of water to the sediment and 1.0 ml of 25% trichloroacetic acid. Mix. Place in water bath and centrifuge. Combine with first supernatant.

Add 1 drop of 0.1% p-nitrophenol indicator solution, and add NH_4OH, drop by drop, until the solution becomes yellow.

Add 1 ml of the buffer solution and enough water to make 15 ml. Mix.

Pipette an aliquot, 10 ml, containing $2\text{-}3\gamma$ of iron into an Evelyn tube, and add 2 drops of thioglycolic acid and mix.

Determine the center setting (100% transmission on the galvanometer scale) for each solution in the colorimeter. Filter is 515.

Add 1 ml of 0.2% a,a'-bipyridine reagent and mix by gentle shaking or tapping of the tube. Read each tube in the colorimeter with the respective center setting previously determined. The galvanometer reading is recorded to the nearest 0.1 of a scale division if the Evelyn colorimeter is used.

CALCULATIONS: Calculate the amount of iron in the solution in each tube by reference to a standard curve; or use the following formula after calculating the L values from the G readings (where $L = 2 - \log G$):

$$\frac{\text{Micrograms iron}}{\text{Aliquot}} = 40.6 \times L \text{ aliquot} - L \text{ reagent blank}$$

5. IRON-BINDING CAPACITY

REFERENCE: Rath, C. E., and Finch, C. A.: J. Clin. Invest. 28:79, 1949.

REAGENTS:

0.9% NaCl.

Iron standard solution. Prepared by diluting 14 mg of ferrous ammonium sulfate plus 0.5 ml of 1 N acetic acid to a total volume of 100 ml. This represents 20γ of iron per ml of standard solution. Each standard solution is checked by direct iron analysis. Each addition of from 0.05 to 2 ml of plasma represents an increment of 50γ/100 ml serum.

PROCEDURE: Fasting venous blood is withdrawn without hemolysis into a syringe coated with mineral oil. The clotted blood is centrifuged at 2,000 rpm for 15 minutes, and the serum obtained is centrifuged again to remove all red cells. A Coleman spectrophotometer Model 11 and cuvettes of 1 cm depth are used. One cuvette is filled with 5 ml of 0.9% NaCl, while the other is filled with 2 ml of serum and 3 ml of 0.9% NaCl. Iron standard solution is added in 0.05 ml lots to both cuvettes, and a glass stirring rod used to mix the contents. Readings of light transmission at 525 mμ are made 2-3 minutes after each mixing. The iron solution is added until there is no change in the per cent transmission after three successive readings.

The data are plotted, and the point of intersection of the two slopes is taken as the amount of iron necessary to saturate the iron-binding protein.

INTERPRETATION: In normal individuals, the serum iron comprises about a third of the total binding capacity.

ELLIPTOCYTOSIS

► 6. MEASUREMENT OF DIAMETER OF ERYTHROCYTES

REFERENCE: Details of this technique are described in Larsen, G.: Acta med. scandinav. vol. 132, supp. 220, 1948.

INTERPRETATION: It is generally agreed that any individual with more than 25% elliptical erythrocytes can be regarded as a carrier, and anyone with less than 10% elliptical erythrocytes can be regarded as normal.

ERYTHROPOIETIC PORPHYRIA

7. FLUORESCENCE MICROSCOPY

REFERENCE: Schmid, R.; Schwartz, S.; and Sundberg, R. D.: Blood 10:416, 1955.

PROCEDURE: Unstained bone marrow slides are prepared from material aspirated from the sternal marrow. For fluorescence microscopy, a specially constructed microspectrometer, an essential part of which is a Steinheil microanalytic spectroscope, is used. As light source, a modified Bal water-cooled high-pressure GE AH-6 mercury vapor lamp is employed with a primary Corning filter No. 5-58 (5113) to isolate the 405 mμ line. An orange Corning filter No. 3-67 (3482) is placed between the objective and the eyepiece of the microscope.

After studying and photographing the unstained bone marrow slides in the fluorescence microscope, the areas of the smear so examined are marked with a Zeiss slide marker and subsequently stained with Wright's stain for detailed morphological study of the individual cells.

8. TOTAL UROPORPHYRINS

REFERENCE: Lockwood, W. H.: Australian J. Exper. Biol. & M. Sc. 31:453, 1953, based on method of Sveinsson, S. L.; Rimington, C.; and Barnes, H. D.: Scandinav. J. Clin. & Lab. Invest. 1:2, 1949.

PROCEDURE: One ml of glacial acetic acid is added to 10 ml of urine, and the coproporphyrin is removed by extraction with 20 ml of ether. The ether is washed twice with a total of 5 ml of water, and the washings are added to the main aqueous layer. To this is added 0.5 ml of saturated $CaCl_2$ solution, and then 40% NaOH, 1.5 ml being added after the first permanent precipitate. The calcium salts are then spun down, washed once with methanol to remove water, and dissolved in methanolic HCl. The solution is allowed to stand for at least an hour and is then passed into saturated sodium acetate overlayered with ether. The ether is washed with H_2O, Na_2CO_3, and extracted three times with a total of approximately 4 ml of 3 N HCl. The optical densities are then read in a 1 cm cuvette at 425 mμ, 407 mμ, and 390 mμ and compared with known standards.

INTERPRETATION: The normal range of uroporphyrin excretion is between 15 and 30 mg/24 hours. The isomers for uroporphyrins (I and III) may be separated by the methods described by Rimington, C., and Miles, P. A.: Biochem. J. 50:202, 1951, and

Watson, C. J.; Schwartz, S.; and Hawkinson, V.: J. Biol. Chem. 157:345, 1945.

► 9. TOTAL URINARY COPROPORPHYRIN

REFERENCE: Schwartz, S.; Zieve, L.; and Watson, C. J.: J. Lab. & Clin. Med. 37:843, 1951.

COLLECTION OF URINE: A 24 hour urine collection is made in a bottle containing 5 Gm of Na_2CO_3.

EXTRACTION OF SAMPLE: To 5 ml of the well-mixed urine in a separatory funnel, add 5 ml of buffered acetic acid solution (prepared by adding four volumes of glacial acetic acid to one volume of saturated aqueous sodium acetate solution), 75-100 ml of ethyl acetate, and 15-20 ml of distilled water. This is shaken well. The aqueous phase is discarded. The ethyl acetate is washed twice with 20-30 ml portions of 1% sodium acetate and once with 0.005% aqueous iodine (prepared fresh by diluting with water, from a refrigerated stock, 1% solution of iodine in alcohol).

The porphyrin is then extracted from the ethyl acetate with four portions of about 5 ml each of 1.5 N HCl. If the fourth extract still has any reddish orange fluorescence when irradiated in the dark with near ultraviolet light, the HCl extracts are continued till no fluorescence shows.

The combined HCl extracts are diluted with 1.5 N HCl to 25 ml or some other convenient volume, and the fluorescence intensity is measured in a sensitive fluorimeter.

The sample is read in a fluorimeter employing a photomultiplier tube (manufactured by Calectron, Inc., 2444 Beverly Road, St. Paul 4, Minn.) and compared with coproporphyrin standards.

INTERPRETATION: The normal values for children are given by Hsia, D. Y. Y., and Page, M.: Proc. Soc. Exper. Biol. & Med. 85:86, 1954; and for adults, by Schwartz *et al.*: J. Lab. & Clin. Med. 37:843, 1951.

The ratio of urinary coproporphyrin isomers (I and III) can be determined by a fluorescence-quenching technique described by Schwartz, S.; Hawkinson, V.; Cohen, S.; and Watson, C. J.: J. Biol. Chem. 168:133, 1947.

10. PORPHOBILINOGEN

REFERENCES: Modification of method by Watson, C. J., and Schwartz, S.: Proc. Soc. Exper. Biol. & Med. 47:393, 1941. A more detailed technique is described by Westall, R. G.: Nature 170:614, 1952.

REAGENT: Ehrlich's reagent (2% dimethyl amino benzaldehyde in 6.0 N HCl).

PROCEDURE: Into a 10 ml volumetric flask place 0.1 ml of urine, 4.9

ml of H_2O, and 5.0 ml of Ehrlich's reagent. A color develops whose density (between 0.05 and 0.10 in a cell 1 cm long) is read at 535µ in a Beckman spectrophotometer exactly 5 minutes after adding the reagent. The color which is developed from the porphobilinogen is equivalent to a molar extinction of 36,000 under these conditions, where

$$\text{Molar extinction} = \log_{10}\frac{I_0}{I} \times \frac{1}{\text{cm} \times \text{mol/L}}$$

Chapter 4

DEFICIENCIES OF PLASMA PROTEIN FRACTIONS

AGAMMAGLOBULINEMIA

► 11. SERUM GAMMA GLOBULIN

REFERENCE: Preparation of antiserum and precipitation in agar is given in Gitlin, D.: Paper 3 in *Serological Approaches to Studies of Protein Structure and Metabolism* (W. H. Cole, ed.) (New Brunswick, N. J.: Rutgers University Press, 1954).

PROCEDURE: The serum of the patient is simply placed over the antiserum-agar in the tube and allowed to stand at room temperature for 18-24 hours. Sterile conditions are not observed.

INTERPRETATION: The presence of a band of precipitate in the agar indicates the presence of gamma globulin in the patient's serum. The distance the precipitation band has migrated from the interface between the agar and the patient's serum is also a good indication of the concentration of gamma globulin.

CERULOPLASMIN DEFICIENCY

12. CERULOPLASMIN

(a) SPECTROPHOTOMETRIC METHOD

REFERENCES: Holmberg, C. G., and Laurell, C. B.: Acta chem. scandinav. 2:550, 1948; Scheinberg, H., and Gitlin, D.: Science 116:484, 1952.

PROCEDURE: Plasma is clarified by Seitz filtration, and light absorption is measured in a Beckman spectrophotometer from 540µ to 660 mµ. A cell with a 5.0 cm path length is required. When successive measurements of the spectral curve show no change with time, a solution of buffered ascorbate is added to make the plasma concentration 0.27%. Spectra are measured hourly for 5 hours at room temperature. The concentration of ceruloplasmin is estimated by dividing the decrease in optical density, corrected for dilution by the extinction coefficient $E_{1\%}^{5m}$, 610 mμ equals 3.4.

INTERPRETATION: Normal range, 10-20 mg/100 ml ceruloplasmin. In Wilson's disease, it is less than 2 mg/100 ml.

(b) SERUM COPPER ENZYME METHOD

REFERENCE: Holmberg, C. G., and Laurell, C. B.: Scandinav. J. Clin. & Lab. Invest. 3:103, 1951.

REAGENTS:

Acetate buffer, pH 6.0.

Paraphenylendiamine (ppd), 5 mg per ml, pH 6.0.

PROCEDURE: Serum, 0.3 ml, is dialyzed at +4° C against acetate buffer for 12 hours. This is placed in the side arm of a Warburg vessel. One ml of ppd solution and 0.6 ml of acetate buffer are placed in the main chamber of the Warburg flask, and the oxygen uptake is measured in the Warburg flask at 37° C. On all occasions, a control sample, using 0.3 ml of distilled water, is used to correct for the oxygen uptake of ppd which occurs in the absence of ceruloplasmin.

INTERPRETATION: Normal range, 3-4.5 μM/ml/hr; in Wilson's disease, 0.5-1.5 μM/ml/hr.

(c) IMMUNOCHEMICAL METHOD

REFERENCES: Described in Scheinberg, H., and Gitlin, D.: Science 116:484, 1952; Markowitz, H., et al.: J. Clin. Invest. 10:1498, 1955.

13. DIRECT-REACTING PLASMA COPPER

REFERENCE: Gubler, C. J., et al.: J. Clin. Invest. 32:405, 1953.

REAGENTS:

Saturated solution of sodium pyrophosphate.

0.1% aqueous solution of sodium diethyldithiocarbamate.

PROCEDURE: To 1.0 ml of plasma, 0.5 ml of a saturated solution of sodium pyrophosphate and 2.5 ml of redistilled water are added. The optical density (D1) is measured with a spectrophotometer (Beckman DU or B with cells having a 1.0 cm light path) at a wavelength of 440 mμ. Then 0.2 ml of diethyldithiocarbamate solution is added, and the optical density (D2) again read after a suitable time interval. A reagent blank containing 3.5 ml of water,

0.5 ml of pyrophosphate, and 0.2 ml of carbamate is prepared, and the optical density (D3) determined.

The μg of direct-reacting copper per 100 ml of plasma is calculated from the following formula:

$$D2 - (D1f + D3) \times K \times 100$$

where f is 0.952 and K is constant derived from the standard curve.

INTERPRETATION: Normal range, 0-20 μg/100 ml; in Wilson's disease, 20-40 μg/100 ml.

► 14. PLASMA COAGULATION (QUALITATIVE)

REFERENCE: Frick, P. G., and McQuarrie, I. J.: Pediatrics 13:44, 1954.

PROCEDURE: Plasma is mixed with equal volumes of any of the following reagents:

CaCl$_2$ (¼-1/80 M).
CaCl$_2$ (¼-1/80 M) plus rabbit brain thromboplastin.
Bovine thrombin (conc. 1-5,000 units/cc).

With normal plasma, a fibrin clot will form. With plasma from a patient with congenital afibrinogenemia, no clot will form.

15. PLASMA FIBRINOGEN LEVEL

REFERENCE: Cullen, G. E., and Van Slyke, D. D.: J. Biol. Chem. 41:587, 1920.

REAGENTS:

0.8% NaCl.
CaCl$_2$ solution made up by dissolving 2.5 Gm of anhydrous CaCl$_2$ in 100 ml of water.
Conc. H$_2$SO$_4$.
K$_2$SO$_4$.
Copper sulfate.

PROCEDURE: Blood is collected in a tube containing 0.5% potassium oxalate, and the plasma is separated by centrifugation. Five ml of plasma is added to 150 ml of 0.8% NaCl and 5 ml of the CaCl$_2$ solution. This is allowed to stand for 10-15 minutes until complete coagulation takes place. The solution is filtered with filter paper and washed with 0.8% NaCl five times, allowing each washing to remain in contact with the fibrin for 10 minutes by clamping the outlet of the funnel for that period.

The filter paper containing the fibrin clot is transferred to a Kjeldahl flask; and 20 ml of concentrated H$_2$SO$_4$, 12 Gm of K$_2$SO$_4$, and a crystal of copper sulfate are added. The nitrogen of the fibrin is determined in the usual way. The plasma fibrinogen level can be calculated from the nitrogen content of the fibrin clot.

INTERPRETATION: Normal range, 200-400 mg/100 ml. Patients with afibrinogenemia show no detectable fibrinogen.

Chapter 5

DEFICIENCIES OF CLOTTING FACTORS

PREPARATIONS

Oxalated plasma.—Fresh whole blood, 4.5 ml, is mixed with 0.5 ml of 0.1 M sodium oxalate solution. The blood is centrifuged at 1,000 rpm for 5 minutes. The supernatant is taken off as oxalated plasma. The blood must be fresh.

Serum.—Freshly drawn blood is permitted to clot. Several hours later, the clot is centrifuged and the serum removed. The sample is kept for 24 hours at room temperature and then decalcified with one-fifth volume of 0.1 M sodium oxalate.

Aged plasma.—Oxalated plasma is kept in the refrigerator for a month and then used, provided that the one-stage prothrombin time is over 180 seconds.

Adsorbed plasma.—A suspension of 50 mg of $BaSO_4$ powder is added to each ml of freshly oxalated plasma. After mixing for 10 minutes and centrifuged, the clear supernatant plasma is prothrombin free. This must be freshly prepared for use.

TESTS

► 16. CLOTTING TIME

REFERENCE: Lee, R. I., and White, P. D.: Am. J. M. Sc. 145:495, 1913.

PROCEDURE: One ml of blood is withdrawn from an arm vein and the time is noted. The needle is removed, and the contents of the syringe are transferred into a small glass tube (about 8 mm in diameter) which has previously been rinsed out with normal saline solution. The tube is rotated endwise every 30 seconds; and that point at which the rotated blood no longer flows from its position but maintains its surface contour when inverted is taken as the end-point.

INTERPRETATION: The normal range for clotting time by this method is 5-8 minutes.

▶ **17. PLASMA CLOTTING OR RECALCIFICATION TIME**

PROCEDURE: Oxalated plasma, 0.2 ml, is mixed with 0.2 ml of 0.02 M $CaCl_2$ solution and the stop watch is started. The tube is dipped in and out of a water bath at 37° C until a fibrin clot appears. The test is done in triplicate, and the results are averaged.

INTERPRETATION: The normal range for plasma clotting time is 100-200 seconds.

▶ **18. PROTHROMBIN COMPLEX TIME (ONE-STAGE)**

REFERENCE: Quick, A. J.: Am. J. Clin. Path. 15:560, 1945.

REAGENTS:

Thromboplastin (acetone-dried rabbit brain). Each day, a fresh solution is prepared by dissolving 0.2 Gm of the material in 5 ml of normal saline solution and incubating for 15-20 minutes at 50° C. The solution should then be kept in a 37° C water bath until used.

$CaCl_2$, 0.02 M solution.

PROCEDURE: The determination is carried out in a small Pyrex tube placed in a 37° C water bath. To 0.1 ml of oxalated plasma, 0.1 ml of thromboplastin is added. $CaCl_2$, 0.1 ml, is blown forcibly into the mixture and the stop watch started. The tube is shaken lightly in the water bath to within a few seconds of the expected clotting time. For the accurate timing of the end-point, it is essential to tilt the tube very gently.

INTERPRETATION: Normal prothrombin time is 12 seconds.

19. TWO-STAGE PROTHROMBIN DETERMINATION

REFERENCE: Details of the method are given in Ware, A. G., and Seegers, W. H.: Am. J. Clin. Path. 19:471, 1944.

▶ **20. ANTIHEMOPHILIC FACTOR (AHF)**

REFERENCE: Langdell, R. D.; Wagner, R. H.; and Brinkhous, K. M.: J. Lab. & Clin. Med. 41:637, 1953.

REAGENTS:

Citrated hemophilic plasma as substrate.

Cephalin, 0.015%. Prepared from 0.3% stock solution.

Calcium-imidazole reagent. Prepared by mixing 7 parts of 0.11 M $CaCl_2$; 6 parts imidazole buffer, pH 7.2; and 5 parts 0.9% NaCl.

PROCEDURE: The oxalated control or test plasma is treated with $BaSO_4$ and then diluted with oxalated saline to 1, 2.5, 5, and 10%, respectively. During testing, the reagents are kept in a 28° C water bath except for the hemophilic plasma substrate, which is kept in an ice bath.

For each clotting test, the following are added, *in the order listed*, to a 10 × 75 mm dry glass tube: 0.1 ml citrated hemophilic plasma, 0.1 ml diluted control or test plasma, 0.1 ml cephalin, and 0.1 ml calcium imidazole solution. Clotting times for each dilution of plasma are determined in triplicate and the mean determined. The mean clotting times are plotted against the per cent of the test or control plasma used, the latter being indicated on a log scale. By interpolation, the dilution of the test plasma which could give the same clotting times as 1, 2.5, and 5% control plasmas are determined and the AHF activity determined:

$$\frac{\%\ \text{control plasma}}{\%\ \text{test plasma}} \times 100 = \%\ \text{AHF activity in test plasma}$$

INTERPRETATION: In classical hemophilia, the AHF activity is markedly decreased to below 10%.

► 21. PROTHROMBIN UTILIZATION TEST

REFERENCE: Details of this method are given in Langdell, R. D.; Graham, J. D.; and Brinkhous, K. M.: Proc. Soc. Exper. Biol. & Med. 74:424, 1950.

22. PARTIAL THROMBOPLASTIN TIME

REFERENCES: Langdell, R. D.; Wagner, R. H.; and Brinkhous, K. M.: J. Lab. & Clin. Med. 41:637, 1953; Brinkhous, K. M., *et al.*, J.A.M.A. 154:481, 1954.

PROCEDURE: The partial thromboplastin time is performed at 37° C by mixing, in this order: 0.1 ml of oxalated plasma, 0.1 ml of partial thromboplastin (either crude cephalin or Asolectin), and 0.1 ml of 0.02 M CaCl$_2$. The concentration of partial thromboplastin is adjusted by dilution to give a clotting time in the range of 40-80 seconds. A 0.3% suspension is usually satisfactory.

► 23. THROMBOPLASTIN GENERATION TEST

REFERENCE: Biggs, R., and Douglas, A. S.: J. Clin. Path. 6:23, 1953.

PREPARATION OF SAMPLE: Venous blood is collected from a normal subject and from the patient. Part of each sample is citrated by adding 1 part of 3.8% sodium citrate to 9 parts of blood. The plasma is separated after centrifugation at 1,000 rpm for 15 minutes. An additional 3 ml of whole venous blood is placed in a tube with three beads. The tube is stoppered and inverted repeatedly until clotting occurs. This process encourages the conversion of prothrombin to thrombin during coagulation. When coagulation is complete, the blood is allowed to stand at 37° C for 2 hours. The serum is then separated and diluted 1:10 with normal saline for use in the test.

REAGENTS:

Deprothrombinization of plasma. To 1 ml of citrated plasma is added 0.1 ml of aluminum hydroxide suspension. The mixture is incubated at 37° C for 3 minutes, and the alumina is separated by centrifugation. The plasma is diluted 1:5 with normal saline.

Platelets and substrate. Normal blood, 20 ml, is collected in two silicone-treated 10 ml graduated centrifuge tubes each containing 1 ml of 3.8% sodium citrate. The blood is centrifuged at 1,500 rpm for 10 minutes and the plasma separated and put into silicone-treated tubes and centrifuged again for 15 minutes at 3,000 rpm. The platelets are deposited, and the clear supernatant plasma is separated and reserved as substrate for the test. The platelets are washed twice with saline solution, the platelet mass being fragmented with a wooden applicator stick and redeposited on each occasion by centrifugation. After the second washing, the platelets are resuspended in a volume of normal saline solution equal to one third of the volume of original plasma from which they were derived.

PROCEDURE: Into each of six small tubes of uniform diameter placed in a water bath at 37° C, 0.1 ml of substrate plasma is pipetted. In an additional tube in the water bath is placed: 0.3 ml of alumina plasma diluted 1:5, 0.3 ml of platelet suspension, and 0.3 ml of serum diluted 1:10. To this is added 0.3 ml of $M/40$ $CaCl_2$, and a stop watch is started. At intervals of 1 minute, 0.1 ml of the mixture is withdrawn into a graduated Pasteur pipette; and, using the other hand, 0.1 ml of $M/40$ $CaCl_2$ is withdrawn with a second pipette. The contents of the two pipettes are then discharged simultaneously into one of the tubes containing 0.1 ml of substrate. The clotting times of the substrate samples are recorded. This can be represented in terms of thromboplastin concentration, using a thromboplastin dilution curve.

INTERPRETATION: The results of this test in the hemophiliac are given in the following table:

DIFFERENTIATION OF THE HEMOPHILIAS WITH THE THROMBO-
PLASTIN GENERATION TEST

SOURCE OF TEST REAGENTS			RESULTS OF TGT IN VARIOUS HEMOPHILIACS		
Al(OH)$_3$ or BaSO$_4$ Plasma	Serum	Platelets	AHG	PTC	PTA
Patient	Patient	Normal	Abnormal	Abnormal	Abnormal
Patient	Normal	Normal	Abnormal	Normal	Normal
Normal	Patient	Normal	Normal	Abnormal	Normal

24. TEST FOR AC GLOBULIN

REFERENCE: Quick, A. J., and Stefanini, M.: J. Lab. & Clin. Med. 33:819, 1948.

REAGENTS:

Plasma, stored for 14 days.

Tricalcium phosphate suspension. Prepared by dissolving 158 Gm of trisodium phosphate in 1 liter of water. Separately, 66.6 Gm of anhydrous $CaCl_2$ are dissolved in 1 L of water. The $CaCl_2$ solution is poured into the trisodium phosphate with thorough stirring. The pH is adjusted to 7. The precipitated tricalcium phosphate is washed repeatedly by decantation until the NaCl is removed. The volume is brought to 1 L, making a 0.2 M solution. A 0.008 M solution is prepared by adding 4 ml from the stock solution to 96 ml of distilled water.

PROCEDURE: Nine volumes of fresh blood is collected with one volume of 0.1 M sodium oxalate. The plasma is deprothrombinized by treatment with tricalcium phosphate suspension as follows: 1 ml of 0.008 M suspension is transferred to a small tube and centrifuged. The supernatant water is poured off and drained. One ml of plasma is mixed with the packed tricalcium phosphate. After 10 minutes at room temperature, the adsorbent is separated by centrifugation. On adding the treated plasma to stored human plasma, the prothrombin time by the Quick method can be reduced from 60-70 seconds to 10-11 seconds.

INTERPRETATION: The absence of this ability to reduce prothrombin time suggests Ac-globulin deficiency.

25. SPCA

REFERENCE: DeVries, A.; Alexander, B.; and Goldstein, R.: Blood 4:247, 1949.

PROCEDURE: Normal oxalated plasma, 0.05 ml, is mixed with 0.9 ml of $BaSO_4$-treated plasma, and the prothrombin activity (expressed as per cent from a graph) is determined. The patient's serum prothrombin activity is then estimated, and 0.05 ml of this serum is added to the diluted plasma and the prothrombin time determined on 0.1 ml of the mixture.

The SPCA is calculated by subtracting the algebraic sum of the individual prothrombin activities of the serum and plasma components from the observed prothrombin activity of the mixture. The value thus obtained divided by the algebraic sum gives the percentage enhancement of prothrombin activity.

INTERPRETATION: The failure of enhancement of prothrombin activity would suggest SPCA deficiency.

Chapter 6

DISTURBANCES IN AMINO ACID METABOLISM

PHENYLKETONURIA

26. PHENYLPYRUVIC ACID

▶ *(a)* QUALITATIVE METHOD

REAGENTS:
1 N HCl.
10% ferric chloride.

PROCEDURE: A few drops of 10% ferric chloride are added to a specimen of urine previously acidified with a few drops of 1 N HCl. If phenylpyruvic acid is present, the urine will turn an intense green color.

COMMENT: Although this test is simple and serves as an excellent screening device, the presence of large quantities of urates or phosphates may interfere with its sensitivity.

▶ *(b)* QUANTITATIVE METHOD

REFERENCE: Kropp, K., and Lang, K.: Klin. Wchnschr. 33:482, 1955.

REAGENTS:
10% ferric citrate.
10% citric acid.

PROCEDURE: A 1:10 dilution is made of urine. To 5 ml of the diluted urine, 0.5 ml of 10% ferric citrate and 0.5 ml of 10% citric acid are added. The color reaction is read in 3 minutes in a photoelectric colorimeter at 630μ. The unknowns can be compared with standard solutions of phenylpyruvic acid treated in the same manner.

INTERPRETATION: Normal range, 0 mg/24 hours; in phenylketonuria, 500-1,000 mg/24 hours.

▶ 27. DETERMINATION of *l*-PHENYLALANINE

REFERENCE: Modification of method by Udenfriend, S., and Cooper, J. R.: J. Biol. Chem. 203:953, 1953.

REAGENTS:
Acetone-dried powder of Streptococcus faecalis (R).
0.7 M citrate buffer, pH 5.5.
10 N NaOH.

0.001 M *l*-phenylalanine standard.

Chloroform containing 3.3% isoamyl alcohol. The solvents are washed successively with 1 N NaOH, 1 N HCl, and twice with water before mixing.

Methyl orange reagent. Methyl orange, 500 mg, is dissolved in 100 ml of warm water. The resulting solution is washed several times with an equal volume of chloroform. The methyl orange reagent is made by diluting this solution with an equal volume of saturated boric acid solution.

PROCEDURE: To prepare the filtrate, 0.2 ml of 1 N HCl is mixed with 2.0 ml of plasma and placed in a 100° C water bath for 3 minutes. The solution is then neutralized with 0.2 ml of 1 N NaOH, and the supernatant is separated by centrifugation.

The following reagents are placed in a stoppered glass tube of 15 ml capacity:

> 0.2 ml of 0.7 M citrate buffer, pH 5.5.
>
> 0.2 ml of Strep. faecalis suspension. (This is prepared by mixing 8-25 mg of powder with 0.2 ml of water for each tube, depending on activity of enzyme.)
>
> 0.2 ml of standard or filtrate of unknown (0.03-0.3 μM *l*-phenylalanine).
>
> 0.9 ml of water.

The tubes are incubated for 2 hours in a 37° C water bath with occasional shaking.

After cooling, 0.2 ml of 10 N NaOH and 5 ml of chloroform-isoamyl alcohol reagent are added into each tube. The solutions are shaken vigorously for 5 minutes and centrifuged for 2 minutes.

The aqueous phase is removed by aspiration with a fine-tipped pipette.

Two ml of chloroform extract is transferred to a 2 ml volumetric tube which has a glass stopper. Methyl orange reagent, 0.2 ml, is added and the mixture shaken up and centrifuged.

The tubes are warmed in a beaker of water (to remove clouding) and are read directly in a Coleman Junior colorimeter at 430μ.

CALCULATIONS:

$$l\text{-Phenylalanine } (\mu M/ml) = \frac{\text{Reading unknown}}{\text{Reading 0.1 } \mu M/ml \text{ standard}} \times \frac{1.2}{10} \times \frac{1}{0.2}$$

INTERPRETATION: Normal range, 0.02-0.14 μM/ml; in phenylketonuria, 1.2-2.4 μM/ml.

TYROSINOSIS

28. p-HYDROXYPHENYLPYRUVATE

► (a) MILLON REACTION

REFERENCE: Folin, O., and Ciocalteu, V.: J. Biol. Chem. 73:627, 1927.

REAGENTS:

15% $HgSO_4$ in 6 N H_2SO_4.
2 N H_2SO_4.
2% $NaNO_2$.

PROCEDURE: Into a 15 ml centrifuge tube, place 2.5 ml of urine and 2 ml of 15% $HgSO_4$ in 6 N H_2SO_4. This mixture is allowed to stand for 1 hour and then centrifuged. The supernatant liquid is poured into a 50 ml centrifuge tube, the original tube being drained carefully and its sides washed with a few drops of distilled water. A standard solution is prepared in the same manner.

Ten ml of 2 N H_2SO_4 is added. The mixture is then boiled for 15 minutes. A second portion of 10 ml of 2 N H_2SO_4 is added. The liquid is allowed to stand for 30 minutes. If a slight cloudiness appears, the tubes should be centrifuged again. The contents are then poured into a 50 ml volumetric flask. One ml of 2% $NaNO_2$ is added, and the contents are diluted to volume. This is then read at once in a colorimeter.

INTERPRETATION: This reaction measures both tyrosine and tyrosine derivatives but is not specific for p-hydroxyphenylpyruvate. However, it is useful as a screening device for tyrosinosis.

► (b) ALPHA KETO ACID TEST

REFERENCES: Bucher, T., and Kirberger, E.: Biochim. et biophys. acta 8:401, 1952; Knox, W. E., and Pitt, B. M.: J. Biol. Chem. 225:675, 1957.

REAGENTS:

2 N sodium arsenate, pH 6.
2 N sodium arsenate with borate, pH 6.

PROCEDURE: Urine, 0.1 ml, is added to each of two cells, one of which contains 2 ml of sodium arsenate and the other 2 ml of sodium arsenate-borate. The cells are read 5 minutes later in a Beckman DU spectrophotometer, with the first acting as a blank. p-Hydroxyphenylpyruvate gives a characteristic peak at 310μ.

INTERPRETATION: This test is useful in measuring both phenylpyruvic and p-hydroxyphenylpyruvic acid. The former can be ruled out by the ferric chloride test. p-Hydroxyphenylpyruvic acid is not a significant component of normal urine.

ALKAPTONURIA

29. HOMOGENTISIC ACID

▶ *(a)* QUALITATIVE SCREENING TESTS

1. Alkalizing the urine with NaOH or ammonia will turn the urine either dark brown or black.

2. Homogentisic acid will reduce Benedict's solution, giving rise to a yellow or orange precipitate and a brown or black supernatant. To differentiate homogentisic acid from glucose: homogentisic acid will not ferment yeast or rotate a beam of polarized light, while glucose will.

3. When ferric chloride is added dropwise to the urine, an evanescent blue color appears. When strong alkali is added and the specimen is shaken, the solution promptly turns dark.

(b) QUANTITATIVE TESTS

REFERENCE: Lanyar, F., and Lieb, H.: Ztschr. physiol. Chem. 203:135, 1931.

INTERPRETATION: Homogentisic acid is not present in normal urine.

MAPLE SUGAR URINE DISEASE AND H DISEASE

30. AMINO ACID METHODS

▶ *(a)* MEASUREMENT OF TOTAL FREE
ALPHA AMINO NITROGEN

REFERENCES: Van Slyke, D. D., *et al.*: J. Biol. Chem. 141:627, 1941; Hamilton, P. B., and Van Slyke, D. D.: J. Biol. Chem. 150:231, 1943; Van Slyke, D. D.; MacFadyen, D. A.; and Hamilton, P. B.: J. Biol. Chem. 150:251, 1943.

BACKGROUND: The method depends on the fact that alpha amino acids, when boiled in water with an excess of ninhydrin at low pH's, evolve CO_2 of their carboxyl groups quantitatively in a few minutes, in the following manner:

$$RCH(NH_2) COOH \longrightarrow RCHO + NH_3 + CO_2$$

(Proline and hydroxyproline yield their carboxyl CO_2 in the same manner as the amino acids with primary NH_2 in the alpha position.)

PROCEDURE:

1. *Preparation of sample:*

   (a) Plasma.—Two ml of plasma is precipitated in 10 ml of 1% picric acid solution. The precipitate is removed by both

centrifuging and filtration. The supernatant is used for testing.

(b) *Urine.*—Two ml of urine (preserved with thymol) is placed in a ninhydrin reaction vessel, and the pH adjusted to a little over 6. A crystal of thymol and 0.2 ml of 1% urease solution are added, and the vessel is left overnight for removal of urea. The pH is then brought down to about 3 the next day, and the sample is used for testing.

2. *Reaction with ninhydrin.*—The picric acid filtrate of plasma or the urease-treated urine is placed in a ninhydrin reaction vessel; the excess CO_2 is removed by boiling over a microburner; and the solution is chilled in an ice bath. Next 100 mg of ninhydrin is added; the vessel is closed and evacuated; and it is then immersed completely in boiling water and allowed to remain for 20 minutes, with the water boiling vigorously all the time. The vessel is then removed from the water and cooled to room temperature.

3. *Measurement of CO_2.*—The CO_2 is measured in a Van Slyke-Neill manometer by absorption in 0.5 N NaOH and by release of the gas on the addition of 2 N lactic acid.

4. *Calculation.*—The pressure pCO_2 from amino acid groups is calculated as follows:

$$pCO_2 = p_1 - p_2 - c$$

where p_1 represents the initial pressure after release of CO_2; p_2 represents the final pressure after the gas has been reabsorbed by 6 N NaOH and c represents the ninhydrin blank.

The alpha amino N is calculated as follows:

$$\text{Mg alpha amino N/100 cc} = pCO_2 \times \text{Factor} \times V$$

where V is cc of filtrate equivalent to 100 cc, which for plasma is 120 and urine is 50.

INTERPRETATION:

Plasma.—Normal range: 3.4-5.5 mg/100 ml (Hamilton, P. B., and Van Slyke, D. D.: J. Biol. Chem. 150:231, 1943).

Serum.—Normal range: 4.9-7.0 mg/100 ml (MacFadyen, D. A.: J. Biol. Chem. 145:387, 1942).

Urine.—Normal range: 0.75-0.95 mg/lb/24 hours (Hsia, D. Y. Y., and Gellis, S. S.: J. Clin. Invest. 33:1603, 1954).

▶ (b) DETERMINATION OF SPECIFIC AMINO ACIDS BY PAPER CHROMATOGRAPHY

REFERENCES: Consden, R.; Gordon, A. H.; and Martin, A. J. P.: Biochem. J. 38:224, 1944; Dent, C. E.: Lancet 2:637, 1946; Dent, C. E.: *Recent Advances in Clinical Pathology* (2d ed., 1952), p. 238; Woolf, L. I.: Great Ormond St. J. 1:61, 1951; Block, R. J., *et al., Paper chromatography: A laboratory manual* (New York Academic Press, Inc., 1954); Smith, E. L., and Tuller, E. F.: Arch. Biochem. 54:114, 1955.

BACKGROUND: The resolution of mixtures of solutes on filter paper may depend on surface absorption, on ion exchange, or on partition between solvents. Substances absorbed to filter paper were separated by passing through the paper or solvent which would preferentially elute each substance in the mixture; and on this basis, paper-partition chromatography was conceived.

APPARATUS:

Chromatographic chamber.
Desalting apparatus.
Equipment for evaporation in vacuo.
Micropipettes.
Drying oven.
Spraying equipment.

PROCEDURE:

1. *Preparation of sample:*
   (a) Urine:

   Desalting.—Approximately 10 ml of urine (preserved with thymol) is desalted. This can be done by shaking with resins or, with a desalting apparatus, by electrolysis. Such an apparatus can be made in the laboratory (see Consden, Gordon, and Martin) or purchased commercially. (Although some authors feel that this step can be omitted, our experience indicates that the interference of the "salt effect" causes so much distortion and blurring that it makes identification of the amino acid spots very difficult.)

   Evaporation in vacuo.—The desalted urine is then evaporated to dryness at low boiling temperatures, using suction and dry ice. The precipitate is redissolved in water to one fourth of the original volume and is used for spotting on paper.

   (b) Plasma:

   Deproteinization.—The plasma is deproteinized by a solution of sodium tungstate and N-ethylmendelamine. The supernatant is then desalted and evaporated in vacuo, as above.

2. *Application of sample to paper.*—Between 15 and 50 μl of the sample is spotted in the lower right-hand corner of the paper. The sample should be accurately measured with a self-filling micropipette (manufactured by Microchemical Specialties Co.), and not more than 5 μl should be applied at one time. The paper should be thoroughly dried before another sample is

applied. A hair dryer or heat lamp will greatly accelerate the drying process.

3. *Running of chromatogram.*—The chromatogram may be run by a variety of methods, depending on the type of problem and personal preference. The following variables may be used:

Method: ascending, descending, ascending-descending.
Chambers: one-way, two-way, fish tank.
Dimensions: one or two dimensions.
Solvents: phenol, butanol-acetic, collidine-lutidine, etc.
Paper: Whatman No. 1 or 4, S & S, others.

In our laboratory, we have employed two-dimensional ascending chromatography, using a metal rack in a fish tank. The chromatograms have been made with Whatman No. 4 paper, using phenol water in one direction for 12 hours and butanol-acetic in the other direction for 18 hours.

4. *Analysis of data.*—The data may be analyzed by one of the following methods:

(*a*) Densitometer.—The photoelectric densitometer made by Photovolt is excellent for one-dimensional work but is difficult to use and interpret with two-dimensional data.

(*b*) Direct analysis of ninhydrin spray.—The papers are sprayed with ninhydrin, dried in an oven, and analyzed immediately. Each of the amino acids is identified by superimposing using Rf values; and the results are tabulated semiquantitatively by grading against an arbitrary standard, judged under constant lighting conditions.

(*c*) The spots can be cut out and diluted after identification on a duplicate sheet, and the solution measured by addition of ninhydrin on a photoelectric colorimeter.

INTERPRETATION:

Plasma.—Normally, between 19 and 21 amino acids can be identified in the plasma with paper chromatography.

Urine.—Normally, alanine, glutamine, glycine, histidine, and serine are present in measurable quantities. The appearance of other amino acids in excessive quantities is abnormal.

(c) DETERMINATION OF SPECIFIC AMINO ACIDS BY COLUMN CHROMATOGRAPHY

REFERENCES: Stein, W. H., and Moore, S.: Cold Spring Harbor Symposia Quant. Biol. 14:179, 1950; Stein, W. H.: J. Biol. Chem. 201:45, 1953; Stein, W. H., and Moore, S.: J. Biol. Chem. 211:915, 1954; Huisman, T. H. J.: Pediatrics 14:245, 1954.

PROCEDURE: A few ml of specially prepared amino acids from urine or plasma are added to the top of a starch column. The sample is allowed to drain with the starch; and fresh solvent, containing no amino acids, is added and run through under slight pressure. The packed column is mounted over an automatic fraction collector which has been designed to collect continuously small fractions of specific volume. The amino acid concentration in each of the tubes is determined by a simple photometric ninhydrin method. The data obtained permit the construction of effluent curves, which reveal the detailed behavior and full resolving power of the column.

(d) DETERMINATION OF SPECIFIC AMINO ACIDS BY CHEMICAL OR MICROBIOLOGICAL METHODS

REFERENCES:

Amino Acid	References (see below)
Glutamine	1, 2, 4, 5, 17
Alanine	3, 7, 14, 19
Lysine	11, 13, 14, 15, 19
Valine	11, 13, 14, 15, 19
Cysteine-cystine	10
Glycine	3, 6, 11, 14, 19
Proline	14, 19
Leucine	11, 13, 14, 15, 19
Arginine	8, 12, 13, 14, 15
Histidine	11, 13, 14, 15
Threonine	11, 12, 13, 14, 15, 18
Isoleucine	11, 13, 14, 15, 19
Phenylalanine	14, 15, 19
Tryptophane	11, 14, 15, 19
Serine	19
Tyrosine	9, 11, 14, 15, 19
Glutamic acid	4, 5, 17
Methionine	13, 14, 16, 19
Aspartic acid	14, 19

1. Archibald, R. M.: J. Biol. Chem. 154:643, 1944.

2. Hamilton, P. B.: J. Biol. Chem. 158:375, 1945.

3. Christensen, H. M., *et al.*: J. Biol. Chem. 168:191, 1947.

4. Krebs, H. A.; Eggleston, L. V.; and Hems, R.: Biochem. J. 44:159, 1949.

5. Waelsch, H.: Advances Prot. Chem. 6:305, 1951.

6. Alexander, B.; Landwehr, G.; and Seligman, A. M.: J. Biol. Chem. 159:9, 1945.

7. Alexander, B., and Seligman, A. M.: J. Biol. Chem. 159:9, 1945.

8. Huberman, H. D.: J. Biol. Chem. 167:721, 1947.

9. Bernhart, F. W., and Schneider, R. W.: Am. J. M. Sc. 205:636, 1943.

10. Hutchins, M. E., *et al.*: J. Biol. Chem. 185:839, 1950.

11. Hofstatter, L.; Ackermann, P. G.; and Kountz, W. B.: J. Lab. & Clin. Med. 36:259, 1950.
12. Henderson, L. M., and Snell, E. E.: J. Biol. Chem. 172:15, 1948.
13. Kirsner, J. B.; Sceffner, A. L.; and Palmer, W. L.: J. Clin. Invest. 28:716, 1949.
14. Steele, B. F.; Reynolds, M. S.; and Baumann, C. A.: J. Nutrition 40:145, 1950.
15. Hier, S. W., and Bergein, O.: J. Biol. Chem. 163:129, 1946.
16. Harper, H. A.; Kinsell, L. W.; and Barton, H. D.: Science 106:319, 1947.
17. Harper, H. A.: Arch. Biochem. 15:433, 1947.
18. Horn, M. J., et al.: J. Biol. Chem. 169:739, 1947.
19. Steele, B. F., et al.: J. Biol. Chem. 177:533, 1949.

Chapter 7

DISTURBANCES IN CARBOHYDRATE METABOLISM

PENTOSURIA

31. *l*-XYLULOSE

(a) QUALITATIVE SCREENING TEST

One ml of urine is added to 5 ml of Benedict's qualitative reagent, mixed, and placed in a test tube in a water bath at 55° C for 10 minutes. The appearance of a yellow precipitate under these conditions is very suggestive of xylulose.

► (b) PAPER CHROMATOGRAPHY

This may be performed using a 3:2:1.5 mixture of *n*-butanol-pyridine-water solvent (Horrocks, R. H., and Manning, G. B.: Lancet 1:1042, 1949). The sugar spots show up with the *p*-phenylenediamine reagent of Flynn (Flynn, F. V.; Harper, C.; and DeMayo, P.: Lancet 2:698, 1953).

(c) OSAZONE FORMATION

REFERENCE: Enklewitz, M., and Lasker, M.: J. Biol. Chem. 110:443, 1935.

PROCEDURE: Recrystallized phenylhydrazine and sodium acetate are added directly to the urine in the proportion of 4 Gm:6 Gm:1

Gm of total reducing bodies. This is heated for 1¼ hours in a boiling water bath and then cooled in air. In urine which contains a large amount of xylulose, a precipitate, osazone, begins to form in the hot solution. This is filtered off as soon as the solution is cold.

The osazone is allowed to stand overnight and is then dried and recrystallized several times. The phenylhydrazine is identified as *l*-xylosazone by (1) its gross and microscopic appearance and its solubility, (2) its melting point at 162° C, (3) the formation of *dl*-xylosazone, (4) its optical activity, and (5) its nitrogen content.

INTERPRETATION: *l*-Xylulose is not a component of normal urine.

FRUCTOSURIA

32. FRUCTOSE

PROCEDURE: Fructose may be identified in the urine by the following methods:

1. In an acid urine, the reducing sugar must be present and active at room temperature.
2. The urine must ferment with ordinary yeast.
3. The urine must be levorotatory, and the levorotation must disappear upon fermentation.
4. The Selivanoff test must be positive:

   Reagent.—Selivanoff's reagent is prepared by dissolving 0.05 Gm of resorcinol in 100 ml of dilute 1:2 hydrochloric acid.

   Method.—A few drops of urine are added to 5 ml of Selivanoff's reagent and heated to boiling. The presence of fructose is indicated by the production of a red color, which may or may not lead ultimately to the separation of a red precipitate. The latter is dissolved in alcohol to impart a striking red color.

5. Preparation of methylphenylosazone.—This is prepared by adding urine to 4 Gm of methylphenylhydrazine and enough alcohol to clarify the solution. Four ml of 50% acetic acid is added, and the mixture is heated for 5-10 minutes in a boiling water bath. When the mixture has stood for 15 minutes at room temperature, crystallization begins, and is completed in 2 hours. The crystals have a melting point of 153° C. The osazone can be compared with that prepared from fructose by paper chromatography.

▶ 6. Paper chromatography.—Fructose can be identified by paper chromatography, using butanol-ethanol-ammonia as solvents and aniline phthalate as developer.

INTERPRETATION: Fructose is not a component of normal urine.

33. FRUCTOSE TOLERANCE TEST

This test is performed by giving 50 Gm of fructose by mouth after an 18 hour fast. Samples of blood are taken both before the test and at 30, 60, 90, 120, and 240 minutes after ingestion. Fructose is determined by the method described by Roe (J. Biol. Chem. 107:15, 1934).

REAGENTS:

0.1% alcohol-resorcinol solution.

30% HCl.

PROCEDURE: The blood is precipitated with zinc sulfate and NaOH, and the filtrate is added to tubes containing 2 ml of 0.1% alcohol-resorcinol solution and 6 ml of 30% HCl. The tubes are shaken vigorously and kept in a water bath at 80° C for 8 minutes. The color is compared colorimetrically with known standards.

INTERPRETATION: Levels of fructose in excess of 40 mg/100 ml are suggestive of fructosuria. The presence of fructose in the urine after the test is also highly suggestive of the diagnosis.

GALACTOSEMIA

▶ 34. GALACTOSE IN URINE

PROCEDURE: Galactose may be identified in the urine by the following methods:

1. Mucic acid test.—Urine, 50 ml, and concentrated nitric acid, 12 ml, are heated in a water bath and cooled overnight. A fine white precipitate of mucic acid will form if lactose or galactose is present. These crystals can be identified under the microscope and by their melting point (217°-218° C).

2. Osazone test.—Clarified and concentrated urine, 25 ml, is mixed with phenylhydrazine hydrochloride and sodium acetate and heated in a water bath for 45 minutes. The crystals that appear can be compared with the osazone prepared from pure galactose. After three recrystallizations the crystals should melt constantly at 182° C; and when mixed with a known specimen containing galactosazone, there should be no depression of the melting point. The osazone can also be compared with that prepared from galactose by paper chromatography.

3. Paper chromatography.—Galactose can be identified in the urine by using one-dimensional chromatograms with butanol-

ethanol-ammonia as solvent and aniline phthalate as developer and comparing the unknown with known galactose standards.

INTERPRETATION: Galactose is not a component of normal urine.

▶ 35. GALACTOSE TOLERANCE TESTS

The galactose tolerance can be determined by two different methods: the oral and intravenous.

1. For the oral galactose tolerance test, 1.75 Gm/kg body weight of galactose is given by mouth on a fasting stomach. Duplicate 0.2 ml capillary blood samples are collected both prior to feeding and at 30, 60, 90, 120, and 240 minutes after feeding.

2. For the intravenous galactose tolerance test, 1.2 Gm/kg body weight of galactose is injected intravenously and duplicate blood samples are taken both before injection and at 15, 30, 45, 60, and 75 minutes after injection.

BLOOD GALACTOSE DETERMINATION

REFERENCES: Hartmann, A.: J. Pediat. 43:1, 1953; Somogyi, M.: J. Biol. Chem. 117:771, 1937.

REAGENTS:

Fresh baker's yeast.

Copper reagent, made up of 25 Gm of Na_2CO_3, 25 Gm of Rochelle salt, 4 Gm of $CuSO_4 \cdot 5H_2O$, 20 Gm of $NaHCO_3$, 200 Gm of Na_2SO_4 (anhydrous, analytic grade), 1.5 Gm of KI, and 6 ml of 1 N KIO_3 diluted to 1 L.

Iodide and iodate solution, prepared by adding 2 Gm of Na_2CO_3 dissolved in 50 ml of 0.1 N $KICO_3$ and diluted to 1 L.

1 N H_2SO_4.

0.005 N thiosulfate solution.

1% starch solution.

PROCEDURE: One of the duplicate samples is precipitated with zinc sulfate and sodium hydroxide. The other sample is first treated with fresh baker's yeast (0.2 ml of blood is added to 5.8 ml of 10% suspension of washed fresh yeast), allowed to stand 5 minutes, then precipitated with zinc sulfate and NaOH in the same manner.

Five ml of filtrate is placed into a Pyrex tube containing 5 ml of the copper reagent. The tube is stoppered with a glass bulb and placed in a boiling water bath for 20 minutes and cooled. If the solution to be tested contains more than 0.50 mg of glucose, then 5 ml of iodide and iodate solution is added. (This is equivalent to an additional 0.50 mg of glucose.)

Five ml of 1 N H_2SO_4 is then added. After standing 5-10 minutes with occasional agitation, the solution is rinsed and titrated with

0.005 N thiosulfate solution. One ml of 1% starch solution is added toward the end-point.

The amount of sugar present is calculated from the amount of thiosulfate solution added minus the amount added to the blank tube made with water. If titration is less than 1 ml of thiosulfate, the result is doubtful because of the reagent's approach to capacity. The difference between the yeast-treated tube and the untreated tube represents the galactose level in the blood.

INTERPRETATION: Galactose levels in excess of 50 mg/100 ml by either test are abnormal.

► 35a. GALACTOSE-1-PO₄ URIDYL TRANSFERASE ACTIVITY

REFERENCES: Anderson, E. P.; Kalckar, H. M.; Kurahashi, K.; and Isselbacher, K. J.: J. Lab. & Clin. Med. 50:469, 1957; and Tentative Technical Bulletin No. 600, Sigma Chemical Co., St. Louis 18, Missouri.

REAGENTS*:

0.9% NaCl.

Uridine diphosphoglucose (UDPG), 5 μM/ml.

Galactose-1-PO$_4$, 7.5 μM/ml (barium free).

Tris glycine buffer, 0.2 M, pH 8.1.

UDPG dehydrogenase, 800 units/ml.

PROCEDURE: Approximately 5 ml of blood is collected in heparinized tubes. The red cells are washed twice with a double volume of 0.9% NaCl and hemolyzed by the addition of an equal volume of cold distilled water. The hemolysate (0.25 ml) is then incubated with UDPG, galactose-1-PO$_4$, and tris glycine buffer for 30 minutes at 37° C. For each sample, a control is run where no galactose-1-PO$_4$ is added to the substrate. After incubation, UDPG is determined in heat-inactivated hemolysates by means of UDPG dehydrogenase. The difference between the measurements of UDPG in the sample and the control represents the amount of UDPG consumed through the activity of Gal-1-P-uridyl transferase. Uridine diphosphoglucose pyrophosphorylase activity is also determined to assure that the blood sample and the hemolysate are properly handled.

INTERPRETATION: The means of Gal-1-P-uridyl transferase activity were found to be 4.5 ($\pm$0.47) and 0.5 ($\pm$0.04)/Gm Hgb for the normal and galactosemic patients, respectively.

---

*All reagents may be obtained from Sigma Chemical Company, St. Louis 18, Missouri.

GLYCOGEN STORAGE DISEASE

36. EPINEPHRINE RESPONSE

An injection of 0.1-0.2 ml of epinephrine should normally cause a rise of 40-70 mg/100 ml in the blood sugar at the end of 1 hour. This rise does not occur in patients with glycogen storage disease Type I (of the liver and kidneys) and is reduced in Types III and IV*a*.

► 37. GLUCOSE-6-PHOSPHATASE OF THE LIVER

REFERENCE: Technique is described in Cori, G. T., and Cori, C. F.: J. Biol. Chem. 199:661, 1952.

PROCEDURE: The obtained livers are frozen within 4 hours. Samples were not allowed to thaw before use. Small pieces (0.3-4 mg) are chiseled off the frozen livers, weighed, and homogenized immediately in ice-cold water in a cold stainless-steel homogenizer, or ground in a cold mortar without sand. For 1 part of liver, 2 parts of water is used.

The homogenates are filtered through gauze to remove small amounts of fibrous tissue, yielding a filtrate which can be pipetted without difficulty.

Several dilutions of the same homogenate are incubated with glucose-6-PO_4 in order to test proportionality to enzyme concentration.

The samples are deproteinized with trichloroacetic and the filtrates analyzed for inorganic phosphate, by the method of Fiske and Subbarow.

Each experiment includes samples incubated without the addition of glucose-6-PO_4. The amount of inorganic phosphate formed after incubation without substrate is deduced from that formed in the presence of substrate. In all instances, only small amounts of phosphate were formed on incubation without substrate.

The reaction mixture consists of:

    0.3 ml   0.1 M potassium citrate, pH 6.8
    0.5 ml   0.01 M potassium-glucose-6-PO_4, pH 6.8
             (or 0.5 ml H_2O for blanks)
    0.2 ml   homogenate (equivalent to 4-33 mg of liver)
    ———
    1.0 ml   Total volume

The reaction mixture is incubated for 1 hour at 30° C and removed at the end of 1 hour and placed in ice. It is deproteinized with 1 ml of 10% TCA (ice cold), and the inorganic phosphate on 1 ml of the filtrate is determined.

38. CHARACTER OF GLYCOGEN

REFERENCES: Technique is described in Illingworth, B.; Larner, J.; and Cori, G. T.: J. Biol. Chem. 199:631, 1952; and in Larner, J.; Illingworth, B.; Cori, G. T.; and Cori, C. F.: J. Biol. Chem. 199:641, 1952.

HEREDITARY SPHEROCYTOSIS

► 39. OSMOTIC FRAGILITY

REFERENCE: Shen, S. C., and Ham, T. H.: New England J. Med. 229:701, 1943.

PROCEDURE: Accurately measured 0.1 ml samples of blood are pipetted into a series of tubes containing 1.0 ml amounts of the following solutions: hypertonic NaCl (2.0, 1.5, and 1.0%), isotonic NaCl (0.85%), and hypotonic NaCl (0.8-0.1%) and distilled water. The samples are mixed and centrifuged. The supernatant fluid is poured into a separate set of clean tubes, and 0.5 ml of the supernatant solutions are diluted to 10 ml with distilled water in Evelyn colorimetric tubes. One drop of NH_4OH is added to each tube, and the samples are read and the hemoglobin determined in an Evelyn colorimeter, using a 540 mμ filter. The colorimetric values observed in the hypertonic salt mixtures are averaged as the "blank" and subtracted from each value obtained in the hypotonic range to give a corrected figure for hemolysis.

The per cent hemolysis of each salt concentration is then calculated by dividing the corrected figure for the hemolysis by the corrected figure for complete hemolysis produced in distilled water. The results can then be plotted with the hemolysis in per cent as the ordinate and tonicity of the hypotonic mixture as the abscissa.

► 40. MECHANICAL FRAGILITY

REFERENCE: Shen, S. C.; Castle, W. B.; and Fleming, E. M.: Science 100:387, 1944.

PROCEDURE: Defibrination is performed under aseptic conditions in 50 ml Erlenmeyer flasks containing glass beads. The fibrin clot is then removed with sterile applicators. The hematocrit of the specimen is adjusted to 35% by adding or removing plasma, and 0.5 ml of the corrected specimen is placed in a 50 ml Erlenmeyer flask with 8 glass beads and rotated for 60 minutes at 100 rpm. in a rotator with the center of the flask 3.25 cm from the center of the wheel.

Of the remaining portion of the corrected specimen, 0.1 ml is added to 1.0 ml of distilled water (complete osmotic lysis) in a centrifuge tube; another 0.1 ml is added to 1 ml of 1.25% NaCl (no osmotic lysis) in a second tube. The amounts of free hemoglobin in the supernatant of these tubes are determined in an Evelyn photoelectric colorimeter; and the results are designated H (complete lysis) and O (no lysis), respectively.

Two 0.1 ml samples from the rotated samples are added to each of two tubes containing 1 ml of 1.25% NaCl solution. These are similarly centrifuged, and the free hemoglobin in the supernatants is determined. Results are designated as S_1 and S_2, respectively.

The mechanical fragility of the sample is then determined by the use of the following formula:

$$MF = \frac{S - O}{H - O}$$

and expressed as a percentage value, where S is the average of S_1 and S_2.

INTERPRETATION: Values above 6% are abnormal in adults and in children after the age of 1 week.

41. INCUBATED OSMOTIC AND MECHANICAL FRAGILITY

PROCEDURE: Procedures 40 and 41 are repeated on sterile blood which has been incubated for 24 hours at 37° C.

Chapter 8

DISTURBANCES IN ENDOCRINE METABOLISM

CONGENITAL HYPOTHYROIDISM WITH GOITER

42. RADIOACTIVE IODINE UPTAKE AND KSCN EFFECT

REFERENCE: Techniques are outlined in Stanbury, J. B., and Hedge, A. N.: J. Clin. Endocrinol. 10:1471, 1950.

43. EFFECT OF METHIMAZOLE

REFERENCE: The methods are described in Stanbury, J. B.; Ohela, K.; and Pitt-Rivers, R.: J. Clin. Endocrinol. 15:54, 1955.

44. I^{131}-LABELED MONO- AND DIIODOTYROSINE IN BLOOD AND URINE

REFERENCE: Technique is described in detail in Stanbury, J. B. Kassenaar, A. A. H.; and Meijer, J. W. A.: J. Clin. Endocrinol 16:735, 1956.

► ## 45. PREGNANETRIOL IN URINE

REFERENCE: Bongiovanni, A. M., and Clayton, G. W., Jr.: Bull Johns Hopkins Hosp. 94:180, 1954.

PROCEDURE: A 50 ml aliquot of a freshly collected 24 hour urine specimen is incubated at 37° C with 15,000 units of glucuronidase (obtained from Warner Institute, New York City) and 10 ml of 0.5 M acetate buffer, pH 4.5, for 24 hours. When high levels of steroid metabolites are expected, only 5 ml of urine with proportionately less enzyme and buffer is employed.

The urine is then extracted three times with one-third volume of benzene. The urine is then discarded. The benzene is washed three times with 15 ml of 1.0 N NaOH and three times with water. The benzene is now evaporated on a steam bath with a gentle air blast.

A column is prepared (11.0 mm diameter) with 12 Gm of alumina (Harshaw Chemical Co., Elyria, Ohio) and benzene. The urine residue is dissolved in 5-10 ml benzene with the aid of gentle heat and applied to the column. Two extra washings of the residue with 3-4 ml of benzene are performed to insure quantitative transfer.

A simple three-fraction elution with the following solutions is employed: (a) 100 ml of 0.05% ethanol in benzene (this may be discarded), (b), 150 ml of 2.0% ethanol in benzene, and (c) 100 ml of 10% ethanol in benzene. The second fraction contains the pregnanediol and the third pregnanetriol. A 50 ml aliquot of the second and third fraction is evaporated in a flask with air to dryness. To the dry flasks is added 5.0 ml of ethanol, which is then evaporated to insure complete removal of benzene. To each of the dry flasks is added 10 ml of concentrated H_2SO_4 with swirling, and the resultant chromogens are read in 20 minutes with the Beckman DU spectrophotometer at 325, 390, 425, 440, and 460 mμ.

The results are corrected and calculated as follows:

$$\text{Corrected reading at 425 m}\mu = \text{OD at 425} - \frac{\text{OD 390} + \text{OD 460}}{2}$$

INTERPRETATION: Normal range of pregnanetriol, 0-2.0 mg/24 hours. Patients with adrenal hyperplasia excrete 10-40 mg/24 hours.

46. 17-KETOSTEROIDS IN URINE

REFERENCE: Slightly modified from Drekter, I. J.; Pearson, S.; Bartczak, E.; and McGavack, T. H.: J. Clin. Endocrinol. 7:795, 1947.

PRINCIPLE: A 24 hour urine specimen is collected. An aliquot of the urine is hydrolyzed with HCl and extracted with ether and then washed with NaOH to remove the phenolic compounds. The solvent is evaporated, and the dried residue taken up in alcohol. The resulting color is produced by the coupling of the ketone group at position 17 with *m*-dinitrobenzene in the presence of a strong alkali.

REAGENTS:

Conc. HCl.

5 N KOH (carbonate free).

Absolute ethyl alcohol, aldehyde free.

2% *m*-dinitrobenzene. The *m*-dinitrobenzene should be purified according to the method of Callow *et al.* Dissolve 20 Gm of *m*-dinitrobenzene in 750 ml of 95% alcohol, warm to 40° C to dissolve, and add 100 ml of 2 N NaOH. After 5 minutes, cool the solution and add 2,500 ml of water. Collect the precipitated *m*-dinitrobenzene on a Buchner funnel, wash with large amounts of water, and suck dry. Recrystallize twice in succession from 120 ml and 80 ml of absolute alcohol. The material should be obtained as colorless needles.

From this make the 2% *m*-dinitrobenzene solution in alcohol. It may be preserved in a dark bottle and kept for about 2 weeks.

Standard solution of dehydroisoandrosterone or androsterone containing 50 mg/100 ml in absolute alcohol.

Working standard: 1 ml of the stock standard solution is diluted to 10 cc with absolute alcohol (0.2 ml equals 0.01 mg).

10% NaOH.

Ether.

COLLECTION: A 24 hour urine specimen is collected in a bottle containing 5 ml of concentrated HCl.

HYDROLYSIS: To 5 ml of concentrated HCl in a 50 ml glass-stoppered Erlenmeyer flask, add 20 ml of urine. Place the flask in a water bath at 80° C for 15 minutes and then cool it. This solution may be left for 24 hours in the refrigerator.

EXTRACTION: In a 125 ml separatory funnel put 10 ml of the hydrolyzed urine. Add 20 ml of ether and shake for 1 minute. Remove the aqueous layer. Add 10 ml of 10% NaOH and shake. Remove the aqueous layer. Add 10 ml of distilled water and shake. Remove the aqueous layer. Into a 50 ml glass-stoppered centrifuge tube put the washed ether layer and centrifuge slowly for about 1 minute.

EVAPORATION: Into three test tubes place 5 ml of the ether extract. Evaporate in a water bath at 56° C until all the ether has completely disappeared. (The stored residue may be stored in a desiccator indefinitely.)

COLOR REACTION (Zimmerman reaction): Tubes 1, 2, and 3 are used for duplicate unknowns and a pigment blank. Additional tubes (4 and 5) are used for standard and reagent blank. The arrangement of the tubes is as follows:

UNKNOWN (TUBES 1 AND 2)	PIGMENT BLANK (TUBE 3)	STANDARD (TUBE 4)	REAGENT BLANK (TUBE 5)
0.2 alcohol	0.4 ml alcohol	0.2 ml diluted standard	0.2 ml alcohol
0.2 m-dinitro-benzene	. . . .	0.2 ml m-dinitro-benzene	0.2 ml m-dinitro-benzene
0.2 ml 5 N KOH	0.2 ml 5 N KOH	0.2 ml 5 N KOH	0.2 ml 5 N KOH

Place all tubes in a 25° C water bath for 60 minutes. Immediately add 10 ml of 80% ethyl alcohol and read in a photoelectric colorimeter within 10 minutes, using filter 540 mμ.

Ten ml of 80% alcohol is used as the colorimeter blank.

CALCULATIONS: Corrected:

$$\frac{\text{Optical density of unknown}}{\text{Optical density of standard}} \times 0.01 \times \frac{1}{2} \times 24 \text{ hr urine volume} =$$

Mgm 17-ketosteroids/24 hour specimen

To correct optical density of unknown, subtract optical density of reagent blank plus optical density of pigment blank from optical density of unknown.

To correct optical density of standard, subtract optical density of reagent blank from optical density of standard.

NORMAL RANGE:

Male adults: 10-20 mg/24 hours.

Adult females: 5-15 mg/24 hours.

In children from birth to 8 years, the values are near 0 or less than 1 mg/24 hours. At the age of 12 they are 1.5-5 mg, and then they gradually increase to adult levels at about the age of 16. There is no marked sex difference until the age of 16 years. There is a moderate day and night variation.

47. TETRAHYDRO-S IN URINE

REFERENCE: Technique is described in detail in Eberlein, W., and Bongiovanni, A. M.: J. Clin. Endocrinol. 15:1531, 1955.

Chapter 9

DISTURBANCES IN PIGMENT METABOLISM

CONGENITAL METHEMOGLOBINEMIA

48. METHEMOGLOBIN

REFERENCE: Evelyn, H. T., and Malloy, K. A.: J. Biol. Chem. 126:655, 1938.

REAGENTS:
0.1 M phosphate buffer, pH 6.9.
Sodium cyanide or sodium hydrosulfite solution, dilute.

PROCEDURE: To 16 ml of distilled water, 0.6 ml of blood is added. After the solution has stood for 10 minutes, 8 ml of 0.1 M phosphate buffer is added and the solution centrifuged.

The solution is put into two similar 1 cm Beckman glass cells and first read against a water blank in a Beckman spectrophotometer. The absorption band at 633 mμ is characteristic of methemoglobin. A small amount of sodium cyanide or sodium hydrosulfite is then added to one of the cells, resulting in the disappearance of the band. The differences between the two cells represents the methemoglobin content of the solution.

INTERPRETATION: Methemoglobin levels in excess of 1% of total hemoglobin are abnormal.

49. DIAPHORASE I

REFERENCE: Technique is described in detail in Gibson, Q. H.: Biochem. J. 42:13, 1948.

50. OXYGEN DISSOCIATION CURVE

REFERENCE: Technique is described in detail in Darlington, R. C., and Roughton, F. J. W.: Am. J. Physiol. 137:56, 1942.

HEPATIC PORPHYRIA

51. PORPHOBILINOGEN

See Procedure 10.

52. UROPORPHYRIN

See Procedure 8.

► 53. COPROPORPHYRIN

See Procedure 9.

CONGENITAL FAMILIAL NONHEMOLYTIC JAUNDICE WITH KERNICTERUS

► 54. BILIRUBIN EXCRETION TEST

PROCEDURE: Commercial bilirubin, 5 mg/kg, is dissolved in 0.1 M sterile Na_2CO_3 and injected intravenously. The serum bilirubin is determined at 30 minutes, 1, 2½, 4, and 6 hours after injection. A retention of more than 10% after 6 hours is abnormal.

► 55. BILIRUBIN CONJUGATION WITH GLUCURONIDE BY TISSUE HOMOGENATES

REFERENCE: Grodsky, G. M., and Carbone, J. V.: J. Biol. Chem. 226:449, 1957.

REACTANTS:

Bilirubin solution.—Stock solution consists of 10 mg of bilirubin (Eastman 2101) dissolved in 100 ml of chloroform. Immediately before each experiment, a 10 ml aliquot is extracted by shaking with 5 ml of 0.3% of bovine albumin solution made alkaline by the addition of 0.15 ml of 2.5% NH_4OH; extraction is repeated and the extracts are pooled. The pH is adjusted to 7.4, using N HCl. The final concentration of bilirubin in this solution is approximately 40γ/ml.

Boiled liver extract.—Three Gm of fresh liver tissue is quickly disrupted in an all-glass homogenizer in 2.5 ml of 0.5% KCl; the contents are poured into a large test tube containing 7.5 ml of the KCl solution and boiled for 10 minutes. The volume is readjusted with water, and the supernatant fluid is stored at 6° C during the preparation of the homogenate.

Tissue homogenate.—One Gm of fresh liver or other test tissue is ground in a homogenizer with 10 ml of ice-cold, alkaline KCl (prepared by adding 32×10^{-5} $KHCO_3$ to 0.154 M KCl).

PROCEDURE: One ml each of the above three reactants are added to 25 ml flasks containing 0.3 ml of 0.5 M K_3PO_4 (pH 7.4) and 0.1 ml of 0.3 M $MgCl_2$. Incubation is carried out in air at 37° C. for 30-45 minutes, with shaking. After this period, the flasks are removed quickly, placed in an ice bath, and their contents are removed and centrifuged in a Servall centrifuge for 5 minutes. Three ml of the supernatant fluid is diluted to 10 ml with water. The zero time control flasks are chilled in ice after the addition of all reactants, and "direct" bilirubin is assayed immediately.

BILIRUBIN ASSAY: The "1 minute" bilirubin is used as a measure of conjugation of bilirubin to "direct" bilirubin. The 10 ml samples are divided into two 5 ml portions. To one is added 1 ml of fresh diazo reagent (0.1% sulfanilic acid in 0.18 N HCl plus 0.03 ml of 0.5% sodium nitrite); to the other, 1 ml of blank solution (0.18 N HCl) is added. After one minute, the tubes are read in a spectrophotometer at 535μ. To determine "total" bilirubin, 6 ml of ethanol is added to each tube and the color is read after 30 minutes.

INTERPRETATION: A 4- to 5-fold increase in "direct" bilirubin over that observed in the controls indicates an intact bilirubin-glucuronide conjugating enzyme system in the test tissue.

Chapter 10

OTHER PROBABLE ENZYME DISTURBANCES

HYPOPHOSPHATASIA

56. SERUM ALKALINE PHOSPHATASE ACTIVITY

REFERENCE: Kaplan, A., and Narahara, A.: J. Lab. & Clin. Med. 41:819, 1953.

PRINCIPLE: The phosphatase of the serum liberates phenol from a substrate of disodium phenylphosphate. Therefore, the phosphatase activity is defined as that activity which liberates 1 micromol of phenol per milliliter of serum per hour at 37° C.

REAGENTS:

Substrate: 0.05 M disodium phenylphosphate. Purify by extracting 1.5 Gm with 25 ml portions of hot alcohol. Filter with suction and dry in air. Place 1.09 Gm in a 100 ml volumetric flask and make up to 100 ml volume with water.

Borate buffer, pH 9.8. Dissolve 9.5 Gm of sodium borate in 950 ml of water and add 35-40 ml of N NaOH until the pH of 9.8 is reached as measured with a pH meter. Make up to 1 L.

20% MgCl₂.

Buffered substrate. To 10 ml of substrate solution, add 1 ml of 20% MgCl₂ and make up to 100 ml with borate buffer.

1.5 M formaldehyde.

Saturated alcoholic borax solution. To 150 ml of 95% ethyl alcohol, add 850 ml of water and 35 Gm of sodium borate and shake well. Let the undissolved residue remain in the bottle.

Diazo reagent. Place 100 ml of water in an ice bath and cool below 5° C. Dissolve 0.125 Gm of Red B salt in the cold wate and filter. Add 1 ml of cold, approximately 1.8 N H_2SO_4 an store in the refrigerator.

Standard phenol solution. Dissolve 0.940 Gm of anhydrous phen crystals in water and make up to 100 ml. Phenol concentratio is 100 µM/L.

Working phenol standard, 0.05 µM/ml. Dilute 1 ml of standar phenol solution to 100 ml volume. Transfer 5 ml of this dilute standard to a 100 ml volumetric flask and make up to volun with water. Prepare the working standard on the same day used.

PROCEDURE: Make a 1:100 dilution of serum. Place 2 ml of buffere substrate in a test tube and allow it to come to equilibrium in 37° C water bath. Add 1 ml of the diluted serum, mix, and le stand in the 37° C water bath for 30 minutes. At the end of th time, stop the reaction by adding 2 ml of 1.5 M formaldehyde so lution and remove from the bath.

A blank is run for each serum. Two ml of substrate are heate at 37° C for 30 minutes. Add 2 ml of 1.5 M formaldehyde solu tion, followed by 1 ml of serum.

COLOR DEVELOPMENT: To both test solution and blank, add 4 ml saturated alcoholic borax solution and 1 ml of diazo reagent. M well immediately. This is important, for otherwise the coupling the phenol with the diazotized salt will be incomplete. After 5 mi utes read in a photoelectric colorimeter at a transmission of 490 m

PREPARATION OF STANDARD CURVE: Place 0.5, 1.0, 2.0, 3.0, and 4. ml of phenol working standard containing 0.025, 0.05, 0.10 0.150, and 0.200 µM, respectively, of phenol in a series of te tubes. Add 1 ml of borate buffer and sufficient water to each make a total volume of 5 ml. Develop and measure the color the phenyl dye, as described above, by the addition of alcohol borax solution and diazo reagent. Plot the optical densities again 200 times the concentration of phenol expressed as micromole Thus the serum alkaline phosphatase is obtained directly in uni when the time of the reaction is 30 minutes and 1 ml of a 1:10 dilution of serum is used.

INTERPRETATION: Normal range, 0.8-4.5 µM, with an average of 2 µM.

► 57. PHOSPHOETHANOLAMINE

PROCEDURE: Urine is subjected to two-dimensional chromatograph and the color is developed with ninhydrin, as described in Pr cedure 30 (p. 307). The phosphoethanolamine appears as a lar blue spot whose R_f can be compared with a known sample of phosphoethanolamine.

INTERPRETATION: Phosphoethanolamine is not usually detectable in normal urine.

CYSTIC FIBROSIS OF THE PANCREAS

58. SWEAT ELECTROLYTES

REFERENCE: Shwachman, H., and Leubner, H.: Advances Pediat. 7:297, 1955.

PROCEDURE: No special preparation of the patient is necessary. The back is washed with distilled water and dried. A 3 in. square of gauze is weighed in a container and then placed on the back, care being taken not to touch the area or the gauze with the fingers. A slightly larger square of plastic sheeting is placed over the gauze and taped to the skin. Then the patient is placed in a plastic suit, which is secured about his neck, and wrapped in blankets. At the end of 30-90 minutes, depending on the rate of sweating, he is removed from the bag, the plastic sheeting is removed, and the sweat-soaked gauze is placed in its original container, again taking care not to touch it with the fingers. The container and gauze are weighed, giving the weight of sweat by difference. Forty ml of distilled water is added to the container to elute the sweat. Five ml of the solution is then diluted to 50 ml and the sodium concentration is determined, using the flame photometer.

INTERPRETATION: A sodium value of more than 60 mEq/L is diagnostic of cystic fibrosis of the pancreas.

59. STOOL TRYPSIN TEST

REFERENCE: Shwachman, H.; Patterson, P.; and Laguna, J.: Pediatrics 4:222, 1949.

PROCEDURE: A 1:1,000 dilution of stool is made, placed on the gelatin surface of an x-ray film, and incubated for 1 hour at 38° C.

INTERPRETATION: Three negative results for stool trypsin in the 1:5 or 1:10 dilution should be considered sufficient evidence to justify a tentative diagnosis of cystic fibrosis of the pancreas in a child.

60. DUODENAL FLUID

Duodenal fluid is obtained by intubation following an 8 hour fast. The position of the tube may be checked by x-ray. The specimen should be alkaline.

(a) VISCOSITY

REFERENCE: Shwachman, H., and Leubner, H.: Advances Pedia 7:283, 1955.

PROCEDURE: Using an Ostwald viscosimeter, viscosity is measure immediately after collection of the specimen, without centrifuga tion or filtration.

INTERPRETATION: Viscosity time, in minutes, exceeds 3 minutes i 87% of the patients with cystic fibrosis and complete pancreatic in sufficiency, and in 70% of the patients with cystic fibrosis an partial pancreatic insufficiency.

► (b) TRYPSIN

REFERENCE: Shwachman, H., and Leubner, H.: Advances Pedia 7:286, 1955.

PROCEDURE: Serial dilutions of duodenal fluid with phosphate buffe (pH 8.4) are incubated at 37° C with 2 ml of 7.5% solution c Knox gelatin, in a final volume of 4 ml. After 1 hour the tubes ar chilled, and the end-point is read as the last tube in which th gelatin remained liquid. The result is given as the number of ml c duodenal fluid present in this tube.

INTERPRETATION: Normally, the minimal volume of duodenal juic which gives a positive trypsin result is 0.0025-0.04 ml. An alternat end-point consists of determining the reduction in viscosity of gelatin-enzyme mixture, incubated as above. A unit of trypsin i defined as the amount of enzyme required to reduce the initial vis cosity of the mixture by 20% in 1 hour. Normally, the duodena juice contains 40-400 trypsin units per ml. Values of 0.1-0.3 n by the former end-point method and of less than 20 trypsin uni per ml by the viscosity reduction method signify pancreatic ir sufficiency.

► (c) AMYLASE

REFERENCE: Lawrence, G. (to be published).

PRINCIPLE: Amylase activity is a measure of the ability of the er zyme to reduce a carbohydrate. The results are expressed as th amount of reducing substances formed from a buffered substrat under controlled conditions of pH, temperature, and time.

REAGENTS: Starch or glycogen substrates may be used which ar made up with a buffer.

Phosphate chloride buffer. Dissolve 2.7312 Gm of potassiu acid phosphate and 4.3 Gm of NaCl in 300 ml of distilled wate Add approximately 10 ml of 1 N NaOH and check the pH. Ac just pH to 7.0. Make up to a volume of 500 ml with distilled water.

Starch substrate. Mix 1.0 Gm of soluble starch with a little cold distilled water. Add this slowly to a boiling solution of phosphate chloride buffer and continue heating until the mixture is clear (about 1-5 minutes). Make up the solution to a volume of 100 ml with phosphate chloride buffer.

Glycogen substrate. Add 0.5 Gm of glycogen to 70 ml of phosphate chloride buffer. Mix and make to a volume of 100 ml with phosphate chloride buffer.

NaOH, 0.3 N.

$ZnSO_4$, 5%. These two reagents should be titrated against each other so that 10 ml of $ZnSO_4$ equals 10 ml of 0.3 N NaOH.

Glucose standard. One ml equals 0.05 ml of glucose.

Alkaline copper reagent. Dissolve 14 Gm of anhydrous disodium phosphate and 20 Gm of Rochelle salt in about 350 ml of distilled water. Add 50 cc of 1 N NaOH. With constant shaking, add 40 ml of 10% $CuSO_4$ (• 5 H_2O). Add 90 Gm of anhydrous Na_2SO_4. When this has dissolved, dilute to 500 ml with distilled water.

Arsenomolybdate color reagent. Dissolve 25 Gm of ammonium molybdate in 450 ml of distilled water, add 21 ml of concentrated H_2SO_4, mix, and add 3 Gm of sodium arsenate which has been dissolved in 25 ml of distilled water. Mix and place in an incubator at 37° C for 24-48 hours.

METHOD: Make a 1:250 dilution of the duodenal contents with phosphate chloride buffer solution. This should be done just prior to use. Into two small tubes, marked "1" and "2," put 3 ml of substrate and warm to 37° C for 5 minutes.

Take a few ml of diluted duodenal contents and put into a boiling water bath for 15 minutes and cool.

To tube 1, add 0.2 ml of diluted duodenal contents and incubate at 37° C for 15 minutes.

At the end of the incubation period, immediately add 0.4 ml of 0.3 N NaOH to tubes 1 and 2.

To tube 2, add 0.2 ml of boiled duodenal contents. (This tube represents a blank duodenal tube which has no enzymatic activity, only other reducing substances.)

To both tubes, add 0.4 ml of 5% $ZnSO_4$, shake, and then centrifuge.

In the meantime, prepare a blank for the glucose standard as follows: 3.2 ml of distilled water, 0.4 ml of 0.3 N NaOH, and 0.4 ml of 5% $ZnSO_4$. (If a glucose curve or factor has been established, this step is not necessary.)

Into 25 ml calibrated sugar tubes add the following reagents

	TUBE 1	TUBE 2	STANDARD BLANK	STANDARD (1 ml-0.5 mg GLUCOSE)
Filtrate	0.5 ml	0.5 ml	2 ml	2 ml
Water	1.5 ml	1.5 ml	....	....
Alkaline copper reagent	2 ml	2 ml	2 ml	2 ml

Cover tubes and place in a boiling water bath for 10 minutes Cool in ice bath for 5 minutes.

To all tubes, add 1 ml of color reagent (arsenomolybdate reagent). Mix well and dilute to a volume of 25 ml with distilled water. Read in a colorimeter at 515 mμ.

A distilled water blank is used to set the galvanometer at 100% transmission or zero optical density, and all the tubes are read against a water blank.

CALCULATIONS:

1. Optical density of standard minus optical density of blank equals corrected optical density of standard.
2. Optical density of tube 1 minus optical density of tube 2 equals corrected optical density of unknown.
3. The results are calculated as follows:

$$\frac{\text{Optical density of unknown}}{\text{Optical density of standard}} \times 0.1 \times \frac{20}{0.5} \times 250 = \text{Mg of reducing substances}$$
liberated at 37° C for 15 minutes

INTERPRETATION: Normal range of amylase activity for glycogen substrate: 0.19-0.65 Gm/cc of reducing substances, starch substrate 0.026-0.90 Gm/cc of reducing substance at 37° C and 15 minutes' incubation.

► (d) LIPASE

REFERENCE: Shwachman, H.; Farber, S.; and Maddock, L. L.: Am. J. Dis. Child. 66:418, 1943.

PROCEDURE: Duodenal juice is diluted 1:10 with phosphate buffer. To 2.5 Gm of olive oil in a glass-stoppered Erlenmeyer flask are added: 2 ml of aminoacetic acid buffer, pH 8.9 (prepare 7.505 Gm of glycocoll plus 5.85 Gm of NaCl/L; mix nine volumes with one volume of 0.1 N NaOH), 0.5 ml of CaCl$_2$ (2%), 0.5 ml of egg albumin (3%), and 10 ml of diluted duodenal juice. Shake well, incubate at 37° C for 1 hour and then add 36 ml of an alcohol-ether mixture (4 parts of 95% ethanol to 1 part of ether). Titrate liberated fatty acids against 0.1 N alcohol-KOH, with thymol blue as indicator. Titrate a similar mixture in which enzyme has been inhibited by adding alcohol-ether immediately after adding duodenal juice. Subtract latter number of ml of KOH from number used in titration of incubated sample.

INTERPRETATION: A lipase unit is the amount which splits 24% of 2.5 Gm of olive oil under these conditions.

$$\text{Units}/100 \text{ ml juice} = \frac{\text{ml } 0.1 \text{ N KOH} \times 100}{20.7}$$

Values of 0-10 units are typical of pancreatic cystic fibrosis.

61. MUCOPROTEINS

REFERENCE: Di Sant'Agnese, P. *et al.*: Pediatrics 19:252, 1957.

PROCEDURE: One ml of duodenal fluid (or more) is centrifuged to remove any particles not in solution. To the supernatant fluid is added nine volumes of ethanol-benzene (equal parts of absolute alcohol and petroleum benzene). The mixture is left at 4° C for 2 hours, then centrifuged, supernatant decanted, and precipitate washed twice with ethanol. Distilled water, twice the original volume of duodenal fluid, is added to the precipitate. If solution is not complete, the tube is re-examined after 1 hour at room temperature.

INTERPRETATION: Precipitates from normal persons dissolve easily in water. Considerable insoluble residue remains in cases of cystic fibrosis, dissolving only in 1 N NaOH after heating. Water-insoluble mucoprotein is present in 100% of patients with cystic fibrosis and complete pancreatic achylia, in 58% (8/14) of patients with cystic fibrosis and partial pancreatic achylia, and in an occasional person without cystic fibrosis.

DEFICIENCY OF GLUCOSE-6-PO$_4$ DEHYDROGENASE

61a. DETERMINATION OF GLUCOSE-6-PO$_4$ DEHYDROGENASE

REFERENCE: Zinkham, W. H.; Lenhard, R. E., Jr.; and Childs, B.: Bull. Johns Hopkins Hosp. 102:169, 1958.

REAGENTS:

0.14 M NaCl.

0.3 M MgCl$_2$, pH 7.0.

0.19 M tris (hydroxymethyl aminomethane) buffer, pH 8.0.

0.02 M dipotassium glucose-6-PO$_4$, pH 7.0.

0.002 M TPN (triphosphopyridine nucleotide), pH 6.8.

PROCEDURE: Five ml of venous blood is collected in a test tube containing 1.0 mg of sodium heparin. The specimen is immediately centrifuged in the cold at 3,000 rpm for 10 minutes. The supernatant plasma, white-cell layer, and a small portion of the red cells are aspirated, and the remaining red cells are washed three times in the cold with chilled 0.14 M NaCl. Most of the saline is removed after the last washing, and 0.2 ml of packed red cells is added to 3.8 ml of distilled water. A hematocrit is done on the remainder of the red-cell sediment. The red-cell and water mixture is left standing at 26° C for 10 minutes, and the solution is vigorously shaken before and after the period of incubation. The resulting hemolysate is centrifuged in the cold at 3,000 rpm for 10 minutes, and the supernatant is withdrawn.

An assay for glucose-6-PO$_4$ dehydrogenase activity is done in the 1 cm cell of the model DU Beckman spectrophotometer at 340μ. The assay system consists of 0.1 ml of hemolysate, 0.1 ml of MgCl$_2$, 1.0 ml of tris buffer, 0.1 ml of glucose-6-PO$_4$, 0.2 ml of TPN, and 1.5 ml of water. The blank solution contains all these reagents but TPN and glucose-6-PO$_4$. The reaction is started by addition of TPN, and optical density readings are made at 1 minute intervals from 5 to 20 minutes after starting the reaction.

CALCULATIONS: The glucose-6-PO$_4$ dehydrogenase activity is calculated as follows:

$$\frac{\text{Change of OD/Min}}{2.07} \times 20 \times \frac{100}{\text{Hct}} \times 1,000$$
$$= \text{Units of glucose-6-PO}_4 \text{ dehydrogenase/100 ml RBC}$$

INTERPRETATION: Normal adults show a range of 150-215 units/100 ml RBC. Patients with glucose-6-PO$_4$ dehydrogenase deficiency show less than 10 units/100 ml RBC.

61b. GLUTATHIONE STABILITY TEST

REFERENCE: Beutler, E.: J. Lab. & Clin. Med. 49:84, 1957.

REAGENTS:

3.0% metaphosphoric acid solution. Prepared by dissolving 3.0 Gm of reagent acid phosphoric meta (Merck) (35% HPO$_3$) in 100 ml of water.

2% sodium nitroprusside solution. Prepared fresh daily.

Sodium cyanide–sodium carbonate solution. Prepared by adding 328 mg of sodium cyanide and 15.9 Gm of sodium carbonate to 100 ml of water.

Glutathione (GSH) standard.

Acetylphenylhydrazine.

PROCEDURE: 1 ml of whole blood is added to 2 ml of distilled water. After a few minutes, 5 ml of a 3.0% metaphosphoric acid solution is added during constant agitation of the hemolysate with a stirring rod. Approximately 3 Gm of NaCl is added and the test tube sealed with parafilm; then the mixture is shaken for 10 min utes in a Burrell wrist-action shaker, Model BB, set at the maximum amplitude. The suspension is filtered through paper (Whatman No. 2 and S & S No. 595 have both been satisfactory). These manipulations are all carried out at room temperature. Two ml of the filtrate is added to a 25 mm Coleman Junior spectrophotometer cuvette containing 6 ml of saturated NaCl solution. The mixture is allowed to equilibrate for 10-20 minutes at 21-23° C in a water bath. One ml of the sodium nitroprusside is layered over the filtrate, and 1 ml of the sodium cyanide–sodium carbonate mixture is added immediately. The contents of the cuvette are mixed and measured in a Coleman Junior spectrophotometer against a reagent blank containing 6 ml of saturated NaCl solution, 1 ml of the sodium nitroprusside, and 1 ml of the sodium cyanide–sodium carbonate mixture. The glutathione content is compared with a glutathione standard run simultaneously. The GSH content is calculated according to the linear relationship that exists between optical density of the GSH-nitroprusside complex and the GSH concentration. The GSH content of the red cells equals the whole-blood GSH divided by the hematocrit of the sample.

The stability of the red-cell GSH to acetylphenylhydrazine is determined as follows: Heparinized venous blood samples are used within 3 hours of the time they are drawn. The blood is mixed and oxygenated by shaking vigorously in 24 mm screw-cap vials. After the red-cell glutathione level is determined in the usual manner, 1 ml aliquots of whole blood are added to test tubes containing 5 mg of acetylphenylhydrazine. A glass stirring rod is used to aid in the suspension of the acetylphenylhydrazine, and the tube is agitated by vigorously tapping its bottom against the palm of the hand to assure solution of the acetylphenylhydrazine and adequate oxygenation of the red cells. The tube is incubated at 37° C. The agitation is repeated at the end of 1 hour, and at the end of 2 hours the GSH determinations are made in the usual manner.

INTERPRETATION: A striking fall of GSH content of whole blood after incubation with acetylphenylhydrazine, as compared with before incubation, indicates deficiency of glucose-6-PO_4 dehydrogenase.

SUSCEPTIBILITY TO SUXAMETHONIUM

62. DETERMINATION OF PSEUDOCHOLINESTERASE

REFERENCE: Kalow, W., and Genest, K.: Canad. J. Biochem. & Physiol. 35:339, 1957.

PROCEDURE; Human serum or plasma is diluted 1:100. As a solvent, 1/15 M phosphate buffer, pH 7.4, should always be used. Crystalline benzylcholine chloride (Hoffmann-LaRoche) is stored in a vacuum desiccator over H_2SO_4. For the stock solution of substrate, the concentration is 2×10^{-4} M. The stock solution of inhibitor is 4×10^{-5} M dibucaine (Nupercaine®, Ciba).

The spectrophotometric measurements are performed at 240 mμ. Esterase stock solution diluted with equal parts of the buffer is used as the optical blank. For measuring reaction rates, the solutions of benzylcaine and of dibucaine are mixed in equal proportions, and 2 ml of this mixture is added to 2 ml of the stock solution of esterase. The procedure is then repeated, using buffer instead of the solution of dibucaine. Both reactions are recorded for 3 minutes, as timed by a stop watch. Because of the absorbence of dibucaine, the recordings of the inhibited and the uninhibited reaction begins at different levels of absorbence.

Immediately after completion of each recording, while the sample is still in the cell compartment, the temperature is measured by dipping a Thermistor into the solution. If there is a difference of temperature between the inhibited and the uninhibited reaction, the following formula should be used to correct the observed reaction rates to agree with the rate at 26° C:

Reaction rate at 26° C = Observed rate × antilog
[0.0283 × (26° C − Measured degrees C)]

The results are calculated by the following equation:

Dibucaine number = Per cent inhibition

$$= 100 \times 1 - \left(\frac{\text{Decrease of absorbence in presence of dibucaine}}{\text{Uninhibited decrease of absorbence}} \right)$$

INTERPRETATION: A dibucaine number under 70 is probably abnormal.

Chapter 11

RENAL TRANSPORT DEFECTS

NEPHROGENIC DIABETES INSIPIDUS

► 63. TESTS FOR DIABETES INSIPIDUS

REFERENCE: Carter, A. C., and Robbins, J.: J. Clin. Endocrinol. 7:753, 1949.

PROCEDURE: All antidiuretic therapy is stopped, and fluids are withheld for 8 hours preceding the test. The subjects are hydrated with water, 20 ml/kg of body weight, by mouth over a period of 1 hour. Thirty minutes after the hydration is begun, an indwelling catheter is inserted. Urine specimens are collected in 15 minute periods, and urine flow is calculated in ml per minute. After two control periods with an adequate urine flow (i.e., greater than 5 ml/minute), an infusion of 2.5% NaCl is begun. This is administered at the rate of 0.25 ml/kg/minute for 45 minutes. If no decrease in urine flow occurs during the first two post-infusion periods of 15 minutes each, 0.1 unit of Pitressin® is given intravenously and its effect on urine flow observed.

INTERPRETATION: In normal individuals there should be a prompt and marked decrease in urine flow following the infusion of saline. Patients with pituitary diabetes insipidus show continued diuresis during and after the infusion. They will, however, show a decrease of urine flow following Pitressin®. Patients with nephrogenic diabetes insipidus will show no change after Pitressin.®

CYSTINURIA

64. CYSTINE

REFERENCE: Lewis, H. B., Ann. Int. Med. 6:183, 1933.

(a) CYANIDE NITROPRUSSIDE TEST

REAGENTS:
5% sodium cyanide solution, freshly prepared.
5% sodium nitroprusside, freshly prepared.

PROCEDURE: To 5 ml of urine, 2 ml of a 5% sodium cyanide solution is added, and the reaction is allowed to proceed for 10 minutes. A few drops (usually 5 drops delivered from a serological pipette) of a 5% nitroprusside solution are added and thoroughly mixed. Normal urine shows a pale brown or occasionally a very faint flesh color, while urine containing cystine shows a rather stable magenta color.

(b) SULLIVAN REACTION

REAGENTS:
5% aqueous solution of sodium cyanide.
0.5% aqueous solution of 1,2-naphthoquinone-4-sodium sulfonate.
10% solution of anhydrous sodium sulfite in 0.5 N NaOH.
2% solution of $Na_2S_2O_4$ in 0.5 N NaOH.

PROCEDURE: To 5 ml of urine, 2 ml of a freshly prepared aqueous solution of sodium cyanide is added. The solution is thoroughly mixed, and the reduction is allowed to proceed for 10 minutes at room temperature. One ml of 1,2-naphthoquinone-4-sodium sulfonate is added. The contents of the tubes are carefully mixed, and immediately 5 ml of a 10% solution of anhydrous sodium sulfite in NaOH is added. The solutions are mixed, and the reac tion is allowed to proceed for 30 minutes at room temperature After the addition of 1 ml of a 2% solution of $Na_2S_2O_4$ in 0.5 N NaOH, a pure red color is obtained if cystine is present.

▶ **65. AMINO ACIDS BY PAPER-PARTITION CHROMATOGRAPHY**

The techniques are discussed in detail in Procedure 30, b.

66. LYSINE TOLERANCE TEST

REFERENCE: Robson, E., and Rose, G. A.: Clin. Sc. 16:75, 1957.

PREPARATION OF AMINO ACID: The monochloride of l-lysine is dis solved in water which contains sufficient NaOH to give a solution of pH 7.4.

METHOD OF ADMINISTRATION: The test subject is first given 1 L of water, and then 250 ml of water every 15 minutes thereafter.

Four consecutive specimens of urine are collected, as follows

1. After a control period of 40 minutes. Immediately after this, an amino acid solution containing 5 Gm of l-lysin is given intravenously in 1-3 minutes, using a 100 m syringe connected to a polyethylene cannula which had previously been introduced into a suitable vein.
2. After a study period of 15 minutes.
3. After a study period of 30 minutes.
4. After a final study period of 30 minutes.

A venous blood sample is withdrawn from another vein a about the midpoint of each period of urine collection.

PROCEDURE: The plasma ultrafiltrate and urine are examined fo amino acids by the standard paper chromatographic technique described in Procedure 30, b.

INTERPRETATION: Lysine infusions into normal patients cause trar sient increases in the renal clearances of cystine, arginine, an ornithine. Similar infusions in cystinurics and in patients havin Fanconi's syndrome cause little or no increase in renal excretio of cystine, arginine, and ornithine. Unaffected heterozygous car riers of recessive cystinuria and of Fanconi's syndrome behave a do normals following infusion.

CYSTINOSIS

67. CYSTINE CRYSTALS

(a) WOLLASTON'S TEST

PROCEDURE: After the specimen has been dried under alcohol, stron hydrochloric acid will make the hexagonal crystals change int long needles grouped in bundles.

(b) POLARIZED LIGHT

PROCEDURE: The crystals are birefringent and react positively to the sulfur test with an alkaline lead acetate solution.

(c) SULLIVAN REACTION

See Procedure 64, *b.*

(d) PAPER CHROMATOGRAPHY

See Procedure 30, *b.*

Chapter 12

DISTURBANCES IN LIPID METABOLISM

IDIOPATHIC HYPERLIPEMIA AND PRIMARY HYPERCHOLESTEREMIA

68. TURBIDITY OF PLASMA

REFERENCE: Geyer, R. P.; Mann, G. V.; and State, F. J.: J. Lab. & Clin. Med. 33:175, 1948.

REAGENTS:

30% coconut oil emulsion.

5% dextrose.

Conc. NH_4OH.

30% H_2O_2.

PROCEDURE: By means of a hemoglobin pipette, 20 mm^3 of blood is collected and discharged into 2 ml of 5% dextrose solution contained in a 13 × 100 mm Pyrex tube, and the pipette is rinsed in the usual manner. The contents of the tube are well mixed by rotation, and the tube is centrifuged at 1,300 rpm for 10 minutes. The supernatant is decanted into a Klett microtube, care being taken to avoid carry-over of the sedimented cells, and 0.05 ml of concentrated NH_4OH is added; after mixing, 0.05 ml of H_2O_2 is added. The tubes are heated in a water bath at 60°-65° C for 4 minutes and then cooled to room temperature. Any moisture which has condensed on the sides of the tube is removed by gentle tapping. The turbidity is read in the colorimeter, using filter No. 42.

A standard curve is obtained by making various dilutions of the emulsion, using 5% dextrose solution as the diluent. Two ml quantities of each dilution are placed in the microtubes and delivered as above.

► 69. TOTAL SERUM LIPIDS

REFERENCE: Swahn, B.: Scandinav. J. Clin. & Lab. Invest. vol. 5 supp. 9, 1953.

PRINCIPLE: The method consists of the application of 10-20λ of serum to filter paper and subsequent staining of the lipids with a solution of Sudan Black B in 50-55% aqueous ethanol. The dye dissolves physically in lipids, this being the staining mechanism. The coefficient of partition of the dye is enormously in favor of lipid in an aqueous ethanol-lipid system. The concentration of ethanol is so low that its lipid-dissolving effect is minimal and can be disregarded.

REAGENTS:

Saturated solution, Sudan Black B. To about 0.1 Gm of Sudan Black B, add 100 ml of 60% ethanol. Continuously stir the mixture and heat to boiling point. (Owing to evaporation during heating and subsequent filtration, the final ethanol concentration will be 50-55%.) Allow the solution to cool and then filter it (e.g., through Munktell No. 00 filter paper) at least twice to separate off any undissolved dye.

Rinsing fluid, 50% ethanol.

Eluent, 20 vol% glacial acetic acid in absolute ethanol.

TECHNIQUE: Small incisions are made 2.0 cm apart along the longitudinal edge of a strip of Whatman No. 1 filter paper measuring 4.0 × 26.0 cm. To the center of each 2 × 4 cm field is applied 0.02 ml of serum (or, if total lipids are in the range of 3-6 Gm/100 ml, use 0.01 ml). One of the fields is left blank, to serve as a blank on the method. Standard triolein solution* (1,000 mg/100 ml solution in absolute ethanol), 0.02 ml, is applied to one of the fields. This is the reference standard.

The serum and triolein spots are allowed to dry at room temperature. When the spots are dry, the strip is immersed in a dye bath consisting of the dye in a 50-55% ethanol solution, where it is allowed to remain for 3 hours. The paper is removed, and adhering dye solution is allowed to drain from the paper, which is then placed in a washing bath of 50-55% ethanol. This is twice repeated. The filter paper is allowed to dry after the third washing.

The lipid spots appear as blue to blue-black spots on a white to very pale blue-black background. The filter paper strip is cut into strips at the site of each incision. These segments are placed

*Manufactured by California Company for Biochemical Research, Los Angeles 63, Calif.

in tubes containing 4.0 ml of acetic acid-ethanol eluent. Elution time is 30-60 minutes.

The extinction of the blue solution is read in a spectrophotometer at 590 mμ, using 1.0 cm cuvettes. The extinction of the blank is subtracted from that for the sera and the triolein standard. The amount of total lipids in the serum is given by the following formula:

$$\text{Total lipid} = \frac{\text{Lipid content of triolein standard (mg/100 ml)}}{\text{Extinction value for triolein standard}} \times \text{Extinction for serum}$$

70. TOTAL AND FREE CHOLESTEROL

REFERENCES: Schoenheimer, R., and Sperry, W. M.: J. Biol. Chem. 106:745, 1934; Sperry, W. M., and Webb, W.: J. Biol. Chem. 187:97, 1950.

PRINCIPLE: Serum is treated with acetone-ethanol to remove the proteins and extract the lipids. To an aliquot of the extract, digitonin is added, which precipitates free cholesterol as digitonide. For total cholesterol, an aliquot is saponified with KOH and precipitated with digitonin. The precipitates are washed and dried and dissolved in glacial acetic acid. Acetic anhydride-H_2SO_4 reagent (Liebermann-Burchardt reaction) is added, and the tube read in a colorimeter at 625 mμ.

REAGENTS:

Mixture of 1 part acetone and 1 part absolute alcohol redistilled.

Mixture of 1 part acetone and 2 parts ether.

1% digitonin in 50% alcohol.

50% KOH.

10% acetic acid.

Glacial acetic acid.

Stock cholesterol, 100 mg in 100 ml of glacial acetic acid.

Acetic anhydride-H_2SO_4 reagent. This must be prepared immediately before use. Cool 10 ml of acetic anhydride in an ice bath. Add 1 ml of concentrated H_2SO_4 with constant shaking. Put in ice bath for 10 minutes before using. If more than 10 ml of this reagent is used, make up in the ratio of 10:1. Be sure to use the reagent within 30 minutes after it has been made up—never later.

PROCEDURE: If both *total* and *free* cholesterol are to be determined, use the following preparatory procedure for each:

Into a 10 ml volumetric flask put 5 ml of acetone-alcohol mixture. Add 0.5 ml of serum with constant shaking, and warm in boiling water bath until solvent boils. Cool, and make up to volume with acetone-alcohol mixture. Filter the mixture through fat-free cotton or filter paper.

Total cholesterol:

Extraction (for total cholesterol or for a small amount of available serum).—Place 3 ml of acetone-alcohol mixture into a graduated centrifuge tube. Add 0.2 ml of serum with constant shaking. Warm in water bath and cool. Make up to a volume of 5 ml with acetone-alcohol mixture. Cover with foil and centrifuge.

Precipitation.—Put 1 ml of the extract into a graduated centrifuge tube. Add 1 drop of 50% KOH. Mix with a stirring rod and leave rod in tube. Place in a sand bath and incubate at 37°-40° C for 30 minutes. Raise stirring rod and add acetone-alcohol mixture to the 2 ml mark. Add 1 drop of phenolphthalein. Titrate this with 10% acetic acid, about 4-6 drops and 1 drop in excess. Add 1 ml of digitonin to the solution and mix thoroughly. Place the mixture in a sand bath at room temperature for at least 3 hours, or preferably overnight.

Centrifugation.—Remove the stirring rod carefully so that there are no adherent particles. Then place the tubes in a wire rack corresponding to tube numbers and centrifuge for 15 minutes. Decant the supernatant fluid and remove the last drop by touching a paper towel or filter paper. Replace the stirring rod and wash down the sides of the tube with 2 ml of acetone-ether mixture. Remove the stirring rod and centrifuge the tube. Decant the supernatant fluid and repeat the washing, using ether only. Centrifuge the tube, decant it, and replace the rod in the tube.

Color development.—See below.

Free cholesterol:

Extraction.—See above, under Total cholesterol.

Precipitation.—Put 2 ml of the alcohol-acetone extract into a 15 ml centrifuge tube. Add 1 ml of 1% digitonin solution. Mix with a stirring rod. Cover with aluminum foil and let stand in a dark place for 16 hours or overnight.

Centrifugation.—Take out stirring rod and handle as for total cholesterol. Centrifuge. Decant filtrate and wash as for total cholesterol, except wash one more time with ether (total of three washes).

Color development for free and total cholesterol.—Add 0.5 ml of glacial acetic acid and warm in 60° C block until the precipitate has dissolved. *Be careful—too much heat destroys cholesterol.*

Add 3 ml of chloroform and 1 ml of acetic anhydride-H_2SO_4 reagent to all tubes, mix with a stirring rod, let stand for 25 minutes, and read in a Beckman DU spectrophotometer at 625μ wavelength and 0.04 slit width. The blank is prepared in the same manner except that 0.5 ml acetic acid is used in place of the unknown.

CALCULATIONS: The calculations are based on using 1 ml of filtrate for total cholesterol and 2 ml of filtrate for free cholesterol.

Total cholesterol, using 0.2 ml of serum to 5 ml of acetone-alcohol:

Optical density (of unknown) $\times$ Factor $\times$ 25 $\times$ 100
= Mg cholesterol/100 ml serum

Free cholesterol, using 0.2 ml of serum to 5 ml of acetone-alcohol:

Optical density $\times$ Factor $\times$ 12.5 $\times$ 100
= Mg free cholesterol/100 ml serum

INTERPRETATION: Keys has reported that, in males, the average total serum cholesterol increases from an average of about 173 mg/100 ml at 19 years of age to 252 mg/100 ml at 52 years. Values for females are somewhat lower up to the age of menopause.

71. PHOSPHOLIPIDS

PRINCIPLE: The lipids are extracted in an alcohol-ether mixture and digested with H_2SO_4 and H_2O_2. The phospholipid is now present as phosphate and is determined colorimetrically by a method for inorganic phosphorus.

REAGENTS:

Alcohol-ether mixture, 3:1. Mix three volumes of ethyl alcohol with one volume of ether.

10 N H_2SO_4.

30% H_2O_2.

2.5% ammonium molybdate. Dissolve 2.5% ammonium molybdate in distilled water and make up to a volume of 100 ml. Discard when precipitate forms.

Aminonaphthol-sulfonic acid reagent (Fiske-Subbarow). In a 100 ml mixing cylinder place 97.5 ml of 15% sodium bisulphite and 2.5 ml of 20% sodium bisulphite. Add 250 mg of recrystallized 1-amino-2-naphthol-4-sulfonic acid. The fresh solution should always be colorless (on aging it acquires a yellow tinge); discard it when the reagent blank shows an appreciable increase.

PROCEDURE: Into a 20 ml volumetric flask place 18 ml of alcohol-ether mixture. Add 1 ml of plasma or serum slowly, and with agitation, to the mixture. Heat in a boiling water bath until the contents of the flask boils. Cool to room temperature. Adjust to a volume of 20 ml. Mix and filter.

Into a 25 $\times$ 200 mm Pyrex test tube place 2 ml of the filtrate. Evaporate to dryness. Add 0.5 ml of 10 N H_2SO_4. Heat gently over a small flame. As soon as charring occurs or fumes appear, reduce the flame until the digest barely boils, and continue heating until no more charring occurs. Superheating must be avoided and at no time should the flame touch the tube above the level of the fluid. Allow the tube to cool for 30 seconds and add 1 drop of 30% H_2O_2. If the digest does not become colorless, add another drop of 30% H_2O_2 and heat again. Repeat this process until oxidation is complete. Add 2 ml of distilled water and heat to boiling for a few seconds. Cool to room temperature and transfer quantitatively to a 10 ml graduated test tube. (This represents the unknown.)

In another graduated test tube, place 0.5 ml of 10 N H_2SO_4 and 5 ml of distilled water. (This represents the reagent blank.) To both unknown standard and reagent blank, first add 0.5 ml of 2.5% ammonium molybdate and mix; then to both unknown standard and reagent blank, add 0.5 ml of aminonaphthol-sulfonic acid reagent and mix. Dilute all samples to 8 ml with distilled water, mix, and let stand in the dark for 10 minutes. Read in a photoelectric colorimeter at a wavelength of 660 mμ, setting the reagent blank at 100% transmission.

Standard.—A standard may be prepared at the same time in which 5 ml of a solution contains 0.02 mg of phosphorus. Place 5 ml of the standard solution in a graduated tube and add 0.5 ml of 10 N H_2SO_4. Develop the color as for the unknown, starting with the last step.

CALCULATION: Since 2 ml of filtrate represents 0.1 ml of serum and the standard contains 0.02 mg of phosphorus,

$$\frac{\text{Optical density of unknown}}{\text{Optical density of standard}} \times \frac{100}{0.1} \times 0.02 = \text{Mg phospholipid phosphorus/100 ml}$$

To convert into phospholipids, multiply by 25.

INTERPRETATION: Normal values for plasma lipid phosphorus in the postabsorptive state are given as 6-11 mg/100 ml. Phospholipids increase in those conditions in which there is an increase in cholesterol, although the increase is usually smaller. About half of the phospholipid is lecithin.

Chapter 13

THE MUSCULAR DYSTROPHIES

SEVERE GENERALIZED FAMILIAL MUSCULAR DYSTROPHY

► 72. PENTOSE (*l*-XYLULOSE) IN URINE

See Procedure 31.

Chapter 14

MISCELLANEOUS METABOLIC DISORDERS

DIABETES INSIPIDUS

73. RESPONSE TO SALINE AND PITRESSIN®

See Procedure 63.

74. URIC ACID (IN PLASMA OR SERUM)

PRINCIPLE: Uric acid, in a tungstic acid protein-free filtrate, is treated with phosphotungstic acid in the presence of cyanide and urea, to produce a blue color.

SAMPLE:

Plasma or serum from blood withdrawn during postabsorptive state.

Anticoagulant for plasma, lithium oxalate. Avoid an excess.

REAGENTS:

1. Sulfuric acid, volumetric N/12. Add 2.5 ml of concentrated H_2SO_4 (Grasselli, A.C.S.) to 1,000 ml of distilled water and mix well. Titrate against standard 0.1 N alkali, using phenolphthalein as indicator. Adjust accordingly and retitrate (20 ml of N/12 acid requires 16.7 ml of 0.1 N alkali).

2. Sodium tungstate, 10% aqueous. Dissolve 10 Gm of sodium tungstate ($Na_2WO_4 \cdot 2H_2O$—Mallinckrodt, Folin Special) in distilled water and dilute to 100 ml. The solution must be neutral or slightly alkaline to phenolphthalein, not more than 0.4 ml being required to neutralize 10 ml of 0.1 N HCl. Preserve in resistant glass bottle.

3. Cyanide-urea reagent (Newton). Just before use, dissolve 1 Gm of sodium cyanide (NaCN—Merck, A.C.S.) in 20 ml of 20% urea (see below). Discard any excess.

    Urea, 20% aqueous. Dissolve 20 Gm of urea ($[NH_2]_2CO$—Merck, reagent) in distilled water and dilute to 100 ml. If the solution is not crystal clear, allow it to stand for several days and filter through a Schleicher and Schuell No. 576 paper.

4. Phosphotungstic acid reagent (Brown). Into a 1,000 ml Florence flask place 100 Gm of sodium tungstate ($Na_2WO_4 \cdot 2H_2O$ —Mallinckrodt, Folin Special), 20 Gm of anhydrous dibasic sodium phosphate (Na_2HPO_4—Mallinckrodt, AR), and 150 ml of distilled water. Heat until solution is complete. Slowly, and with constant shaking, add 100 ml of warm 25% H_2SO_4 (see

below). Reflux gently for 1 hour. Cool under running tap water to room temperature. Transfer to a 1,000 ml volumetric flask thoroughly rinsing out the original flask with several portion of distilled water and transferring the washings to the volu metric flask. Dilute to volume with distilled water and mix by inversion. Reagent is stable indefinitely at room temperature

Sulfuric acid, 25% aqueous. Slowly add 25 ml of concen trated H_2SO_4 (Grasselli, A.C.S.) to 75 ml of distilled water and mix well. This mixture should be prepared shortly before use and added, as indicated above, while still warm.

5. Uric acid stock standard. Weigh out 100 mg of uric acid and transfer to a 1 L volumetric flask. Dissolve 0.3 Gm of lithium carbonate in 100 ml of water, and filter. Heat the lithium carbonate solution to 60° C and pour onto the uric acid. Shake until all the uric acid dissolves (the solution usually remains slightly turbid). Cool the flask under running water. Add 20 ml of 40% formaldehyde (formalin). Dilute to about 500 ml and add 15 ml of normal H_2SO_4. Mix, dilute to the mark, and transfer to a cool, dark place (refrigerator). (Normal H_2SO_4 is obtained by diluting concentrated acid 1:36.)

6. Working standard (1 ml = 0.01 mg of uric acid). Dilute stock solution 1:10 ml in volumetric flask.

PROCEDURE: To 8 ml of 1/12 N H_2SO_4 add 1 ml of serum and mix. Add 1 ml of 10% sodium tungstate and shake vigorously. Filter or centrifuge. In a 25 ml graduated test tube (sample) place 2.5 ml of protein-free filtrate and 2.5 ml of distilled water; mix. In a second 25 ml graduated test tube (reagent blank) place 5 ml of distilled water. In a third 25 ml graduated test tube (standard) place 1 ml of standard uric acid solution (containing 0.01 mg) and 4 ml of distilled water. To each tube add *from a burette* 3 ml of freshly prepared cyanide-urea reagent (see 3, above), and mix. Add 1 ml of phosphotungstic acid reagent (see 4, above), and mix. Dilute to 15 ml with distilled water and mix by inversion. Allow to stand at room temperature away from direct light for 60 minutes.

Measure the transmittancy of the sample against the reagent blank set at 100% transmission at a wavelength of 700 mμ. Obtain the value for uric acid from the calibration table or prepared standard.

CALCULATION:

$$\frac{\text{Optical density of unknown}}{\text{Optical density of standard}} \times 4 = \text{Mg of uric acid/100 ml}$$

Index